Math Calculations for Pharmacy Technicians
A Worktext

Third Edition

Math Calculations *for* Pharmacy Technicians

A Worktext

Elaine Beale, RPh
Pharmacy Technician Program Director
 and Instructor
Paul D. Camp Community College
Franklin, Virginia

ELSEVIER

ELSEVIER

3251 Riverport Lane
St. Louis, Missouri 63043

MATH CALCULATIONS FOR PHARMACY TECHNICIANS: ISBN: 978-0-323-43088-3
A WORKTEXT, THIRD EDITION

Copyright © 2019 by Elsevier, Inc. All rights reserved.

All rights reserved. No part of this publication may be reproduced or transmitted in any form or by any means, electronic or mechanical, including photocopying, recording, or any information storage and retrieval system, without permission in writing from the publisher, except that, until further notice, instructors requiring their students to purchase Math Calculations for Pharmacy Technicians: A Worktext, Third Edition, by Elaine Beale, may reproduce the contents or parts thereof for instructional purposes, provided each copy contains a proper copyright notice as follows: Copyright © 2019 by Elsevier Inc.

Details on how to seek permission, further information about the Publisher's permissions policies and our arrangements with organizations such as the Copyright Clearance Center and the Copyright Licensing Agency, can be found at our website: www.elsevier.com/permissions.

This book and the individual contributions contained in it are protected under copyright by the Publisher (other than as may be noted herein).

Notices

Knowledge and best practice in this field are constantly changing. As new research and experience broaden our understanding, changes in research methods, professional practices, or medical treatment may become necessary.

Practitioners and researchers must always rely on their own experience and knowledge in evaluating and using any information, methods, compounds, or experiments described herein. In using such information or methods they should be mindful of their own safety and the safety of others, including parties for whom they have a professional responsibility.

With respect to any drug or pharmaceutical products identified, readers are advised to check the most current information provided (i) on procedures featured or (ii) by the manufacturer of each product to be administered, to verify the recommended dose or formula, the method and duration of administration, and contraindications. It is the responsibility of practitioners, relying on their own experience and knowledge of their patients, to make diagnoses, to determine dosages and the best treatment for each individual patient, and to take all appropriate safety precautions.

To the fullest extent of the law, neither the Publisher nor the authors, contributors, or editors, assume any liability for any injury and/or damage to persons or property as a matter of products liability, negligence or otherwise, or from any use or operation of any methods, products, instructions, or ideas contained in the material herein.

Previous editions copyrighted 2013 and 2007.

International Standard Book Number: 978-0-323-43088-3

Content Strategist: Kristin Wilhelm
Content Development Manager: Ellen Wurm-Cutter
Content Development Specialist: Erin Garner
Publishing Services Manager: Jeff Patterson
Project Manager: Lisa A. P. Bushey
Design Direction: Ryan Cook

Printed in Canada

Last digit is the print number: 9   8   7   6   5   4   3

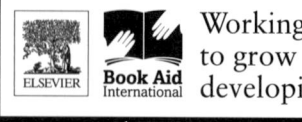

Dedication

To my mom, Gina, my husband, Jim, my brother, Frank, and my children, Eric, Dylan, and Carrie, for their support and understanding.

To my students, past and present, for helping me to understand how people struggle with and eventually master mathematics. Thank you for allowing me to share my love of the subject with you.

To the students who will use this text, I hope that it clarifies and makes the learning process easier for you. I wish you the best of luck in your chosen career.

Elaine Simmons Beale

Reviewers

Sandra Andrews, CPhT, BS
Certified Pharmacy Technician
Patient Care Management
Chambersburg Hospital
Chambersburg, Pennsylvania

Christopher Johnston, PhD
Associate Professor of Mathematics
Lindenwood University
St. Charles, Missouri

Joshua J. Neumiller, PharmD, CDE, FASCP
Vice-Chair & Associate Professor, Department of Pharmacotherapy
Director of Experiential Services
Editor-in-Chief, Diabetes Spectrum
Washington State University, College of Pharmacy
Spokane, Washington

Bobbi Steelman, MAE, CPhT
Director of Education
Daymar Colleges Group
Bowling Green, Kentucky

Preface

Patient safety depends on the ability of health care professionals, especially those responsible for the preparation, distribution, and administration of medication, to correctly calculate doses and dosages. Pharmacy technicians must learn this skill and use it throughout their careers. This text, which meets the guidelines prepared by the American Society of Health-System Pharmacists (ASHP) for accredited pharmacy technician programs, provides the basic mathematical concepts that are applied to pharmacy.

My goal with *Math Calculations for Pharmacy Technicians: A Worktext* is to assist pharmacy technician students in mastering the mathematical calculations necessary to prepare medications safely. It covers calculations used in inpatient settings, as well as outpatient settings, with a chapter covering basic business math for retail practice.

This text includes two basic methods of calculating medicinal dosages and doses: ratio/proportion and dimensional analysis. Even though I present both methods, you will learn that each one has its place in calculations, and you will complete the exercises using the method that works best for you.

The book is organized from basic mathematical calculations (fractions, decimals, percentages) to basic medication calculations to more complicated dose and dosage calculations related to prescriptions and hospital orders. Each chapter builds upon the previous knowledge base to ensure that the student is competent in one skill before adding another. Some students may not need the very basic instructions, but I recommend at least working through the pretests and posttests to make certain you are confident enough to proceed to the next chapter. The final chapter presents routine retail accounting procedures and focuses on business calculations, as well as inventory control.

Because practice is so important, the text includes more than 1800 practice problems covering a wide range of concepts. The concepts of pharmaceutical mathematics build from each chapter, with reinforcement of previous material throughout the text. The worktext format allows students to work at a pace that is right for them and meets the needs of the instructor and course objectives. The time devoted to each chapter may vary depending on the student's mathematical level. For this reason, the student's prior mathematical competence is tested with each chapter. Be sure that calculations are shown for each problem; this allows the person to pinpoint and correct errors.

ORGANIZATION OF MATERIAL

The text is divided into five sections: Section I, Introduction and Basic Math Skills, which includes an assessment of math skills needed in this field, as well as a review of basic math skills; Section II, Measurements and Conversions, which explores the different measurement systems used in pharmacy; Section III, Calculations with Prescriptions and Medication Orders, which focuses on the calculations needed to fill common prescriptions and medication orders; Section IV, Special Medication Calculations, which covers special medications, diverse populations, and less commonly used pharmaceutical calculations; and Section V, Business Math, which covers business math for retail pharmacy.

CHAPTER FEATURES

Learning Objectives and Key Words

Each chapter begins with a set of learning objectives and a list of key words.

OBJECTIVES

1. Know the standard abbreviations, rules for expressing measurements, and basic equivalencies for the household system of measurement.
2. Know the standard abbreviations, rules for expressing measurements, and the basic equivalencies for the metric system of measurement.
3. Know the standard abbreviations, rules for expressing measurements, and the basic equivalencies for the apothecary system of measurement.

KEY WORDS

Apothecary system One of the oldest measurement systems used to calculate drug orders using measurements such as grains and minims

Biologicals Medications that are tested for potency in a biologic system

Electrolytes Elements such as sodium (Na), potassium (K), magnesium (Mg), and calcium (Ca) that are necessary for normal body functions

International System of Units (metric system) Internationally accepted system of measurement of mass, length, and time

International unit/Unit A specific unit of measurement used for biologicals; a measurement of a medication's action as opposed to its weight (as with the units mcg, mg, g); specific to each particular medication

Milliequivalents (mEq) A type of unit used to express the concentration of electrolytes

Specific gravity The ratio of the density of a substance to the density of water when dealing with liquids in pharmacy

Standards An exact quantity agreed on for use in comparing measurements

Unit A general term covering any quantity chosen as a standard; for a measurement to make sense, it must include a number and a unit; examples of units: mg, mL, teaspoon

U.S. customary system (household system) System of measurement based on common kitchen measuring devices

Viscosity Thickness of a substance

Pretest and Posttest

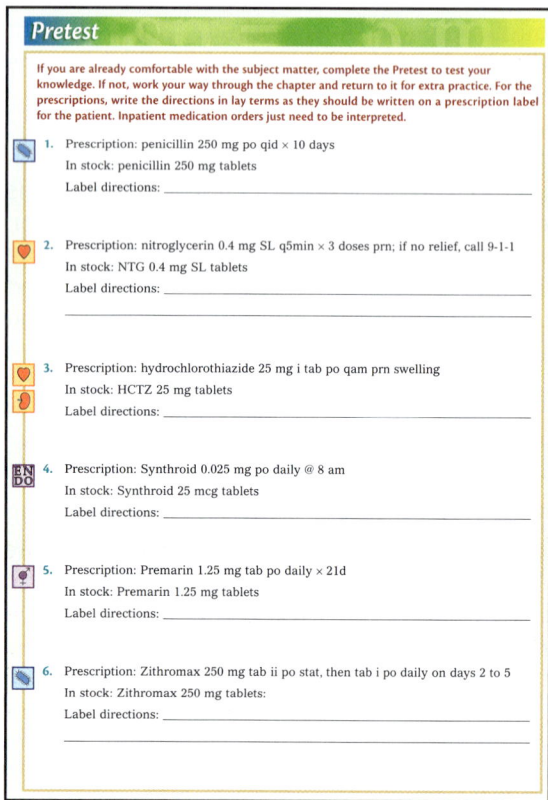

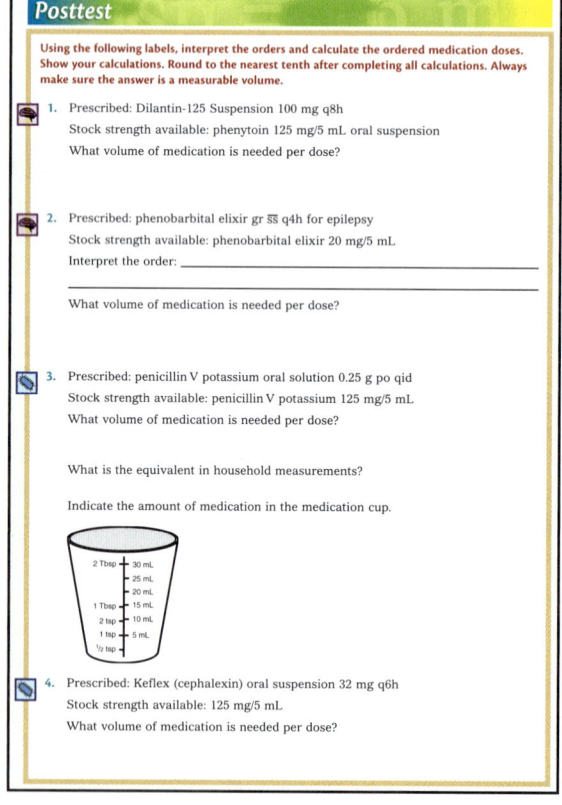

Included in each chapter is a pretest that indicates the level of student understanding of the calculation principles to be presented. If the material presented is understood at a level upon which to build comprehension of future concepts, the student may find that only a brief review in that area is needed. Students should move on to the next chapter only when they feel comfortable with the material presented and have demonstrated that they understand the subject matter.

Students who complete the exercises in each chapter may retake the pretest before taking the posttest at the end of the chapter to ensure that they have mastered the material. A student who continues to have problems with the posttest should study the chapter again. The importance of proper calculations cannot be overemphasized, and a working knowledge of accurate calculations is essential.

Practice Problems

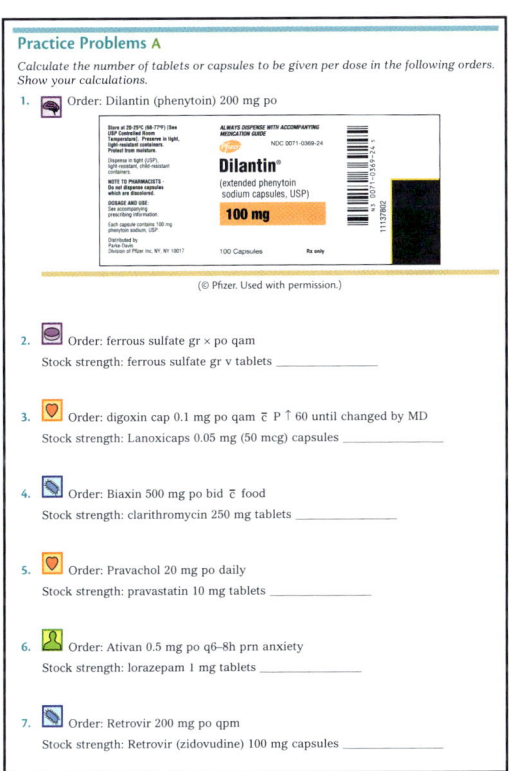

(© Pfizer. Used with permission.)

The practice problems may be used as in-class work, as well as for homework. Be sure the knowledge base for each exercise is understood so any previous mistakes are not made in subsequent calculations. Understanding the basis for pharmaceutical calculations is essential in preventing errors in actual practice. *Always look at your answer and ask yourself if it makes sense.* Then refigure for accuracy. Many errors can be prevented in this manner. Ask for assistance from the pharmacist if needed to ensure patients' safety.

Answer Key

The answers to every third problem are presented in the Answer Key so students can check their individual work and determine if they have completed the calculations correctly. If the answer is incorrect, the student has immediate feedback. Instructors should require students to show all mathematical calculations, so they can see the point at which mistakes occur and can correct the concept before students advance to more difficult calculations.

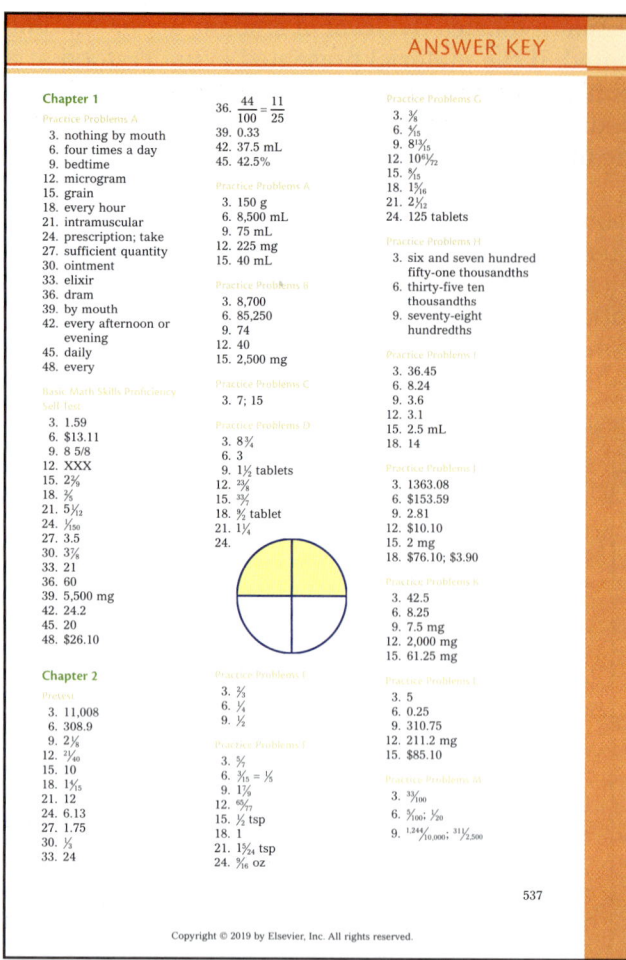

Body System Icons

Throughout the text, when medications are used in practice problems, icons indicate the general use for certain drugs. In this way, students learn mathematical calculations and are also exposed to the medications and their uses. The following icons are included in the text:

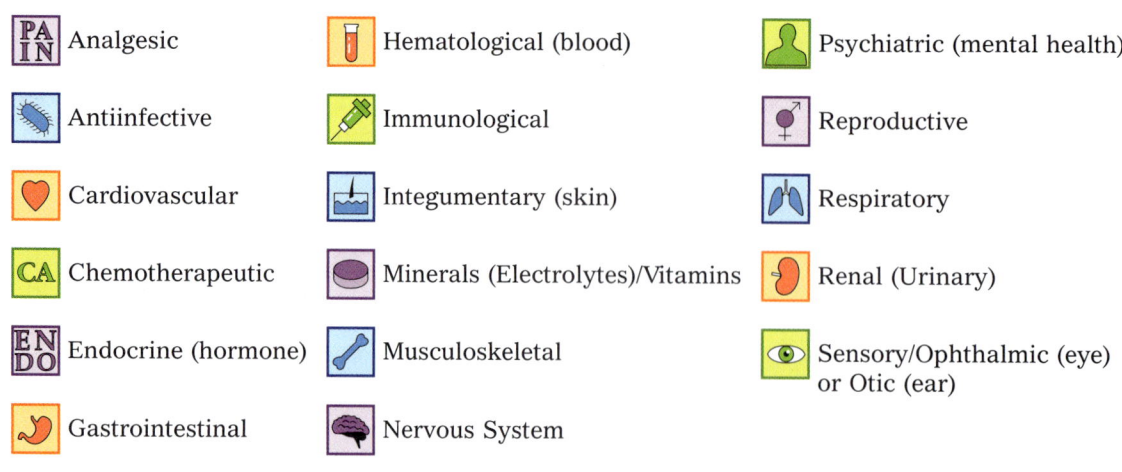

Tech Notes and Tech Alerts

I have included **Tech Notes** boxes to highlight important concepts. Another set of boxes called **Tech Alerts** have been added to assist students in perceiving areas where comprehension is essential to reduce errors and to enhance patient safety.

> **TECH NOTE**
> The generic name should be expressed with a lowercase letter, such as diazepam. The brand name is expressed with a capital letter, such as Valium. If the medication is a generic form of the drug, a trade name will not be found on the label.

> **! TECH ALERT**
> Even though, in most inpatient pharmacies, a pharmacist enters medication orders into the computer, the pharmacy technician still has a responsibility to check as he or she is filling orders and report any concerns to the pharmacist.

Additional Practice Problems Appendix

A new appendix features 528 additional practice problems covering the most difficult sections of the book.

ANCILLARIES

Instructor Ancillaries Available on Evolve

New and Improved TEACH Instructor's Resource: The TEACH Instructor's Resource provides instructors with customizable lesson plans, student handouts, and PowerPoint slides based on learning objectives. With these valuable resources, instructors will save valuable preparation time and create a learning environment that fully engages students in classroom preparation.

ExamView Test Bank: Contains more than 1100 multiple-choice questions.
Instructor Practice Problems: Provide even more practice using these additional problems.
Answer Keys: Allows instructors to easily check answers to every problem in the book.
Image Collection: Includes images in the text so they can be used as teaching aids.

Student Ancillaries Available on Evolve

Student Practice Problems: Enhance calculation skills with additional practice problems that correspond to every chapter in the text.
Comprehensive Posttest: Interactively tests students' knowledge and mastery of all content.

SPECIAL NOTE

To comply with *The Joint Commission's (TJC) official "Do not Use" List*, these abbreviations and recommendations have been clearly identified in this text.

Official "Do Not Use" List[1]

DO NOT USE	POTENTIAL PROBLEM	USE INSTEAD
U, u (unit)	Mistaken for "0", the number "4" or "cc"	Write "unit"
IU (international unit)	Mistaken for IV (intravenous) or the number 10 (ten)	Write "International Unit"
QD, Q.D., qd, q.d. (daily)	Mistaken for each other	Write "daily"
Q.O.D., QOD, q.o.d, qod (every other day)	Period after the Q mistaken for "I" and the "O" mistaken for "I"	Write "every other day"
Trailing zero (X.0 mg)	Decimal point is missed	Write X mg
Lack of leading zero (.X mg)		Write 0.X mg
MS	Can mean morphine sulfate or magnesium sulfate	Write "morphine sulfate"
MSO_4 and $MgSO_4$	Confused for one another	Write "magnesium sulfate"

[1] Applies to all orders and all medication-related documentation
Copyright The Joint Commission, 2012. Reprinted with permission.

In addition, please refer to the *Institute for Safe Medication Practices (ISMP) List of Error-Prone Abbreviations, Symbols, and Dose Designations* at https://www.ismp.org/tools/errorproneabbreviations.pdf and review this listing. This list is also included on pages 2-6 of the text. To realistically teach pharmacy technicians, some of these abbreviations are included throughout this text since they are still frequently used with prescriptions and medication orders.

Elaine Simmons Beale, RPh

Acknowledgements

I would like to thank Robert and Eugenia Fulcher for their earlier editions of this text, which provided me with a guideline for this edition. I would also like to thank the following people from Elsevier: Erin Garner, Content Development Specialist, Lisa Bushey, Project Manager, and Kristin Wilhelm, Content Strategist, for their continual help and guidance, as well as the numerous reviewers and editors.

Most of all, I would like to thank my family, who put up with my countless hours on the computer in my "Mom Cave" as they call it.

Elaine Simmons Beale

Table of Contents

SECTION I Introduction and Basic Math Skills, 1

1. Abbreviations, Symbols, and Basic Mathematical Skills for Pharmacy Technicians, 1
2. Review of Basic Mathematical Skills, 15

SECTION II Measurements and Conversions, 59

3. Conversion of Clinical Measurements of Numbers, Time, and Temperature, 59
4. Measurement Systems, Units, and Equivalencies, 73
5. Conversions Within Measurement Systems, 88
6. Conversions Between Measurement Systems, 104

SECTION III Calculations with Prescriptions and Medication Orders, 119

7. Interpretation of Medication Labels and Orders, 119
8. Calculation of Oral Solid Doses, 149
9. Calculation of Oral Liquid Doses, 164
10. Calculation of Parenteral Doses, 185
11. Unit Calculations With Anticoagulants and Insulin, 211
12. Calculation of Medications by Age, Body Weight, and Body Surface Area, 241
13. Interpreting Physicians' Orders for Dosages and Days' Supply, 281

SECTION IV Special Medication Calculations, 325

14. Calculations With Ratio and Percentage Strengths, 325
15. Calculations for Simple Dilutions, Mixtures, and Compounding, 354
16. Calculation of Medications Used Intravenously, 403

SECTION V Business Math, 453

17   Business Math for Pharmacy Technicians, 453

Appendix: Extra Practice Problems, 486

Answer Key, 543

Glossary, 553

Index, 557

IN SECTION I

1. Abbreviations, Symbols, and Basic Mathematical Skills for Pharmacy Technicians
2. Review of Basic Mathematical Skills

SECTION I
Introduction and Basic Math Skills

CHAPTER 1

Abbreviations, Symbols, and Basic Mathematical Skills for Pharmacy Technicians

OBJECTIVES

1. Introduce The Joint Commission (TJC) Official "Do Not Use" List and the Institute for Safe Medication Practices (ISMP) List of Error-Prone Abbreviations, Symbols, and Dose Designations.
2. Learn medical and pharmaceutical abbreviations.
3. Explain why proficiency in basic math skills is essential for pharmacy technicians, and assess level of basic mathematical skills necessary for pharmaceutical calculations.

KEY WORDS

Active ingredient The ingredient in a medication that has the desired effect on the body

Excipients Medicinally inactive substances that are added to medication formulations; fillers, binders, coloring agents, flavorings, preservatives

Pharmacology Study of drugs, their uses, and their interactions with living systems

INTRODUCTION

Pharmacology is the study of the uses, mechanisms of action, and effects of medications on body systems. Chemicals used as medications, or drugs, are the basis of pharmacology. Medications used to treat conditions and diseases must be dosed, prepared, and administered correctly. Calculating doses correctly is essential for the safety of patients.

Different medicinal preparations contain different amounts of *active ingredients*. Preparations also contain a variety of *excipients*, which are medicinally inactive substances added to the formulation as fillers, binders, coloring agents, flavorings, and preservatives. Each drug has its own specific concentration of active ingredients in a formulation. For example, a tablet may be manufactured in 10 and 20 mg strengths and a liquid may be manufactured in 125 mg/5 mL and 250 mg/5 mL strengths. The safe and effective amount of medication has been tested and recognized as within acceptable limits by the U.S. Department of Health and Human Services' Food and Drug Administration (FDA). The *U.S. Pharmacopeia* and the *National Formulary (USP-NF)* are manuals that provide standards for medication ingredients, preparation, and storage, which are enforced by the FDA. Each medication has its own recommended dose range. The pharmacy technician must have a thorough understanding of both the mathematical skills and the terminology used in medicine.

INTERPRETING PHARMACEUTICAL ABBREVIATIONS AND SYMBOLS

Knowledge of medical terminology and abbreviations is necessary for properly interpreting and dispensing prescription and medication orders, as well as educating patients in taking medications at home. Abbreviations are used to refer to routes of administration, frequency of dosing, and units of measurement within systems, among others.

Some abbreviations that have been used for years have been found to lead to medication errors, which led to the development of The Joint Commission (TJC) Official *"Do Not Use" List* of abbreviations. To comply with this list, none of the included abbreviations have been used in this text.

Official "Do Not Use" List[a,b]

DO NOT USE	POTENTIAL PROBLEM	USE INSTEAD
U, u (unit)	Mistaken for "0," the number "4," or "cc"	Write "unit"
IU (international unit)	Mistaken for IV (intravenous) or the number 10 (ten)	Write "International Unit"
QD, Q.D., qd, q.d. (daily)	Mistaken for each other	Write "daily"
Q.O.D., QOD, q.o.d, qod (every other day)	Period after the Q mistaken for "I" and the "O" mistaken for "I"	Write "every other day"
Trailing zero (X.0 mg)	Decimal point is missed	Write X mg
Lack of leading zero (.X mg)		Write 0.X mg
MS	Can mean morphine sulfate or magnesium sulfate	Write "morphine sulfate"
MSO_4 and $MgSO_4$	Confused for one another	Write "magnesium sulfate"

[a]Applies to all orders and all medication-related documentation.
[b]Copyright The Joint Commission, 2016. Reprinted with permission.

In addition, the Institute for Safe Medication Practices (ISMP) has compiled a *List of Error-Prone Abbreviations, Symbols, and Dose Designations* (https://www.ismp.org/tools/errorproneabbreviations.pdf).

List of Error-Prone Abbreviations, Symbols, and Dose Designations

ABBREVIATION	INTENDED MEANING	MISINTERPRETATION	CORRECTION
μg	Microgram	Mistaken as "mg"	Use "mcg"
AD, AS, AU	Right ear, left ear, each ear	Mistaken as "OD, OS, OU" (right eye, left eye, each eye)	Use "right ear," "left ear," or "each ear"
OD, OS, OU	Right eye, left eye, each eye	Mistaken as "AD, AS, AU" (right ear, left ear, each ear)	Use "right eye," "left eye," or "each eye"
BT	Bedtime	Mistaken as "BID" (twice daily)	Use "bedtime"
cc	Cubic centimeters	Mistaken as "u" (units)	Use "mL" (milliliters)
D/C	Discharge or discontinue	Premature discontinuation of medications if D/C (intended to mean "discharge") has been misinterpreted as "discontinued" when followed by a list of discharge medications	Use "discharge" and "discontinue"

ABBREVIATION	INTENDED MEANING	MISINTERPRETATION	CORRECTION
IJ	Injection	Mistaken as "IV" or "intrajugular"	Use "injection"
IN	Intranasal	Mistaken as "IM" or "IV"	Use "intranasal" or "NAS"
HS	Half-strength	Mistaken as "bedtime"	Use "half-strength" or "bedtime"
hs	At bedtime, hours of sleep	Mistaken as "half-strength"	
IU[a]	International unit	Mistaken as "IV" (intravenous) or "10" (ten)	Use "units"
o.d. or OD	Once daily	Mistaken as "right eye" (OD-oculus dexter), leading to oral liquid medications administered in the eye	Use "daily"
OJ	Orange juice	Mistaken as "OD" or "OS" (right or left eye); drugs meant to be diluted in orange juice may be given in the eye	Use "orange juice"
Per os	By mouth, orally	The "os" can be mistaken as "left eye" (OS—oculus sinister)	Use "PO," "by mouth," or "orally"
q.d. or QD[a]	Every day	Mistaken as "q.i.d.," especially if the period after the "q" or the tail of the "q" is misunderstood as an "i"	Use "daily"
qhs	Nightly at bedtime	Mistaken as "qhr," or every hour	Use "nightly"
qn	Nightly or at bedtime	Mistaken as "qh" (every hour)	Use "nightly" or "at bedtime"
q.o.d. or QOD[a]	Every other day	Mistaken as "q.d." (daily) or "q.i.d." (four times daily) if the "o" is poorly written	Use "every other day"
q1d	Daily	Mistaken as "q.i.d." (four times daily)	Use "daily"
q6PM, etc.	Every evening at 6 PM	Mistaken as "every 6 hours"	Use "daily at 6 PM" or "6 PM daily"
SC, SQ, sub q	Subcutaneous	"SC" mistaken as "SL" (sublingual); "SQ" mistaken as "5 every"; the "q" in "sub q" has been mistaken as "every" (e.g., a heparin dose ordered "sub q 2 hours before surgery" misunderstood as "every 2 hours before surgery")	Use "subcut" or "subcutaneously"
ss	Sliding scale (insulin) or ½ (apothecary)	Mistaken as "55"	Spell out "sliding scale"; use "one-half" or "½"
SSRI	Sliding scale regular insulin	Mistaken as "selective-serotonin reuptake inhibitor"	Spell out "sliding scale (insulin)"
SSI	Sliding scale insulin	Mistaken as "strong solution of iodine" (Lugol's)	
i/d	One daily	Mistaken as "tid"	Use "1 daily"
TIW or tiw	3 times a week	Mistaken as "3 times a day" or " twice in a week"	Use "3 times weekly"
U or u[a]	Unit	Mistaken as the number "0" or "4," causing a 10-fold overdose or greater (e.g., 4U seen as "40" or 4u seen as "44"); mistaken as "cc," so dose given in volume instead of units (e.g., "4u" seen as "4 cc")	Use "unit"

ABBREVIATION	INTENDED MEANING	MISINTERPRETATION	CORRECTION
UD	As directed ("ut dictum")	Mistaken as "unit dose" (e.g., diltiazem 125 mg IV infusion "UD" misinterpreted as meaning to give the entire infusion as a unit [bolus] dose)	Use "as directed"
DOSE DESIGNATIONS AND OTHER INFORMATION	**INTENDED MEANING**	**MISINTERPRETATION**	**CORRECTION**
Trailing zero after decimal point (e.g., 1.0 mg)[a]	1 mg	Mistaken as "10 mg" if the decimal point is not seen	Do not use trailing zeros for doses expressed in whole numbers
"Naked" decimal point (e.g., .5 mg)[a]	0.5 mg	Mistaken as "5 mg" if the decimal point is not seen	Use zero before a decimal point when the dose is less than a whole unit
Abbreviations such as mg. or mL. with a period following the abbreviation	mg mL	The period is unnecessary and could be mistaken as the number "1" if written poorly	Use "mg," "mL," etc. without a terminal period
Drug name and dose run together (especially problematic for drug names that end in "L" such as Inderal 40 mg; Tegretol 300 mg)	Inderal 40 mg Tegretol 300 mg	Mistaken as "Inderal 140 mg" Mistaken as "Tegretol 1300 mg"	Place adequate space between the drug name, dose, and unit of measure
Numerical dose and unit of measure run together (e.g., 10 mg, 100 mL)	10 mg 100 mL	The "m" is sometimes mistaken as a zero or two zeros, risking a 10- to 100-fold overdose	Place adequate space between the dose and unit of measure
Large doses without properly placed commas (e.g., 100000 units; 1000000 units)	100,000 units 1,000,000 units	100000 has been mistaken as 10,000 or 1,000,000; 1000000 has been mistaken as 100,000	Use commas for dosing units at or above 1,000, or use words such as 100 "thousand" or 1 "million" to improve readability
DRUG NAME ABBREVIATIONS	**INTENDED MEANING**	**MISINTERPRETATION**	**CORRECTION**

To avoid confusion, do not abbreviate drug names when communicating medical information. Examples of drug name abbreviations involved in medication errors include the following:

APAP	acetaminophen	Not recognized as acetaminophen	Use complete drug name
ARA A	vidarabine	Mistaken as "cytarabine (ARA C)"	Use complete drug name
AZT	zidovudine (Retrovir)	Mistaken as "azathioprine" or "aztreonam"	Use complete drug name
CPZ	prochlorperazine (Compazine)	Mistaken as "chlorpromazine"	Use complete drug name
DPT	Demerol-Phenergan-Thorazine	Mistaken as "diphtheria-pertussis-tetanus" (vaccine)	Use complete drug name

ABBREVIATION	INTENDED MEANING	MISINTERPRETATION	CORRECTION
DTO	Diluted tincture of opium, or deodorized tincture of opium (Paregoric)	Mistaken as "tincture of opium"	Use complete drug name
HCl	hydrochloric acid or hydrochloride	Mistaken as "potassium chloride" (the "H" is misinterpreted as "K")	Use complete drug name unless expressed as a salt of a drug
HCT	hydrocortisone	Mistaken as "hydrochlorothiazide"	Use complete drug name
HCTZ	hydrochlorothiazide	Mistaken as "hydrocortisone" (seen as HCT 250 mg)	Use complete drug name
$MgSO_4$[a]	magnesium sulfate	Mistaken as "morphine sulfate"	Use complete drug name
MS, MSO_4[a]	morphine sulfate	Mistaken as "magnesium sulfate"	Use complete drug name
MTX	methotrexate	Mistaken as "mitoxantrone"	Use complete drug name
NoAc	Novel/new oral anticoagulant	No anticoagulant	Use complete drug name
PCA	procainamide	Mistaken as "patient-controlled analgesia (PCA)"	Use complete drug name
PTU	propylthiouracil	Mistaken as "mercaptopurine"	Use complete drug name
T3	Tylenol with codeine No. 3	Mistaken as "liothyronine"	Use complete drug name
TAC	triamcinolone	Mistaken as "tetracaine, Adrenalin, cocaine"	Use complete drug name
TNK	TNKase	Mistaken as "TPA"	Use complete drug name
TPA or tPA	Tissue plasminogen activator, alteplase (Activase)	Mistaken as "tenecteplase (TNKase)," or less often as another tissue plasminogen activator, "retaplase (Retavase)"	Use complete drug names
$ZnSO_4$	zinc sulfate	Mistaken as "morphine sulfate"	Use complete drug name
STEMMED DRUG NAMES	**INTENDED MEANING**	**MISINTERPRETATION**	**CORRECTION**
"Nitro" drip	nitroglycerin infusion	Mistaken as "sodium nitroprusside infusion"	Use complete drug name
"Norflox"	norfloxacin	Mistaken as "Norflex"	Use complete drug name
"IV Vanc"	intravenous vancomycin	Mistaken as "Invanz"	Use complete drug name
SYMBOLS	**INTENDED MEANING**	**MISINTERPRETATION**	**CORRECTION**
ℨ	Dram	Symbol for dram mistaken as "3"	Use the metric system
♏	Minim	Symbol for minim mistaken as "mL"	Use the metric system
x3d	For 3 days	Mistaken as "3 doses"	Use "for 3 days"

SYMBOLS	INTENDED MEANING	MISINTERPRETATION	CORRECTION
> and <	Greater than and less than	Mistaken as opposite of intended; mistakenly use incorrect symbol; "< 10" mistaken as "40"	Use "greater than" or "less than"
/ (slash mark)	Separates two doses or indicates "per"	Mistaken as the number "1" (e.g., "25 units/10 units" misread as "25 units and 110" units)	Use "per" rather than a slash mark to separate doses
@	At	Mistaken as "2"	Use "at"
&	And	Mistaken as "2"	Use "and"
+	Plus or and	Mistaken as "4"	Use "and"
°	Hour	Mistaken as a zero (e.g., q2° seen as q 20)	Use "hr," "h," or "hour"
Φ or ∅	zero, null sign	Mistaken as numerals "4," "6," "8," and "9"	Use 0 or zero, or describe intent using whole words

ᵃThese abbreviations are included on The Joint Commission's "minimum list" of dangerous abbreviations, acronyms, and symbols that must be included on an organization's "Do Not Use" list, effective January 1, 2004. Visit www.jointcommission.org for more information about this Joint Commission requirement.

© ISMP 2015. Permission is granted to reproduce material with proper attribution for internal use within health care organizations. Other reproduction is prohibited without written permission from ISMP.

The following is a list of some common abbreviations and symbols that you should know. Although some of the following are included in one or both of these lists, you should still be aware of them and their preferred substitutes. Some may still be included on the PTCE—the national pharmacy technician certification examination.

Route of Administration

ID—intradermal
IM—intramuscular
IT—intrathecal
IV—intravenous
PO—by mouth
PR—rectal
PV—vaginal
*SC, SQ, sub q—subcutaneous—use **"SUBCUT"**
SL—sublingual (under the tongue)
TOP—topical

Frequency of Administration

qh—every hour
q2h—every 2 hours
q4h—every 4 hours
q6h—every 6 hours
q8h—every 8 hours
q12h—every 12 hours
*†qd—once a day—use **"daily"**
bid—twice a day
tid—three times a day
qid—four times a day
*†qod—every other day—use **"every other day"**
q week—every week
q month—every month

Times of Administration

ac—before meals
pc—after meals
am—morning
pm—evening
noc—night
*hs—hour of sleep—use *"bedtime"*
prn—as needed
ASAP—as soon as possible
STAT—at once, immediately

Dosage Forms

SOLIDS
cap—capsule
tab—tablet

LIQUIDS
fl, f—fluid
liq—liquid
susp—suspension
syr—syrup

SEMISOLIDS
cr—cream
lot—lotion
supp—suppository
ung/oint—ointment

Measurement Systems

METRIC SYSTEM
mcg—microgram
mg—milligram
g—gram
kg—kilogram
mL—milliliter
L—liter
m—meter

HOUSEHOLD SYSTEM
gtt—drop(s)
tsp, Tsp, t—teaspoon
tbsp, Tbsp, T—tablespoon
c, C—cup
oz—ounce
pt—pint
qt—quart
gal—gallon
#, lb—pound
", in—inch
', ft—foot

APOTHECARY SYSTEM—ABBREVIATIONS AND SYMBOLS

gr—grain
*ʒ/dr—dram—recommendation from ISMP is "use metric system"
ʒ/oz—ounce
*♏—minim—recommendation from ISMP is "use metric system"
*flʒ/fl dr—fluid dram
fl ʒ/fl oz—fluid ounce

MISCELLANEOUS MEDICATION MEASUREMENTS

mEq—milliequivalent
*†IU/U—international unit/unit—use **"international units"** or **"units"**

Ears and Eyes

*AD—right ear—use **"right ear"**
*AS—left ear—use **"left ear"**
*AU—each ear—use **"each ear"**
*OD—right eye—use **"right eye"**
*OS—left eye—use **"left eye"**
*OU—each eye—use **"each eye"**

General Abbreviations

ā—before
p̄—after
c̄—with
s̄—without
=—equal to
≠—not equal to
*<—less than use **"less than"**
*>—greater than, more than - use **"greater than"**
↑—higher than, increase
↓—lower than, decrease
āā—of each
ad lib—as desired
DAW—dispense as written
NKA—no known allergies
NKDA—no known drug allergies
non rep—do not repeat
NPO, npo—nothing by mouth
OTC—over the counter
qs—sufficient quantity
rep—repeat
℞—prescription, treatment, take this drug
TO—telephone order
*UD—ut dict—use **"as directed"**
VO—verbal order

*These abbreviations are found on the ISMP List of Error-Prone Abbreviations, Symbols, and Dose Designations due to medication safety issues. They should not be used but may still appear in the pharmacy setting.
†Indicates terms on TJC Official "Do Not Use" list.

Practice Problems A

Interpret the following abbreviations.

1. #, lb _____
2. ↓ _____
3. npo _____
4. ↑ _____
5. gtt _____
6. qid _____
7. q4h _____
8. mL _____
*9. hs _____
10. fl _____
11. tbsp, T _____
12. mcg _____
*13. U _____
14. cap _____
15. gr _____
16. OTC _____
17. bid _____
18. qh _____
19. q2h _____
20. kg _____
21. IM _____
22. IV _____
23. ad lib _____
24. ℞ _____

*These abbreviations are found on the TJC Official "Do Not Use" list and ISMP List of Error-Prone Abbreviations, Symbols, and Dose Designations due to medication safety issues. They should not be used but may still appear in the pharmacy setting.

25. tid _____ *26. qod _____

27. qs _____ 28. prn _____

29. tab _____ 30. ung _____

31. syr _____ 32. supp _____

33. elix _____ 34. aa _____

*35. ʒ _____ *36. ʒ _____

37. qam _____ 38. tsp, t _____

39. po _____ 40. p̄ _____

41. ā _____ 42. qpm _____

43. stat _____ 44. q12h _____

45. qd _____ 46. s̄s̄ _____

47. TO _____ 48. q _____

49. s̄ _____ 50. c̄ _____

*These abbreviations are found on the TJC Official "Do Not Use" list and ISMP List of Error-Prone Abbreviations, Symbols, and Dose Designations due to medication safety issues. They should not be used but may still appear in the pharmacy setting.

THE NEED FOR A PHARMACY TECHNICIAN TO MASTER MATHEMATICAL SKILLS

Pharmacy technicians are involved in the calculations of the amount of medication necessary to provide correct doses. They must also ensure that there are a sufficient number of doses for the desired length of therapy prescribed by the physician. Mathematics is used daily in the preparation of medications in both retail and institutional pharmacies. The responsibility that accompanies the preparation of medications is one that must be taken seriously so that effective drug levels are reached and dangerous drug levels are not reached. They must be familiar with acceptable limits—both minimums and maximums—of medications. They are responsible for the medications they prepare, although a pharmacist is required to double-check everything before it leaves the pharmacy.

Technicians are responsible for their actions, which are heavily dependent on mathematical skills. The course of pharmacology covers the skills required to master acceptable dosages and the expected results of medications. This text deals with the mathematical skills necessary for the safe preparation of the amount of medication prescribed for the patient.

The basic fundamental math skills necessary for pharmaceutical calculations include manipulation of fractions, decimals, and whole numbers to calculate the correct amount of medication needed. These skills are used for dose and dosage calculations in three measurement systems—household measurements such as teaspoons and tablespoons, which are used in the United States; metric system measurements such as grams, liters, and meters, which are commonly used throughout the rest of world; and apothecary system measurements such as grains, drams, and ounces, which were the basis of pharmacology but have now been mostly replaced by metric measurements. It is essential to understand these systems of measurement and be able to convert between them to prepare prescriptions for administration.

Additional mathematical conversions are also necessary, such as the conversion between 12-hour and 24-hour (military) time, because military time is used in inpatient settings for medication administration. The standard 12-hour time with AM and PM designations is used in most outpatient settings, so the ability to give the correct time in either situation is necessary. Conversions between Fahrenheit and Celsius temperatures and the use of Arabic and Roman numerals are also important in pharmacy.

BASIC MATH SKILLS USED IN PHARMACY

Basic math skills are necessary for safe and accurate dosage calculations. Understanding whole numbers, fractions, decimals, and percentages is crucial to pharmaceutical calculations. This knowledge is put to use in solving addition, subtraction, multiplication, and division problems on a basic algebra level. Many of the calculations will involve properly setting up and solving ratio and proportion equations. Knowing your multiplication tables without the use of a calculator is very helpful for keeping up with the pace of work in a pharmacy. A calculator will be available but most pharmacists will expect you to do simple calculations without one.

Practicing math skills without a calculator will increase your analytical math skills—skills that enable you to solve equations and take components of a whole to form relationships among its parts. Analysis of pharmacologic problems is an important step in ensuring accurate calculations with each medication order. Always ask yourself if your answer makes sense and check it.

The following is an assessment to help determine your strengths and weaknesses. It is also an indicator of your readiness to proceed through the text. Chapter 2 focuses on basic skills that you may need to review. Proficiency in basic math skills is extremely important.

SELF-TEST OF BASIC MATH SKILLS

Directions

1. Figure decimals to three places, then **round** the answer to the hundredths place; for example, 1.454 would become 1.45 and 7.5685 would become 7.57.
2. Express fractions in their lowest possible terms; for example, $\frac{4}{8}$ should be reduced to $\frac{1}{2}$.
3. Express ratios in their lowest possible terms; for example, 5:10 should be expressed 1:2.
4. Do your work on paper, without a calculator, and keep your paperwork attached so that if you made an error, you can return to the paper and find the mistake.

Basic Math Skills Proficiency Self-Test

1. Express the following sum in Arabic numerals: XXV + LX = _____
2. 156.90 + 368 = _____
3. 4.65 − 3.056 = _____
4. 3.50 × 43.5 = _____
5. $12.56 + $152.47 + $4.98 + $68.08 = _____
6. $52.43 × 0.25 = _____
7. 0.7 ÷ 0.0035 = _____
8. 78 + 0.186 = _____
9. $\frac{3}{4} + 7\frac{7}{8} =$ _____
10. 25 − 13 = (express in Roman numerals) _____
11. $15.43 × 25 = _____
12. 5,025 − 4,995 = (express in Roman numerals) _____
13. 1,932 ÷ 102 = _____
14. $\frac{1}{5} + \frac{4}{10} + \frac{3}{15} + \frac{5}{6} =$ _____
15. $\frac{5}{6} \div \frac{3}{8} =$ _____
16. $\frac{1}{200} \times 150 =$ _____
17. 6% of 36 = _____
18. Express 0.4 as a fraction. _____
19. Express 0.006 as a %. _____
20. 0.25% of 20 = _____

Copyright © 2019 by Elsevier, Inc. All rights reserved.

21. $1\frac{1}{3} + 3\frac{3}{4} =$ _____

22. $9\frac{1}{4} - 6\frac{3}{8} =$ _____

23. $1\frac{3}{8} \div \frac{1}{4} =$ _____

24. Which fraction has the greatest value? $\frac{1}{150}, \frac{1}{200}, \frac{1}{500}$ _____

25. Which decimal has the least value? 0.012, 0.12, 0.0125 _____

26. Change ¾ to a percentage. _____

27. Change 3½ to a decimal. _____

28. $\frac{2.2}{4.4} \times 60 =$ _____

29. $\frac{12.75}{2.25} =$ _____

30. Which has the greatest value? 3.75, 3¾, 3⅞ _____

31. One stock bottle of medication contains 20 tablets. How many tablets are in stock if the current inventory is 2½ bottles? _____

32. A prescription is written for 150 tablets. How many 50-tablet containers will it take to fill the prescription? _____

33. A prescription is written for 3 capsules a day for 1 week. How many capsules are needed to fill the entire prescription? _____

34. 1 inch equals 2.54 cm. How many centimeters are in 10 inches? _____

35. Express 70:350 in its lowest terms. _____

36. Solve for x. $\frac{50}{25}x = 120$ _____

37. Solve for x. $\frac{1}{100} \times 350 = x$ _____

38. $7 \times -5 =$ _____

39. 1 g = 1,000 mg. How many milligrams are in 5.5 g? _____

40. 1 kg equals 2.2 lb. How many kg are in 88 lb? _____

41. There are 400 prescriptions to fill on one shift, and you have completed 25% of them. How many are left to fill? _____

42. 1 kg equals 2.2 lb. How many pounds are in 11 kg? _____

43. Express 4% as a ratio in its lowest term. _____

44. Solve for x. $\frac{25}{75} = \frac{x}{15}$ _____

45. A stock bottle of medicine contains 500 tablets. How many prescriptions of 25 tablets can be filled with that bottle of medication?

46. Subtract the following and express in Roman numerals.
XIX − XIV =

47. 3.6 ÷ 0.0005 =

48. $4.28 + $5.65 + $0.78 + $15.39 =

49. 195.46 − 35.86 =

50. What is the least common multiple between 4, 6, and 8?

Pharmaceutical calculations incorporate basic algebra skills that are easy to learn as long as one has a good understanding of basic math skills. Continue working on these basic skills in Chapter 2 if needed. Spending the time necessary to become comfortable with the basic skills and information in the first two chapters of the text will make progression through the following chapters much easier. It is exciting to see how these skills lead to an interesting career as a pharmacy technician!

CHAPTER 2

Review of Basic Mathematical Skills

OBJECTIVES

1. Add, subtract, multiply, and divide whole numbers.
2. Add, subtract, multiply, and divide fractions, reduce fractions to the lowest terms, and discuss mixed numbers.
3. Add, subtract, multiply, and divide decimals, and round them to a specific number place value.
4. Convert between fractions, decimals, and percentages.
5. Express numbers in ratio and proportion, and solve for unknowns.

KEY WORDS

Complex fractions Fractions in which the numerator, denominator, or both are fractional units

Convert Change from one form to another

Decimal Representation of a fraction where the denominator is a power of 10 and the numerator is a number placed to the right of a decimal point

Decimal place Place values found to the right of the decimal point

Denominator Bottom number of a fraction

Dividend Number being divided in division

Divisor Number by which another number is divided

Fraction Part of a whole number with a numerator and denominator

Improper fraction Fraction in which the numerator is equal to or greater than the denominator; a fraction that is equal to or greater than 1

Invert To turn upside down or switch positions

Leading zero A zero placed before the decimal point in a number that is less than 1; necessary in pharmacy to reduce possible dosing errors

Least common denominator (LCD) The smallest whole number that can be divided evenly by all denominators of fractions within a problem; necessary for addition and subtraction of fractions; also known as least common multiple (LCM)

Lowest term Form of a fraction in which no common number will divide into both the numerator and denominator evenly

Mixed number Number containing a whole number and a fraction

Numerator Top number found in a fraction

Percent A means of expressing a portion of 100 parts

Product Number obtained by multiplying two numbers together

Proper fraction Fraction in which the numerator is less than the denominator; value is less than 1

Proportion Comparative relationship among the parts; one or more ratios that are compared

Quotient Answer of a division problem

Ratio A means of describing the relationship between two numbers; for example, 1:2

Remainder The amount left over after division

Round To express a number to its nearest place value such as ones, tenths, hundredths, etc.

Scored tablet Tablet containing an indentation for ease of breaking into equal parts

Trailing zero A zero in the farthest right place of a number following the decimal; not used in pharmacy due to the increased potential for dosing errors

Whole number Numeral consisting of one or more digits; number that is not followed by a fraction or decimal

Copyright © 2019 by Elsevier, Inc. All rights reserved.

Pretest

Answer the following and show your work. Do not use a calculator. Round all decimals to the hundredths place.

1. $154 + 1063 + 25 + 376 =$ _____

2. $163 - 69 =$ _____

3. $256 \times 43 =$ _____

4. $256 \div 16 =$ _____

5. $25.6 + 456 + 35.67 =$ _____

6. $354.29 - 45.390 =$ _____

7. $12.56 \times 65.031 =$ _____

8. $655.08 \div 1.2 =$ _____

9. $\dfrac{1}{2} + \dfrac{3}{4} + \dfrac{7}{8} =$ _____

10. $\dfrac{5}{8} - \dfrac{1}{6} =$ _____

11. $\dfrac{1}{8} + \dfrac{5}{12} + \dfrac{5}{6} =$ _____

12. $\dfrac{3}{5} \times \dfrac{7}{8} =$ _____

13. $\dfrac{5}{8} \div \dfrac{1}{4} =$ _____

14. $\dfrac{2}{3} \times \dfrac{14}{15} =$ _____

15. $16 \times \dfrac{5}{8} =$ _____

16. $36 \div \dfrac{4}{9} =$ _____

17. $12\dfrac{1}{2} - 11\dfrac{5}{6} =$ _____

18. $2\dfrac{3}{5} - 1\dfrac{1}{3} =$ _____

19. $4\dfrac{1}{10} \times 2 =$ _____

20. $\dfrac{2}{9} \times 3\dfrac{3}{5} \times \dfrac{5}{6} =$ _____

21. $3 \div \dfrac{1}{4} =$ _____

Pretest, cont.

Round the following decimals to the nearest hundredth.

22. 75.0023 _____

23. 12.015 _____

24. 6.12753 _____

Change the following fractions to decimals.

25. $\dfrac{3}{5}$ _____

26. $1\dfrac{3}{25}$ _____

27. $1\dfrac{3}{4}$ _____

28. $\dfrac{7}{20}$ _____

Reduce to lowest terms.

29. $\dfrac{34}{68}$ _____

30. $\dfrac{25}{75}$ _____

31. $\dfrac{12}{96}$ _____

Solve the following proportions.

32. $\dfrac{x}{3} = \dfrac{15}{30}$ $x =$ _____

33. $\dfrac{5}{15} = \dfrac{8}{x}$ $x =$ _____

34. $\dfrac{3}{x} = \dfrac{11}{33}$ $x =$ _____

35. $\dfrac{1}{50} = \dfrac{x}{40}$ $x =$ _____

Continued

Pretest, cont.

Write the following percents as fractions and simplify.

36. 44% _____

37. 0.5% _____

38. 125% _____

Change the following percents to decimals.

39. 33% _____

40. 0.04% _____

41. 132% _____

42. A prescription calls for 15 mL of water to reconstitute a medication in a 20-mL vial. How many milliliters of water would be needed proportionally to reconstitute 50-mL vial of the same medication?

43. A pharmacist is able to fill six prescriptions in 10 minutes with the assistance of a pharmacy technician. How many prescriptions can be completed in 1 hour?

44. A pharmacy offers a 10% discount for senior citizens. How much will a senior save off of a $25 prescription?

45. 85 is what percent of 200?

INTRODUCTION

In calculation of medications, accuracy is extremely important for patient safety. The patient depends on your calculations and the pharmacist expects you to correctly make those calculations. Answers must be precise; partially correct answers are unacceptable and may endanger patient safety. Basic math skills are essential in pharmacy. Always look at your answer and ask, "Does it make sense?" Use estimation and your knowledge of normal medication doses to be sure your answer is within a normal range.

Review the following concepts and skills, paying close attention to the ones you have the most difficulty understanding. **Do not use a calculator** for this chapter so that you really learn the basic skills. Once you have performed the calculations, you can use a calculator to check your answers. These skills and concepts are the basis for pharmacy calculations.

WHOLE NUMBERS

A whole number is a numeral consisting of one or more digits that is not followed by a decimal or fraction. The digits used in math are 0, 1, 2, 3, 4, 5, 6, 7, 8, and 9. Numbers may also be written in words, such as one, two, ten, one hundred, one hundred thirty, and so on. Commas are recommended to be used on medication doses greater than 999, according to the Institute for Safe Medication Practices (ISMP) (see http://www.ismp.org/tools/guidelines/standardordersets.pdf). Therefore a dose of one thousand units of heparin should be written 1,000 units.

A whole number is always to the left of a decimal point. The numeral 0 is a whole number with the decimal understood to be at the right side of the zero. When adding, subtracting, or multiplying whole numbers, the answer will always be a whole number. This is not always the case when dividing whole numbers. Any number that remains when numbers are not exactly divisible is called a remainder and is expressed as a fraction or decimal. For example, 10 divided by 2 is 5, but 11 divided by 3 is $3\frac{2}{3}$ or $3.66\overline{6}$; 11 and 3 are whole numbers, but they are not evenly divisible and the answer is expressed including a fraction or decimal.

Adding and Subtracting Whole Numbers

When adding or subtracting whole numbers, align the digits from the right and then add or subtract one set of digits at a time starting from the right (from ones to tens to hundreds, etc.).

Addition is finding a sum or total of numbers. Subtraction is finding the difference between two numbers.

EXAMPLE 2.1

$$\begin{array}{cccc} 25 & 236 & 1302 & 10584 \\ +\ 5 & -\ 24 & +\ 205 & -10263 \\ \hline 30 & 212 & 1507 & 321 \end{array}$$

Practice Problems A

Add or subtract the following. Show your work and state measurement units as appropriate.

1. 25 + 56 = _____

2. 105 + 235 = _____

3. 50 g + 100 g = _____

4. 25 mg + 90 mg = _____

5. 125,000 units + 250,000 units = _____

6. 7,500 mL + 1,000 mL = _____

7. 285 − 168 = _____

8. 1549 − 1374 = _____

9. 725 mL − 650 mL = _____

10. 525 g − 175 g = _____

11. 156# − 48# = _____

12. 350 mg − 125 mg = _____

13. 266 kg − 15 kg = _____

14. A bottle of antibiotic needs to be reconstituted with 100 mL of distilled water. You have a 50 mL graduate. How many times will you have to fill it with water to reconstitute the medication?

15. A vial of anesthetic contains 10 mL. The pharmacist asks that you add 30 mL of distilled water to prepare an anesthetic compound for mouth ulcers. How many milliliters will be in the bottle of prepared medication?

Multiplying Whole Numbers

When multiplying whole numbers, align the numbers or factors as you would for addition or subtraction. The use of "×" or "•" denotes that the numbers should be multiplied to find a **product**. Remember that a number multiplied by zero is zero.

First multiply the number on top of the problem by the number at the far right of the bottom of the equation. Place the ones digit of this answer under the line and carry the tens digit to the next place. Multiply the remaining numbers in the subsequent digits, moving from right to left, keeping the numbers in alignment. Move to the next number to the left in the bottom number and repeat the process. Remember that the second number is already in the tens place, so it must be placed one space to the left of the first answer. Sometimes it is helpful to place a zero in the ones place to keep the alignment (place holder shown in **bold** in the following examples). Finally, add the numbers that have been multiplied to obtain the product.

EXAMPLE 2.2

$$\begin{array}{r} 125 \\ \times\, 15 \\ \hline 625 \\ +\, 125\mathbf{0} \\ \hline 1875 \end{array}$$

EXAMPLE 2.3

$$\begin{array}{r} 225 \\ \times\, 10 \\ \hline 000 \\ +\, 225\mathbf{0} \\ \hline 2250 \end{array}$$

Be sure to maintain the alignment!

Dividing Whole Numbers

Division is represented by either "÷" or ")". The number being divided is called the **dividend**, and the number used to divide is the **divisor**. The result of division is the **quotient**.

$$\text{divisor} \overline{)\text{dividend}}^{\text{quotient}}$$

EXAMPLE 2.4

$$\begin{array}{r} 11 \\ 25{\overline{\smash{\big)}\,275}} \\ \underline{-25} \\ 25 \\ \underline{-25} \\ 0 \end{array}$$

In this example, 25 cannot be divided into 2, so move to 27 to divide by 25. Be sure to place the 1 *directly above* the 7 and maintain the correct alignment.

General rules to remember with division:

Any number divided by itself equals 1: $7 \div 7 = 1$
Any number divided by 1 equals that same number: $7 \div 1 = 7$
Zero divided by any number remains zero: $0 \div 7 = 0$
Zero can *never* be the divisor: $7 \div 0$ is undefined

Practice Problems B

Multiply or divide the following. Show your work. Estimate first.

1. $56 \times 10 =$ _____

2. $76 \bullet 11 =$ _____

3. $100 \times 87 =$ _____

4. $3500 \times 265 =$ _____

5. $\begin{array}{r} 653 \\ \times\ 30 \end{array} =$ _____

6. $\begin{array}{r} 275 \\ \times\ 310 \end{array} =$ _____

7. $105 \div 5 =$ _____

8. $840 \div 40 =$ _____

9. $296 \div 4 =$ _____

10. $1125 \div 15 =$ _____

11. $150 \div 15 =$ _____

12. $15{\overline{\smash{\big)}\,600}} =$ _____

13. $12{\overline{\smash{\big)}\,276}} =$ _____

14. $150 \text{ mg} \times 4 =$ _____

15. A prescription is written for ten 250 mg tablets. What is the weight of the medication in the total prescription?

16. The manufacturer's label states to add 375 mL of water to a medication for reconstitution. How many times do you need to fill a 125-mL graduated cylinder to reconstitute the medication?

FRACTIONS

When a whole number or unit is divided into parts, the parts are called **fractions**. Fractions may be expressed in the form a/b or $\dfrac{a}{b}$, with the latter being preferred with pharmaceutical calculations for ease of keeping track of units and reducing numbers. The "a" is called the **numerator** (top number found in a fraction). The "b" is the **denominator** (bottom number of a fraction). Both numbers must be whole numbers, and the denominator can never be 0, which is undefined. The denominator tells how many times the whole unit has been divided.

The circle graph pictured shows a proper fraction. The shaded area shows the part of a whole. There are 3 (numerator) parts out of 4 (denominator) shaded, or ¾.

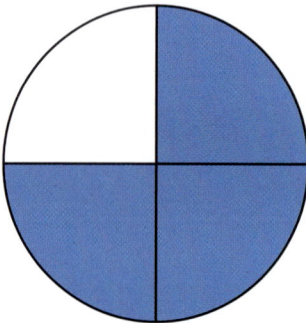

In the next picture, the numerator is 5 and the denominator is 6.

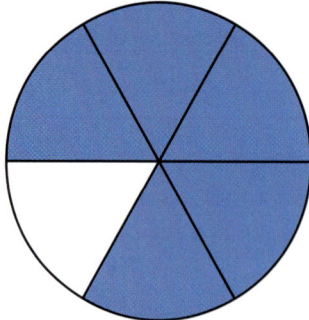

TECH NOTE
Fractions are used in pharmacy in both the household and apothecary systems, but not with the metric system.

Practice Problems C

In the following examples, indicate the numerator and the denominator.

1. $\dfrac{5}{7}$ Numerator _____   Denominator _____

2. $\dfrac{8}{11}$ Numerator _____   Denominator _____

3. $\dfrac{7}{15}$ Numerator _____   Denominator _____

4. $\dfrac{135}{356}$ Numerator _____   Denominator _____

5. $\dfrac{5}{6}$ Numerator _____   Denominator _____

TECH NOTE
Whole numbers are actually fractions in which the numerator is an exact multiple of the denominator.

A **proper fraction** is one in which the numerator is less than the denominator and is part of a whole, such as $\frac{2}{3}$ and $\frac{5}{8}$. Its value is always less than 1. An **improper fraction** is a fraction in which the numerator is greater than or equal to the denominator, making the fraction equivalent to or greater than 1, such as $\frac{9}{8} = 1\frac{1}{8}$ and $\frac{14}{7} = 2$. If the numerator and denominator are the same, the value is 1, such as $\frac{9}{9} = 1$ and $\frac{10}{10} = 1$.

An improper fraction can be changed into a **mixed number** (a whole number and a fraction). Because a fraction indicates division, the numerator divided by the denominator, when $\frac{a}{b}$ or $\frac{a}{b}$ is written, the fraction actually means a ÷ b. To **convert** or change an improper fraction to a mixed number, divide the numerator by the denominator. Any remainder is written over the denominator.

EXAMPLE 2.5

Convert the improper fraction $\dfrac{43}{8}$ to a mixed number.

43 ÷ 8 = 5 with a remainder of 3

$\dfrac{43}{8}$ as a mixed number is $5\dfrac{3}{8}$.

The remainder is the amount that is left over after the whole number has been divided into the numerator the maximum number of times. An improper fraction should always be changed to a mixed number after calculations have been completed.

To change a mixed number to an improper fraction, multiply the whole number by the denominator and add the amount found in the numerator.

EXAMPLE 2.6

Convert $4\frac{1}{8}$ to an improper fraction.

$$4 \cdot 8 = 32$$

Add the 1 found in the numerator of the fraction: $32 + 1 = 33$

The denominator remains the same, so the improper fraction is $\frac{33}{8}$

Practice Problems D

Show your work. Indicate measurements as appropriate.
Convert the following improper fractions to mixed numbers or whole numbers.

1. $\frac{16}{3} =$ _____

2. $\frac{24}{7} =$ _____

3. $\frac{35}{4} =$ _____

4. $\frac{223}{110} =$ _____

5. $\frac{16}{15} =$ _____

6. $\frac{21}{7} =$ _____

7. gr $\frac{5}{4} =$ _____

8. $\frac{9}{8}$ c = _____

9. $\frac{3}{2}$ tab = _____

10. $\frac{6}{6}$ tab = _____

Convert the following mixed numbers to improper fractions.

11. $3\frac{1}{2} =$ _____

12. $2\frac{7}{8} =$ _____

13. $3\frac{1}{4} =$ _____

14. $10\frac{9}{10} =$ _____

15. $4\frac{5}{7}$ = _____

16. $2\frac{1}{2}$ c = _____

17. $6\frac{3}{4}$ qt = _____

18. $4\frac{1}{2}$ tab = _____

19. $3\frac{1}{3}$ c = _____

20. $5\frac{1}{4}$ c = _____

Indicate the fraction or mixed number for the following shaded areas.

21. 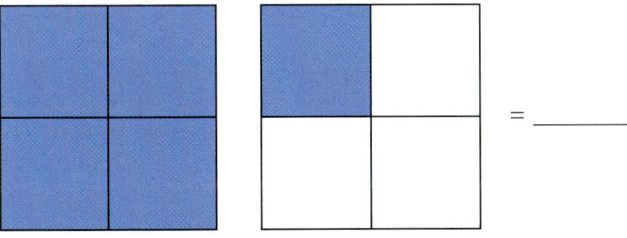 = _____

22. 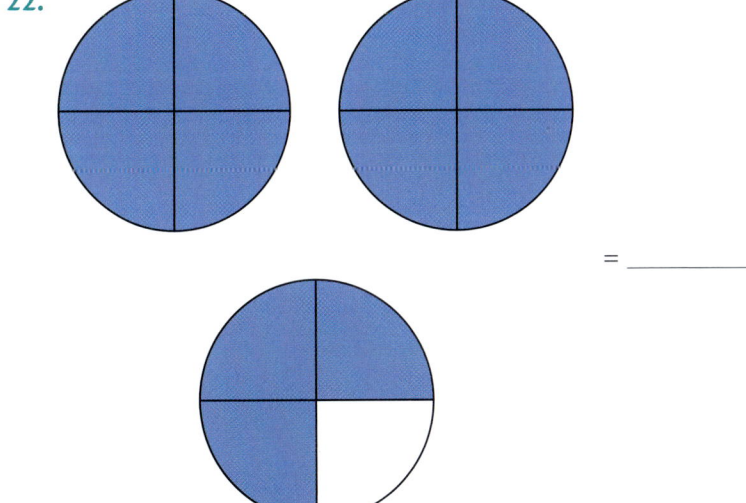 = _____

23. A pharmacist has a medicine cup that is divided into eight equal sections. She fills to the line to indicate five parts. What is the fractional amount that the pharmacist has filled?

24. A customer asks you to show him how to divide a tablet (i.e., a **scored tablet** that is divided into four equal parts) into one-half of a tablet. Fill in the following tablet to indicate this fraction.

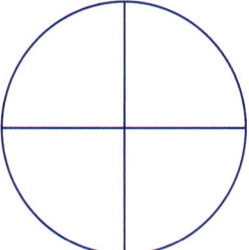

Reducing Fractions to the Lowest Term

Some fractions, called equivalent fractions, have the same value. The fraction ½ is equivalent to ²⁄₄, ³⁄₆, or ⁵⁰⁄₁₀₀. With ²⁄₄, the numerator and denominator can both be divided by 2 to give ½; with ³⁄₆, both parts of the fraction can be divided by 3 to give ½; with ⁵⁰⁄₁₀₀, both components of the fraction can be divided by 50 to give ½. Each of these fractions is actually one-half of the total number of equivalent parts of a whole.

When reducing fractions, the numerator and the denominator must be divided by the same nonzero number. For example, ³⁄₁₂ can be reduced to ¼ by dividing the numerator and denominator by 3. Dividing by ³⁄₃ is the same as dividing by 1, so it does not change the *value* of the fraction. A fraction is reduced to the **lowest term** when no common number will divide into both the numerator and denominator evenly.

Practice Problems E

Reduce the following fractions to the lowest terms. Show your calculations and indicate measurements as appropriate.

1. $\dfrac{3}{6} =$ _____

2. $\dfrac{6}{9} =$ _____

3. $\dfrac{8}{12} =$ _____

4. $\dfrac{25}{125} =$ _____

5. $\dfrac{7}{35} =$ _____

6. $\dfrac{27}{108} =$ _____

7. $\dfrac{6}{48} =$ _____

8. $\dfrac{125}{750} =$ _____

9. A pharmacist has a bottle of medication that contains 90 tablets. He dispenses 45 tablets. What is the fractional use?

10. A medication states to add the first 40 mL out of 60 mL of water and shake. What fraction of the water is added first?

Adding and Subtracting Fractions

When adding or subtracting fractions, the denominators must be the same. Once the denominators are the same number, the numerators may be either added or subtracted. The denominator remains the same.

EXAMPLE 2.7

$$\frac{3}{5} + \frac{1}{5} = \frac{4}{5}$$

EXAMPLE 2.8

$$\frac{3}{5} - \frac{1}{5} = \frac{2}{5}$$

Finding Common Denominators

If the denominators are not the same, the smallest whole number that can be divided evenly by both denominators within the problem is needed: the **least common denominator** (LCD). Sometimes the LCD is easily found because one denominator can be divided by the other. Since 15 is divisible by 5, it is a common denominator for $\frac{3}{5} + \frac{2}{15}$.

To change fractions to their equivalent fractions for adding or subtracting, first find the lowest common denominator. Then multiply the numerator and denominator of each fraction by the fraction *equaling 1* that will make the denominators equal to the LCD. Then add or subtract the fractions by adding or subtracting the numerators and leaving the denominator the same.

EXAMPLE 2.9

$$\frac{3}{10} - \frac{2}{15}$$

The smallest number that both 10 and 15 can divide into equally is 30—the LCD.
10 times 3 equals 30, so multiply the first fraction by $\frac{3}{3}$.

$$\frac{3}{10} \times \frac{3}{3} = \frac{9}{30}$$

15 times 2 equals 30, so multiply the second fraction by $\frac{2}{2}$.

$$\frac{2}{15} \times \frac{2}{2} = \frac{4}{30}$$

Remember that both $\frac{3}{3}$ and $\frac{2}{2}$ equal 1, so the *values* of the fractions are unchanged. Rewrite the equation and solve:

$$\frac{9}{30} - \frac{4}{30} = \frac{5}{30}$$

Reduce the answer by dividing the numerator and denominator by 5:

$$\frac{5}{30} \div \frac{5}{5} = \frac{1}{6}$$

$\frac{5}{5}$ equals 1, so the *value* of the answer is unchanged.

If a mixed number is in the expression, the mixed number should be converted to an improper fraction before finding the common denominator. Then convert both fractions to the lowest common denominator and add or subtract as indicated.

EXAMPLE 2.10

$$\frac{3}{4} + 3\frac{5}{8}$$

3 times 8 is 24 plus 5 equals 29.

$$3\frac{5}{8} = \frac{29}{8}$$

Because 4 times 2 is 8, multiply the numerator and denominator of the first fraction by $\frac{2}{2}$:

$$\frac{3}{4} \times \frac{2}{2} = \frac{6}{8}$$

The problems becomes:

$$\frac{6}{8} + \frac{29}{8} = \frac{35}{8}$$

35 divided by 8 equals 4 with a remainder of 3, so the answer is $4\frac{3}{8}$.

If the LCD is not readily apparent, multiply the denominators and use that number as the common denominator (e.g., if the denominators are 5 and 7, one common denominator will always be 35 because $5 \times 7 = 35$). This method may not provide the least common denominator, but it can be used. It may require further reducing of the answer.

Practice Problems F

Add or subtract the following. Reduce to lowest terms. Show your calculations. Indicate measurements as appropriate.

1. $\frac{1}{3} + \frac{1}{3} =$ _____

2. $\frac{3}{8} + \frac{4}{8} =$ _____

3. $\frac{2}{7} + \frac{3}{7} =$ _____

4. $\frac{5}{8} - \frac{1}{8} =$ _____

5. $\frac{8}{9} - \frac{5}{9} =$ _____

6. $\frac{13}{15} - \frac{10}{15} =$ _____

7. $\dfrac{3}{8}c + \dfrac{2}{8}c = $ _____

8. $\dfrac{5}{6}c - \dfrac{1}{6}c = $ _____

9. $1\dfrac{1}{3} + \dfrac{4}{9} = $ _____

10. $3\dfrac{2}{3} + 1\dfrac{3}{5} = $ _____

11. $1\dfrac{3}{16} + 2\dfrac{3}{8} = $ _____

12. $\dfrac{4}{7} + \dfrac{3}{11} = $ _____

13. $\dfrac{5}{12} + \dfrac{3}{4} = $ _____

14. $\dfrac{2}{3}c + \dfrac{1}{6}c = $ _____

15. $\dfrac{1}{3}$ tsp $+ \dfrac{1}{6}$ tsp $= $ _____

16. $2\dfrac{1}{2}$ qt $+ \dfrac{1}{4}$ qt $= $ _____

17. $\dfrac{1}{8}$ qt $+ \dfrac{3}{4}$ qt $= $ _____

18. $3\dfrac{1}{4} - 2\dfrac{1}{4} = $ _____

19. $4\dfrac{1}{5} - 2\dfrac{9}{10} = $ _____

20. $1\dfrac{7}{8}c - 1\dfrac{3}{16}c = $ _____

21. $2\dfrac{3}{8}$ tsp $- 1\dfrac{1}{6}$ tsp $= $ _____

22. $4\dfrac{3}{4}$ qt $- \dfrac{1}{16}$ qt $= $ _____

23. $3\dfrac{5}{16}\# - 1\dfrac{3}{8}\# = $ _____

24. A bottle of medication granules contains $12\dfrac{1}{2}$ oz of the desired medication. A newer medication container holds $11\dfrac{15}{16}$ oz of the medication. What is the difference in the amount of medication in the two bottles?

25. You have $3\dfrac{3}{4}$ oz of a specific medication. In 1 day, you have used $2\dfrac{3}{16}$ oz of that medication. How much medication will you have left for use to fill prescriptions the next day?

Multiplying Fractions

To find the product of fractions, multiply the numerators *and* the denominators. The product should then be reduced to the lowest term. Multiplication of fractions *does not* require a common denominator.

EXAMPLE 2.11

$$\frac{5}{6} \cdot \frac{3}{5} = \frac{15}{30}$$

Both the numerator and denominator are divisible by 15, so divide the answer by $^{15}/_{15}$ to get $½$.

With multiplication of fractions, any number from either numerator can be reduced with any number in either denominator before multiplying, if possible. The previous example can be viewed as if the line extends over both fractions: $\frac{5 \cdot 3}{6 \cdot 5}$.

The 5 in the numerator of the first fraction could be reduced with the 5 in the denominator of the second fraction, both to 1. The 3 could also have been reduced to 1 and the 6 to 2 before doing any multiplying: $\frac{1 \cdot 1}{2 \cdot 1} = \frac{1}{2}$.

> **TECH NOTE**
> To multiply (or divide) mixed numbers, change the mixed number to an improper fraction first.

Dividing Fractions

Dividing fractions involves **inverting** the divisor (the *second* number in the expression, which is the number to the right of the division sign) so that the numerator becomes the denominator and the denominator becomes the numerator. In simpler terms, the numbers switch places. For example, if $⅘$ is inverted, the fraction would become $5⁄4$. After inverting the numerator and denominator of the fraction to the *right* of the division sign, continue with the steps as for multiplication—multiply the numerators and multiply the denominators, placing the products with the numerators over the denominators. Finally, reduce the resultant fraction to the lowest possible terms.

EXAMPLE 2.12

$\frac{4}{5} \div \frac{5}{10}$ $\frac{5}{10}$ is the fraction to be inverted, so the problem becomes $\frac{4}{5} \cdot \frac{10}{5} = \frac{40}{25}$.

40 divided by 25 equals 1 with 15 left over, so the answer is changed to $1\frac{15}{25}$.

The fraction can be reduced by dividing the numerator and denominator by 5 for the quotient $1\frac{3}{5}$.

As with the previous example, once the multiplication problem has been set up, numbers may be reduced before multiplying. The 5 in the first fraction can be reduced with the 10 in the second fraction, resulting in $\frac{4}{1} \cdot \frac{2}{5} = \frac{8}{5}$. This can be converted in one step to $1\frac{3}{5}$.

CHAPTER 2   Review of Basic Mathematical Skills   31

TECH NOTE
When dividing fractions, invert the fraction to the **right** of the division sign and multiply.

Practice Problems G

Perform the multiplication or division and then reduce the fractions to the lowest terms. Show calculations and indicate measurements as appropriate.

1. $\dfrac{2}{3} \times \dfrac{3}{5} = $ _____

2. $\dfrac{1}{8} \times \dfrac{6}{9} = $ _____

3. $\dfrac{3}{5} \times \dfrac{5}{8} = $ _____

4. $\dfrac{3}{25} \times \dfrac{15}{21} = $ _____

5. $\dfrac{1}{3} \times \dfrac{3}{4} = $ _____

6. $\dfrac{1}{3} \times \dfrac{4}{5} = $ _____

7. $\dfrac{7}{12} \times \dfrac{5}{9} = $ _____

8. $\dfrac{3}{8} \times \dfrac{1}{3} = $ _____

9. $2\dfrac{1}{3} \times 3\dfrac{4}{5} = $ _____

10. $5\dfrac{6}{7} \times \dfrac{7}{8} = $ _____

11. $4\dfrac{3}{4} \times 3\dfrac{5}{9} = $ _____

12. $1\dfrac{3}{8} \times 7\dfrac{8}{9} = $ _____

13. $8\dfrac{1}{9} \times 2\dfrac{3}{4} = $ _____

14. $\dfrac{9}{10} \div \dfrac{2}{5} = $ _____

15. $\dfrac{2}{5} \div \dfrac{3}{4} = $ _____

16. $3 \div \dfrac{1}{3} = $ _____

17. $\dfrac{1}{4} \div 3 = $ _____

18. $\dfrac{3}{4} \div \dfrac{4}{7} = $ _____

Copyright © 2019 by Elsevier, Inc. All rights reserved.

19. $4 \div \dfrac{3}{4} =$ _____

20. $5\dfrac{1}{3} \div \dfrac{2}{6} =$ _____

21. $4\dfrac{1}{3} \div 2\dfrac{2}{25} =$ _____

22. $7\dfrac{2}{3} \div 2\dfrac{2}{5} =$ _____

23. $4\dfrac{3}{4} \div 3\dfrac{1}{6} =$ _____

24. Your stock bottle of medication contains 500 tablets. You have used ¾ of the bottle. How many tablets do you have left in stock for filling future prescriptions?

25. A bottle of liquid antibiotic contains 150 mL of medication, or 30 teaspoons. If each dose is 1½ tsp, how many doses are in the bottle? If the medication is given four times a day, how many days will it last?

Complex fractions are fractional expressions in which the numerator, denominator, or both are expressed as fractions or decimals. This will be covered again in later chapters. Solving these fractions can be approached in a couple of different ways.

Complex Fractions
EXAMPLE 2.13

$\dfrac{¼}{½}$ can be multiplied by $\dfrac{4}{4}$ to convert it to $\dfrac{1}{2}$.

$\dfrac{¼}{½}$ can be written $\dfrac{1}{4} \div \dfrac{1}{2}$ and then inverted and multiplied: $\dfrac{1}{4} \times \dfrac{2}{1} = \dfrac{2}{4} = \dfrac{1}{2}$.

$\dfrac{0.4}{60}$ can be multiplied by $\dfrac{10}{10}$ to form the fraction $\dfrac{4}{600}$, which reduces to $\dfrac{1}{150}$.

$\dfrac{0.4}{60}$ can be written $\dfrac{4}{10} \div \dfrac{60}{1}$ and then inverted and multiplied: $\dfrac{4}{10} \times \dfrac{1}{60} = \dfrac{4}{600} = \dfrac{1}{150}$.

DECIMALS

Decimal are actually fractions with a denominator of 10, 100, 1000, or any multiple of 10. Decimal numbers may include a whole number, a decimal point, and the decimal fraction. The metric system, the most frequently used measurement system in the medical field, uses decimals. Examples of decimals include $0.1 = \dfrac{1}{10}$, $0.01 = \dfrac{1}{100}$, or $0.001 = \dfrac{1}{1000}$.

To avoid errors in the medical field, a decimal less than 1 should always be written with a **leading zero**, a zero in front of the decimal point. For example, the decimal .25 should be written as 0.25, and .5 as 0.5. A medical professional should never write ".25" or ".5" because the decimal could be overlooked. Such an inaccuracy, interpreting a highly increased dosage, could be deadly to the person taking the medicine.

To write decimals using word names, the number to the left will be a whole number and the decimal point becomes the word "and," with the number to the right of the **decimal place** followed by the place values of the decimal ending with "th."

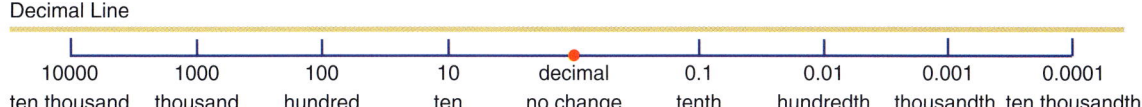

Decimal Line

3.07 is three and seven hundredths.

Three	The number to the left of the decimal point
And	The decimal point
Seven	The number to the right of the decimal point
Hundredths	The place value of the decimal

AND

1.250 is one and two hundred fifty thousandths.

One	The number to the left of the decimal point
And	The decimal point
Two hundred fifty	The number to the right of the decimal point
Thousandths	The place value of the decimal

Zeros at the end of a decimal, **trailing zeros**, do not change the *value* of the number. Trailing zeros are on The Joint Commission's "Do Not Use" list and will *not* be used in pharmaceutical calculations because of possible interpretation errors.

1.250 has the same value as 1.25, so it can also be read as one and twenty-five hundredths.

Practice Problems H

Write the following decimal numbers in words.

1. 4.34 _____
2. 3.5 _____
3. 6.751 _____
4. 90.54 _____
5. 954.6 _____
6. 0.0035 _____
7. 4.02 _____
8. 0.26 _____

9. 0.78 _____

10. 0.175 _____

Comparing Decimals

To compare a decimal, the decimal amounts must be aligned at the decimal point and zeros should be added so that the numbers following the decimal point contain the same number of decimal places. This is important in the comparison of medications in the metric system of measurement.

EXAMPLE 2.14

Compare 0.125, 0.25, and 0.5.

0.125 may appear to be the largest number, but when the numbers are aligned and the proper zeros are added for numbers to have equal decimal places to the right of the decimal point, this proves to be incorrect.

0.125	One-hundred twenty-five thousandths
0.250	Two-hundred fifty thousandths
0.500	Five-hundred thousandths

Adding or removing trailing zeros does not change the value, but it makes the numbers easier to compare. The largest number is really 0.5 and not 0.125, which might not seem apparent without the added zeros. Note that the decimals are less than 1, so a leading zero was added to ensure that the decimal point was not overlooked.

Rounding Decimals

When calculating doses of medication, decimals may need to be rounded to a specific place value. Accuracy in calculating to a particular decimal place is necessary in some circumstances, whereas **rounding** or approximating is acceptable in others. For example, if 18 units of subcutaneous insulin U-100 are ordered, the volume given must be 0.18 mL. It cannot be rounded to 0.2 mL. If an oral medication dose is calculated to be 3.99 mg and a 4-mg tablet is available, the patient would receive one tablet by rounding to the whole number 4.

> **TECH NOTE**
> Determining the appropriate place value when rounding medication doses depends on the potency, the amount, and the route of administration.

> **! TECH ALERT**
> Only round the **final** answer when performing multiple step calculations.

Steps for Rounding

Step 1: Underline the digit in the place for rounding.
Step 2: Look at the digit to the right of the underlined digit:

If it is greater than or equal to 5, round the underlined digit to the next highest number and drop all digits to the right.
If it is less than 5, drop all digits to the right of the underlined digit and keep it the same.

EXAMPLE 2.15

Round 1.16 to the tenths place.

   1.1<u>6</u>: The 6 indicates that the number to its left be rounded up to 1.2.

Round 1.14 to the tenths place.

   1.1<u>4</u>: The 4 indicates that the number to its left is to stay the same or 1.1.

Practice Problems I

Round to the nearest hundredth.

1. 2.356 = _____
2. 5.652 = _____
3. 36.445 = _____
4. 2.984 = _____
5. 0.1245 = _____
6. 8.2374 = _____
7. 6.116 g = _____

Round to the nearest tenth.

8. 3.45 = _____
9. 3.64 = _____
10. 3.26 = _____
11. 12.14 = _____
12. 3.05 = _____
13. 12.49 mg = _____
14. 1.46 mg = _____
15. 2.54 mL = _____

Round the following to the nearest whole number.

16. 9.64 = _____
17. 10.08 = _____
18. 14.16 = _____
19. 125.3 mg = _____
20. 275.1 mL = _____

   Estimating answers to addition, subtraction, multiplication, and division problems involving decimals can be done by rounding to whole numbers to get an approximate answer. This is a good way to check that the decimal is in the correct position in your final answer. For example, the problem 10.3578 divided by 2.15 can be estimated to be around 5 by dividing 10 by 2. Therefore if your final answer is near 0.5 or 50, you know that you have misplaced the decimal.

Adding and Subtracting Decimals

Adding and subtracting decimals requires aligning whole numbers and decimal points. After aligning the decimal points, add zeros at the end of the decimal fraction until all decimal numbers are to the same decimal place. Then just add or subtract as you would for whole numbers, remembering to correctly place the decimal point in the answer.

EXAMPLE 2.16

3.4678 − 2.34

$$\begin{array}{r} 3.4678 \\ -\,2.34\mathbf{00} \\ \hline 1.1278 \end{array}$$

Practice Problems J

Add or subtract as indicated. Show your work. Round final answers to the nearest hundredth and indicate measurements as appropriate.

1. 2.35 + 3.1 + 4.678 = _____
2. 5.7 + 18.25 + 95.37 = _____
3. 2.38 + 14.7 + 1346 = _____
4. 6.002 + 3.23 + 9.1 = _____
5. 12.5 mg + 6.25 mg = _____
6. $12.50 + $0.42 + $140.67 = _____
7. $5.67 + $136.99 + $89.09 = _____
8. 2.76 − 1.98 = _____
9. 4.8 − 1.987 = _____
10. 75.3 − 16.95 = _____
11. 125 − 0.125 = _____
12. $15.75 − $5.65 = _____
13. $17.49 − $5.05 = _____
14. 0.2 g − 0.02 g = _____
15. 12.5 mg − 10.5 mg = _____

16. A prescription costs $25.50. The customer gives you two $20 bills. How much change do you owe the customer?

17. A stock bottle of medication contains 500 mg of drug used in compounding other medications. You used 125 mg for one prescription, 62.5 mg for a second prescription, and 25.25 mg for the third.

    What quantity of medication was used?

    What quantity of the original medication is left?

18. A customer has three prescriptions—one costing $35, the second costing $17.50, and the third costing $23.60.

What is the total cost of the prescriptions?

If the customer gives you four 20-dollar bills, how much should you return?

Multiplying Decimals

Multiplying decimals is similar to multiplying whole numbers. The alignment of the numbers is identical, without regard to the placement of the decimal. The difference is the proper placement of the decimal *after* the product has been calculated. After the product is calculated, count the number of places to the right of the decimal points in both of the numbers that were multiplied. Finally, place a decimal point in the product by counting from right to left the number of decimal places found in both elements of the problem.

EXAMPLE 2.17

$$
\begin{array}{r}
37.25 \\
\times\ 1.5 \\
\hline
18,625 \\
+ 37,250 \\
\hline
55,875 \\
55.875
\end{array}
$$

- 37.25 (two decimal places)
- × 1.5 (one decimal place)
- 18,625 (this is the product of 5 × 3,725)
- +37,250 (this is the product of 10 × 3,725)
- 55,875 (count in three decimal places from the right)
- 55.875 Round to the nearest hundredth for 55.88 or tenth for 55.9

Because trailing zeros may be removed from a decimal number without changing the value, remove them and then multiply. This simplifies the multiplication. For example, if multiplying 7.350 × 0.20, drop the zeros at the ends so that the problem is 7.35 × 0.2 for an answer of 1.470. The trailing zero in the answer can then be dropped to give the final answer of 1.47.

If a number is multiplied by 10 or a multiple of 10, a shortcut in multiplying is to move the decimal of the number as many places to the right as there are zeros in the multiplier. With 12.2 × 10, move the decimal point one space to the *right* for the answer of 122. If the multiplier is 100, the decimal would be moved two places for the answer of 1,220; if the multiplier is 1,000, the decimal would be moved three places for the answer of 12,200; and so on.

Practice Problems K

Multiply the following. Show your work. Drop trailing zeros, round final answers to hundredths if necessary, and indicate measurements as needed.

1. 65.3 × 10 = _____
2. 13.2 × 100 = _____
3. 4.25 × 10 = _____
4. 0.004 × 100 = _____
5. 0.2 × 1000 = _____
6. 16.5 × 0.5 = _____

7. $23.52 \times 0.5 =$ _____

8. $0.35 \times 0.45 =$ _____

9. $1.25 \text{ mg} \times 6 =$ _____

10. $2.5 \text{ mg} \times 2 =$ _____

11. $250 \text{ mg} \times 3 =$ _____

12. $500 \text{ mg} \times 4 =$ _____

13. A physician orders 2.5 mg of a drug taken daily for 10 days. What is the total amount of the drug the patient will take?

14. A mother gives her child 2.5 mL of an antipyretic every 4 hours for fever. How many milliliters of medication will the child receive in 1 day?

15. One bottle of medication contains 12.25 mg. Five bottles of the medication are in stock. How many total milligrams of medication are available for dispensing?

Dividing Decimals

Dividing decimals is much like dividing whole numbers. Write the problem as for long division. If a decimal appears in the divisor, move the decimal to the right until the divisor is a whole number. Then move the decimal point in the dividend the same number of places to the right.

EXAMPLE 2.18

Divide 2.5 by 1.25

Add a terminal zero to 2.5, then move the decimal two places to the right on *both* terms.

$1.25 \overline{)2.50}$

$1.25 \overline{)2.50}$

$125 \overline{)250}$

Place a decimal point on the quotient (answer) line directly above the decimal point in the dividend and divide as usual. The answer is 2.

EXAMPLE 2.19

$1 \div 5$

$5 \overline{)1}$

$5 \overline{)1.0}$

By placing the decimal point directly above the decimal point in the dividend and then dividing, the answer is 0.2.

Remember, in medicine, if the decimal number is less than 1, a zero *must* be added in front of the decimal point to decrease the likelihood of medication errors.

EXAMPLE 2.20

$$40.44 \div 0.4$$

$$0.4 \overline{)40.44}$$

Move the decimal in the divisor and the dividend one place to the right to make the divisor a whole number.

$4\overline{)404.4}$ The answer is 101.1.

In some cases division does not come out evenly, such as when 3 is divided into 1. The answer is $0.33\overline{3}$ to the number of places that zeros are added to the dividend. In these cases, the number may be shown as $0.\overline{3}$, with the line indicating that 3 is a repeating number.

If the divisor is 10 or a multiple of 10, a shortcut in dividing is to move the decimal as many places to the *left* as there are zeros in the divisor. With $122 \div 10$, move the decimal point one space to the left to the answer of 12.2. If the divisor is 100, the decimal would be moved two places; 1000, three places; and so on.

Practice Problems L

Divide the following. Show your work. Add a leading zero and round final answers to hundredths if necessary, and indicate measurements as appropriate.

1. $268.4 \div 4 =$ _____
2. $125 \div 0.25 =$ _____
3. $1.5 \div 0.3 =$ _____
4. $19.95 \div 10.5 =$ _____
5. $33.03 \div 0.03 =$ _____
6. $25.2 \div 100 =$ _____
7. $225.4 \text{ mg} \div 4 =$ _____
8. $2.5 \text{ g} \div 2 =$ _____
9. $1864.5 \div 6 =$ _____
10. $\$124.80 \div 4 =$ _____
11. $1.25 \text{ g} \div 5 =$ _____
12. $844.8 \text{ mg} \div 4 =$ _____
13. $2{,}025 \text{ mL} \div 100 =$ _____

14. A pharmacist needs to divide 1 mL of medication into five equal parts. How many milliliters will be in each?

15. A customer comes to the pharmacy to purchase an expensive medication, which costs $255.30 for a 90-day supply. She asks to purchase it as three separate prescriptions of 30 days each. How much will she pay for each prescription?

Converting Decimals to Fractions

A decimal point separates the whole number that appears to the left and the decimal fraction that is found on the right. To convert a decimal to a fraction, the numerator is the number following the decimal point and the denominator is a power of 10 dependent on the number of digits following the decimal. For example, 3.7 is $3\frac{7}{10}$. The 7 is placed over 10 because there is one place value after the decimal in 3.7. The decimal 0.71 would be $\frac{71}{100}$ because there are two place values after the decimal.

Whereas trailing zeros do not need to be counted as place values, zeros following the decimal point and zeros *between* two whole numbers of a decimal fraction must be counted as place values. For example, 0.05 has two place values, so the fractional equivalent is $\frac{5}{100}$, and 0.505 has three place values, so the fractional equivalent is $\frac{505}{1,000}$.

TECH NOTE
Decimals are used in medication calculations in the metric system and calculations of dollars and cents in business math. $1.25 actually means one dollar and twenty-five hundredths of a dollar, $10.50 is 10 dollars and fifty hundredths of a dollar, and so on.

Practice Problems M

Change the following decimals to fractions. Do not reduce 1 through 5. Reduce 6 through 10 to lowest terms.

1. 0.125 = _____ _____
2. 0.55 = _____ _____
3. 0.33 = _____ _____
4. 0.525 = _____ _____
5. 0.625 = _____ _____
6. 0.05 = _____ _____
7. 0.150 = _____ _____
8. 0.95 = _____ _____
9. 0.1244 = _____ _____
10. 0.042 = _____ _____

CHAPTER 2 Review of Basic Mathematical Skills

Converting Fractions to Decimals

To convert fractions to decimals, divide the numerator by the denominator.

EXAMPLE 2.21

$\frac{1}{2}$ is 1 ÷ 2, which becomes 1.0 ÷ 2 because 2 cannot divide into 1, giving the answer of 0.5.

$\frac{3}{4}$ is 3 ÷ 4, which becomes 3.0 ÷ 4, giving the decimal answer of 0.75.

TECH NOTE
When converting a mixed number to a decimal, the whole number will stay the same and the fractional portion is added after the decimal point once it is converted to a decimal. For example, $1\frac{1}{2} = 1.5$.

Practice Problems N

Convert the following fractions to decimals. Round to the nearest hundredth if necessary.

1. $\frac{1}{2}$ = _____
2. $\frac{7}{8}$ = _____
3. $\frac{4}{5}$ = _____

4. $1\frac{2}{3}$ = _____
5. $7\frac{1}{3}$ = _____
6. $\frac{5}{6}$ = _____

7. $\frac{2}{9}$ = _____
8. $\frac{4}{9}$ = _____
9. $\frac{5}{8}$ = _____

10. $2\frac{1}{2}$ = _____

PERCENT

A **percent** is a part of 100 as a fraction (such as $\frac{1}{100}$) and hundredths as a decimal (such as 0.01). Percents are used to describe medication strengths, to determine the amount of solute in a solvent when preparing medications, to determine the amount of medication that has been administered over a given amount of time, and to determine discounts and markups in retail pharmacy.

Converting a Percent to a Fraction

To convert a percent to a fraction, drop the % sign and write the number over 100. The denominator will *always* be 100. Reduce the fraction to its lowest terms.

POINTS TO REMEMBER
DECIMALS
- Always place a zero before a decimal if no whole number is present.
- When adding or subtracting decimals, align decimal points and add terminal zeros as necessary to make decimal places the same length.
- When multiplying decimals, multiply the numbers, count the number of decimal places in the numbers multiplied, and finally place the decimal point in the product.
- To divide decimal fractions, form a whole number in the divisor by moving the decimal point to the right, then move the decimal point in the dividend (number to be divided) the same number of decimal places to the right. Place the decimal point in the quotient (answer) directly over the decimal point in the dividend and divide as if the numbers are whole numbers.
- When multiplying by 10 or multiples of 10 (e.g., 100 or 1000), the only step necessary is to move the decimal point in the other number to the right by the number of zeros in the multiplier.
- To divide by 10 or a multiple of 10, the decimal point in the dividend, the number being divided, may be moved to the left by the number of zeros in the divisor.

EXAMPLE 2.22

Change 16% to a fraction.

16% becomes $\frac{16}{100}$ and reduces to $\frac{4}{25}$

If the percent is written as a mixed number, the mixed number becomes the numerator and 100 the denominator. The mixed number must be changed to an improper fraction first.

EXAMPLE 2.23

Change to a fraction.

$2\frac{2}{5} = \frac{12}{5}$ Place the fraction over 100

$\frac{12/5}{100}$ or $\frac{12}{5} \div \frac{100}{1}$

To divide fractions, invert and multiply.

$\frac{12}{5} \times \frac{1}{100} = \frac{12}{500} = \frac{3}{125}$

EXAMPLE 2.24

Change 0.5% to a fraction.

$\frac{0.5}{100}$

A decimal cannot be left in a numerator or denominator, so multiply by the smallest fraction that is equal to 1 that will remove the decimal:

$\frac{0.5}{100} \times \frac{2}{2} = \frac{1}{200}$

Another option for solving this is to move the decimal one place to the right in both the numerator and denominator: multiply by $^{10}\!/_{10}$.

$$\frac{0.5}{100} \times \frac{10}{10} = \frac{50}{1,000}$$

This would then reduce to $\frac{1}{200}$.

TECH NOTE
  Any percent over 100 will include a whole number and a fraction.

Practice Problems O

Convert the following percents to fractions. On the first line, drop the percent sign and place the entire number over 100, then simplify. Show your calculations.

1. 12% = _____ _____   2. 60% = _____ _____

3. 125% = _____ _____   4. 33% = _____ _____

5. 75% = _____ _____   6. 80% = _____ _____

7. 0.25% = _____ _____   8. 0.45% = _____ _____

9. 12.5% = _____ _____   10. 0.05% = _____ _____

11. 4% = _____ _____   12. 0.025% = _____ _____

On the first line, show the multiplication equation that will be solved after dropping the percent sign and inverting 100 to multiply (i.e., multiply by $^{1}\!/_{100}$). Write your solution on the second line. Show your reduced answer on the third line if necessary.

13. $\frac{2}{3}$% = _____ _____, _____

14. $\frac{1}{4}$% = _____ _____, _____

15. $1\frac{1}{4}$% = _____ _____, _____

Copyright © 2019 by Elsevier, Inc. All rights reserved.

Converting a Fraction to a Percent

The denominator in a percent is always 100 (because any percent is a part of 100), and the number beside the % sign becomes the numerator. To convert a fraction to a percent multiply the fraction by 100 or by $\frac{100}{1}$ (the fraction for 100) and add the percent sign (%). This is the same as changing the fraction to a decimal and moving the decimal place to the right two places.

EXAMPLE 2.25

Convert to a percent.

$$\frac{1}{5} \cdot 100 = \frac{100}{5} = 20\%$$

If the fraction is a mixed number, change it to an improper fraction first, then multiply by 100.

EXAMPLE 2.26

$$2\frac{3}{5} = \underline{\quad} \%$$

$$2\frac{3}{5} = \frac{13}{5}$$

$$\frac{13}{5} \times \frac{100}{1} = \frac{1300}{5} = 260\%$$

Practice Problems P

Convert the following fractions and mixed numbers to percents. First, write the fraction after multiplying by 100, then show the percent. Round to hundredths as appropriate.

1. $\frac{1}{6}$ = _____ _____ %

2. $\frac{3}{7}$ = _____ _____ %

3. $\frac{2}{5}$ = _____ _____ %

4. $\frac{1}{4}$ = _____ _____ %

5. $\frac{2}{3}$ = _____ _____ %

6. $2\frac{1}{3}$ = _____ _____ %

7. $6\frac{4}{5}$ = _____ _____ %

8. $\frac{9}{40}$ = _____ _____ %

9. $\dfrac{3}{4}$ = _____ _____%

10. $\dfrac{7}{8}$ = _____ _____%

11. $1\dfrac{2}{3}$ = _____ _____%

12. $\dfrac{4}{5}$ = _____ _____%

Converting a Percent to a Decimal

To convert a percent to a decimal, drop the percent sign and divide the number by 100. This can be accomplished by moving the decimal point two places to the left. For example, 25% would become 0.25 by removing the % sign and moving the decimal (.25).

$25\% = \dfrac{25}{100}$ (or $25 \div 100$) $= 0.25$

Zeros may need to be added in front of the number so that two decimal places may be moved.

8% equals $8 \div 100$ or $(0.08) = 0.08$

If the number is already a decimal percent, adding two zeros before the decimal point will allow the change to a decimal; for instance, 0.8% would need two zeros to become a decimal.

0.8% equals $0.8 \div 100$ or $(0.008) = 0.008$

If the percent is over 100%, there will be a whole number before the decimal.

155% equals $155 \div 100$ or $(1.55) = 1.55$

To change a fractional percent to a decimal, first convert the fraction to a decimal, leaving the percent sign as part of the number. Then convert the percent to a decimal by moving the decimal two places to the left (dividing by 100).

EXAMPLE 2.27

Convert ½% to a decimal.

$1 \div 2 = 0.5\%$

Move the decimal two places to the left, adding the necessary zeros, and drop the percent sign.

½% $= 0.5\% = 0.5 \div 100$ or $(0.005) = 0.005$

Practice Problems Q

Convert the following percents to decimals. Do not round.

1. 60% = _____
2. 3% = _____
3. 78% = _____
4. 128% = _____
5. 1.3% = _____
6. 325% = _____
7. 0.05% = _____
8. 0.3% = _____
9. 32% = _____
10. 7% = _____
11. 8.2% = _____
12. 1245% = _____
13. 56% = _____
14. 14.6% = _____
15. 0.06% = _____
16. $\frac{1}{4}$% = _____
17. $\frac{3}{4}$% = _____
18. $\frac{1}{8}$% = _____
19. $2\frac{1}{4}$% = _____
20. $\frac{4}{5}$% = _____

Converting a Decimal to a Percent

To convert a decimal to a percent, multiply by 100, which results in the decimal place being moved two places to the right, and add a percent sign.

EXAMPLE 2.28

Express 0.50 as a percent.

0.50 × 100 moves the decimal two places to the right (0.50).

Add the % sign: 50%.

If the number does not have two places to the right of the decimal point, add zeros so that the decimal point can be moved two places; 0.5 would need a zero added (0.50), and then the decimal point should be moved two places (0.50) so that 0.5 becomes 50%. If the number is a whole number such as 5, two zeros must be added to the number to find the percent. Thus 5 would require two added zeros, becoming 500%.

TECH NOTE
A number greater than 1 is always over 100% because one whole is 100%.

Practice Problems R

Convert the following decimals to percents.

1. 0.25 = _____ %
2. 0.68 = _____ %
3. 0.025 = _____ %

4. 0.6 = _____ %
5. 0.75 = _____ %
6. 5.5 = _____ %

7. 0.7 = _____ %
8. 6 = _____ %
9. 10.4 = _____ %

10. 0.05 = _____ %
11. 105 = _____ %
12. 0.15 = _____ %

13. 21.50 = _____ %
14. 1.025 = _____ %
15. 0.467 = _____ %

The following table contains some common fractions, decimals, and percents for quick reference. Looking at them in this manner may help you see the pattern between the three.

FRACTION	DECIMAL	PERCENT
1/10	0.1	10%
1/4	0.25	25%
1/3	0.3333…	33.3%
1/2	0.5	50%
2/3	0.6666…	66.7%
3/4	0.75	75%
1	1	100%

RATIOS

Expressing Numbers as Ratios

A **ratio** indicates the relationship of one number to another *or* one number to a whole. A ratio expresses a numerator and denominator separated by a colon (:) rather than the division line found in fractions. Numerators are to the left of the colon, and denominators to the right, such as 1:2. The colon is the traditional way to write a division sign in a ratio and is representative of *of, per, to,* or *in*. For example, ¾ as a fractional expression would be 3:4 when written in ratio form. Like a fraction, a ratio may be reduced to lowest terms. Because of the relationship of the numbers in a ratio, the value of the ratio will not be changed if both the numerator and denominator are multiplied or divided by the same number. Multiplication and division are the only numeric operations that can be performed on a ratio without changing its value.

TECH NOTE
A ratio may be written as a fraction, and a fraction may be written as a ratio because each has a numerator and denominator (2:3 or $\frac{2}{3}$).

To express a percent as a ratio, the denominator will always be 100.

$30\% = \frac{30}{100} = 30:100$

To change a decimal to a ratio, express it as a fraction and change the format.

0.09 is $\frac{9}{100}$ or 9:100

When numbers expressed in ratio form are used to compare quantities (one number related to another), they must be expressed in the same units of measure.

EXAMPLE 2.29

Establish a ratio of 3 inches to 1 foot.

1 foot must be changed to 12 inches (12″ = 1 foot).

3″: 12″

Since both sides are reduced by 3″, the unit of inches is canceled and no unit is required in the reduced ratio.

1: 4

When numbers expressed in ratio form are used to describe one number as a part of a whole amount, they *may* have different units of measurements. In pharmacy, ratios are used in this manner. For example, mg is a measurement of weight or mass and mL is a measurement of volume, so one cannot be converted to the other. The relationship is the number of mg "in" or "per" mL.

EXAMPLE 2.30

Establish a ratio for 5 mg per 125 mL and reduce.

5 mg:125 mL   (This is most often written as a fraction.)

1 mg:25 mL

Practice Problems S

Express the following as ratios and then reduce to lowest terms.

1. 2 is to 7 = _____ _____

2. 6 is to 9 = _____ _____

3. 5 is to 25 = _____ _____

4. 36% = _____ _____

5. 125% = _____ _____

6. 95% = _____ _____

CHAPTER 2 Review of Basic Mathematical Skills   49

7. $\dfrac{7}{8}$ = _____ _____

8. $\dfrac{75}{125}$ = _____ _____

9. $3\dfrac{1}{4}\%$ = _____ _____

10. 0.04% = _____ _____

11. 0.08 = _____ _____

12. 0.36 = _____ _____

13. 0.04 = _____ _____

14. 0.1 = _____ _____

15. 6 in:4 ft = _____ _____

16. 50¢:$3.50 = _____ _____

17. 0.25 in:25 in = _____ _____

18. 0.2 mL:5 mL = _____ _____

Include units on the following after reducing.

19. 50 mg:250 mL = _____

20. 2 mg:8 mL = _____

Expressing Ratios as Proportions

A true **proportion** is an expression of equality between two equivalent ratios, such as 4:8 and 6:12. Placing these in a proportional equation, 4:8::6:12, or a fractional equation, $\dfrac{4}{8} = \dfrac{6}{12}$, is read, 4 is to 8 as 6 is to 12. In these pairs of numbers, the relationship between 4 and 8 is that 8 is twice as much as 4 and the relationship between 6 and 12 is that 12 is twice as much as 6. Therefore these ratios are equally proportional to each other, although the numbers are not the same. Both can be reduced to 1:2.

When validating proportional equations such as 4:8::6:12, multiply the two outside numbers, the extremes, and the two inside numbers, the means, so 4 × 12 and 6 × 8. Because both answers are 48, it is a true proportion. The product of the means will equal the product of the extremes in a true proportion.

To verify this equality when written as fractions, cross-multiply $\dfrac{4}{8} \times \dfrac{6}{12}$. Because both answers are 48, it is a true proportion.

When writing the proportion in the form of $\dfrac{a}{b} = \dfrac{c}{d}$, like units of measure must be in positions "a and c" and in positions "b and d." When the proportion is designated in the following manner, $\dfrac{125 \text{ mg}}{5 \text{ mL}} = \dfrac{25 \text{ mg}}{1 \text{ mL}}$, positions "a and c" are in milligrams and "b and d" are in milliliters.

Copyright © 2019 by Elsevier, Inc. All rights reserved.

Practice Problems T

Which of the following are true proportions? Mark with either a yes or a no.

1. $3:9::9:27$ _____
2. $5:25::10:250$ _____
3. $4:12::6:18$ _____
4. $10:90::1:9$ _____
5. $\dfrac{15}{3} = \dfrac{5}{2}$ _____
6. $\dfrac{22}{88} = \dfrac{10}{40}$ _____
7. $\dfrac{1.5}{7.5} = \dfrac{0.25}{1.25}$ _____
8. $\dfrac{2 \text{ mg}}{4 \text{ mL}} = \dfrac{8 \text{ mg}}{16 \text{ mL}}$ _____
9. $\dfrac{2''}{12''} = \dfrac{6''}{24''}$ _____
10. $\dfrac{500 \text{ mg}}{5 \text{ mL}} = \dfrac{100 \text{ mg}}{10 \text{ mL}}$ _____

Solving for Unknowns Using Ratio and Proportion

In the health care field, the ratio and proportion method is often used to calculate different quantities of medication or to calculate dosages. Knowing three of the four parts of the proportion is necessary to solve for the fourth. Proportional equations are used to find the missing or unknown amount, often signified by x. The relationship is set up using the fractional method and solved using cross-multiplication followed by division. This method will be used in the text when it comes to solving for the unknown value. Ratio and proportion calculations are one of the two main methods used in pharmaceutical calculations.

EXAMPLE 2.31

$\dfrac{5}{35} = \dfrac{x}{28}$ cross-multiply

$35x = 5 \cdot 28$

$35x = 140$ divide each side by 35

$x = 4$

A proportion may be verified by substituting the answer in the x position and cross-multiplying to verify that it is a true proportion: $5 \cdot 28 = 140$ and $4 \cdot 35 = 140$.

> **TECH NOTE**
> When three terms of a proportion are known, the sequence of cross-multiplication and division is used to find the unknown term.

Practice Problems U

Solve for the following unknown values. Write as fractions if needed and then cross-multiply and divide. Indicate measurements as appropriate. Show your work.

1. $x:2::14:7$

   $x =$ _____

2. $20:x::5:10$

   $x =$ _____

3. $\dfrac{7}{x} = \dfrac{35}{125}$

   $x =$ _____

4. $\dfrac{x}{11} = \dfrac{2}{2.2}$

   $x =$ _____

5. $\dfrac{2}{24} = \dfrac{x}{36}$

   $x =$ _____

6. $\$0.20:x::\$1.00:\$25$

   $x =$ _____

7. $\dfrac{\$6.00}{8 \text{ capsules}} = \dfrac{x}{36 \text{ capsules}}$

   $x =$ _____

8. $\dfrac{\$75.00}{100 \text{ tablets}} = \dfrac{\$15.00}{x}$

   $x =$ _____

9. $\dfrac{3 \text{ capsules}}{1 \text{ day}} = \dfrac{x}{7 \text{ days}}$

   $x =$ _____

10. $\dfrac{0.4 \text{ g}}{0.15 \text{ g}} = \dfrac{0.16 \text{ g}}{x}$

    $x =$ _____

11. $\dfrac{14 \text{ mL}}{2 \text{ L}} = \dfrac{21 \text{ mL}}{x}$

    $x =$ _____

12. Mr. Smith needs 14 tablets for a week's supply of an antiinflammatory drug. He is going on vacation and needs a 4-week supply. How many tablets are needed to fill the prescription?

13. Periactin liquid is labeled as 5 mg/5 mL. How many mg would be in 25 mL?

14. A medication contains 5 mg per tablet. How many tablets are needed for a 35 mg dose?

15. A cough medication contains 50 mg of active ingredient per mL. The physician orders 100 mg per dose. How many mL are needed for one dose?

16. A physician orders a 250 mg dose of an antibiotic for a child. The pediatric liquid medication contains 125 mg per 5 mL. How many milliliters should the child be given for one dose?

CALCULATIONS WITH PERCENTS

Determining the Percentage of a Quantity

Computation of a given percentage of a quantity may be determined in order to ascertain the part of a whole quantity that is in question. If a percentage of a whole quantity is in question, the known percent is changed to decimal form and multiplied by the whole quantity to provide the needed information. The equation for finding a percentage of a quantity follows:

$$\text{Amount} = \text{Percent required (written as a decimal)} \times \text{Whole amount}$$

EXAMPLE 2.32

What is 3% of 42?

Change the percent to a decimal by dividing by 100 or moving the decimal point two places to the left: 0.03.

$x = 0.03 \cdot 42$

$x = 1.26$

1.26 is 3% of 42.

A few tips on working with percentages of quantities:
- "what" is the unknown, or x
- "is" means "="
- % is the percent (written as a decimal when solving these equations)
- "of" translates to "times" (followed by the whole number)

A question may be presented in three ways:

1. Find the percent: "What is 50% of 15?" $x = 0.5 \cdot 15$.
   Note: remember to change the percent quantity to a decimal

2. Find the whole quantity: "7.5 is 50% of what number?" $7.5 = 0.5 \cdot x$.
   Note: remember to change the percent quantity to a decimal
   Also: "50% of what number is 7.5?" $0.5 \cdot x = 7.5$

3. Find the percent: "7.5 is what percent of 15?" $7.5 = x \cdot 15$.
   Note: remember to change the decimal answer to a percent
   *Also: "What percent of 15 is 7.5?" $x \cdot 15 = 7.5$

Questions 2 and 3 may be asked in a reverse manner, which would result in the equation being written with the sides switched.

EXAMPLE 2.33

15 is 60% of what number?

$15 = 0.6 \cdot x$ Divide both sides by 0.6.

$x = 25$

*15 is 60% of **25.***

EXAMPLE 2.34

15 is what percent of 45?

$15 = x \cdot 45$ Divide both sides by 45.

$x = 0.333$

*15 is **33.3**% of 45.*

Another method of working with percents is to use the knowledge that a percent is always an amount out of 100. One of the three known values will always be 100. A ratio and proportion equation can be set up to solve each of the previous situations as seen in examples 2.35, 2.36, and 2.37:

EXAMPLE 2.35

What is 3% of 42?

$\dfrac{3}{100} = \dfrac{x}{42}$ $100x = 126$ $x = 1.26$

***1.26** is 3% of 42.*

EXAMPLE 2.36

15 is 60% of what number?

$\dfrac{60}{100} = \dfrac{15}{x}$ $60x = 1500$ $x = 25$

*15 is 60% of **25.***

EXAMPLE 2.37

15 is what percent of 45?

$\dfrac{x}{100} = \dfrac{15}{45}$ $45x = 1500$ $x = 33.3$

*15 is **33.3**% of 45.*

> **TECH NOTE**
>
> Percents are used to calculate the amount of active ingredients in a formulation, to compound medications, and to calculate markups and discounts in retail pharmacy.

Practice Problems V

Solve the following problems. Show your work. Indicate measurements as appropriate.

1. What percent of 105 is 35? (Round to tenths.)

2. 25 is what percent of 200?

3. 90% of 50 is what?

4. 105% of 0.9 is what?

5. What percent of 750 is 15?

6. What is 45% of 180?

7. 6 is what percent of 240?

8. What is 15% of $25.40?

9. What is 64% of 8 oz?

10. If you have 100 tablets, what is 5%?

11. What percent of 40 tablets is 22 tablets?

12. If a discount of 15% is applied to a purchase of $25, what is the amount of the discount?

13. If a patient wants 60% of a prescription that is written for 60 tablets, how many tablets will be dispensed to the patient?

14. A customer wants 50% of a prescription that is written for 300 mL. How many mL should be dispensed?

15. 35% of 70 tablets is what?

16. 40 tablets is what percent of 80 tablets?

17. 6 inches is what percent of 24 inches?

18. 120 tablets is what percent of 1,500 tablets?

19. 60% of 360 mL is what?

20. What is 3% of 1,200 mL?

Stop to Check Answers

Before continuing to another problem, **always** ask yourself the following question: "Does this answer make sense?" This is very important in pharmacy math. You will need to use your knowledge of specific medications when asking this question. When an answer is off by only one decimal point, the patient would receive either 10 times too much or 10 times too little medication. This is potentially very dangerous.

In addition to using your knowledge of drug doses, estimation is a good way to check mathematical calculations. To estimate a number, mentally round it to a slightly larger or smaller number containing fewer numerals. Then perform the calculation, mentally knowing that the mental answer will be slightly higher or lower than the actual calculation but will be close to the desired answer. For example, 12.2 times 3.8 could be thought of as 12 times 4, which equals 48. If your answer comes out closer to 5 or 500, you would know you made a decimal placement error. This process can help avoid many calculation errors.

Posttest

Solve the following problems. Round to the nearest hundredth if needed. Indicate measurements as appropriate. Show your calculations.

1. 13 + 24.6 + 36.72 + 0.45 = _____

2. 15.87 − 5.2 = _____

Continued

Posttest, cont

3. $12.76 \times 5.2 =$ _____

4. $25.01 \times 10 =$ _____

5. $25 \div 0.25 =$ _____

6. $16.82 \div 4.02 =$ _____

7. $2 - 1.75 =$ _____

Solve the following fractional equations and then reduce to the lowest terms.

8. $\dfrac{1}{2} + \dfrac{3}{4} + \dfrac{3}{8} =$ _____ _____

9. $\dfrac{5}{6} + \dfrac{7}{12} + \dfrac{5}{8} =$ _____ _____

10. $\dfrac{11}{12} - \dfrac{3}{4} =$ _____ _____

11. $2\dfrac{2}{3} - 1\dfrac{5}{6} =$ _____ _____

12. $\dfrac{1}{5} \times \dfrac{3}{8} =$ _____ _____

13. $\dfrac{8}{9} \times \dfrac{3}{8} \times \dfrac{1}{2} =$ _____ _____

14. $8\dfrac{2}{3} \times \dfrac{1}{3} =$ _____ _____

Posttest, cont

15. $\dfrac{3}{4} \div \dfrac{3}{8} =$ _____ _____

16. $1\dfrac{1}{5} \div \dfrac{6}{7} =$ _____ _____

Solve the following problems.

17. 721 − 0.01 = _____

18. 1.06 + 3.871 = _____

19. 25.5 • 3.2 = _____

20. 12.02 ÷ 6.01 = _____

Convert the following fractions to decimals. Round to the nearest hundredth.

21. $\dfrac{5}{9} =$ _____

22. $2\dfrac{1}{3} =$ _____

23. $\dfrac{16}{25} =$ _____

24. $1\dfrac{5}{6} =$ _____

Convert the following decimals to fractions. Reduce as appropriate.

25. 0.44 = _____ _____

26. 1.64 = _____ _____

27. 5.33 = _____ _____

28. 0.86 = _____ _____

29. 0.8 = _____ _____

Continued

Posttest, cont

Express the following as ratios and then reduce to lowest terms. Show your calculations.

30. $\frac{3}{5}$ _____ _____

31. 10% _____ _____

32. 500 mg in 10 mL _____ _____

33. An antibiotic contains 250 mg in 5 mL of medication. _____ _____

Express the following in proportional equations and then solve for the unknown. Show your calculations. Reduce and indicate measurements as appropriate.

34. One tablet contains 25 mg. How many mg are in three tablets?

35. John takes one tablet twice a day. How many tablets will John need for 2 weeks?

36. Dr. Smith writes a prescription for a 3-month supply of medication for hypertension. A 1-month supply is 60 tablets. How many tablets are needed to fill the prescription?

Solve the following percent problems.

37. Three tablets are what percent of 90? (Round to hundredths)

38. 45% of 1,500 mL is what?

39. What is 15% of 60 tablets?

40. 250 mg is what percent of 1,000 mg?

41. What is 40% of a prescription for 120 tablets?

42. 25 is 20% of how many capsules?

IN SECTION II

3 Conversion of Clinical Measurements of Numbers, Time, and Temperature
4 Measurement Systems, Units, and Equivalencies
5 Conversions Within Measurement Systems
6 Conversions Between Measurement Systems

SECTION II
Measurements and Conversions

CHAPTER 3

Conversion of Clinical Measurements of Numbers, Time, and Temperature

OBJECTIVES

1. Convert between Arabic numerals and Roman numerals.
2. Convert time between standard time and military (or universal) time.
3. Convert temperature between Fahrenheit and Celsius.

KEY WORDS

Arabic numerals The numerals 1, 2, 3, etc.
Celsius (Centigrade) System of measuring temperature; 0° is the freezing point and 100° is the boiling point of water
Fahrenheit System of measuring temperature; 32° is the freezing point and 212° is the boiling point of water

Military time (International Standard Time) System of time that recognizes a 24-hour notation of hours and minutes
Roman numerals Letters from the Roman alphabet that are used to represent numbers, such as I for 1, V for 5, X for 10, etc.

Copyright © 2019 by Elsevier, Inc. All rights reserved.

Pretest

If you are already comfortable with the subject matter, perform the following calculations to test your knowledge. If not, work your way through the chapter and return to them for extra practice. Follow the directions below and show your calculations.

Change the following to Roman numerals.

1. 21 _____
2. 16 _____
3. 54 _____
4. 122 _____

5. 44 _____
6. 95 _____
7. 68 _____
8. 75 _____

Change the following to Arabic numerals.

9. viii _____
10. xix _____
11. lxiv _____
12. xcvii _____

13. ix$\overline{ss}$ _____
14. xvii$\overline{ss}$ _____
15. xxxvii$\overline{ss}$ _____
16. xxiv _____

17. xxiv$\overline{ss}$ _____
18. xliv$\overline{ss}$ _____

Change the following to universal, or 24-hour, time.

19. 7:30 AM _____
20. 5:32 PM _____
21. 12:01 AM _____
22. 11:59 AM _____

23. 1:59 PM _____
24. 1:46 AM _____
25. 8:42 PM _____
26. 9:08 PM _____

Change the following to 12-hour time.

27. 1102 _____
28. 0520 _____
29. 0052 _____
30. 2357 _____

31. 0001 _____
32. 0648 _____
33. 1645 _____
34. 1235 _____

Pretest, cont.

Convert the following temperatures as indicated. Round to the nearest tenth.

35. 98.6° F = _____ C   36. 104.6° F = _____ C   37. 38.6° C = _____ F

38. 29.6° C = _____ F   39. 100.4° F = _____ C   40. 41.8° C = _____ F

41. 41.8° F = _____ C   42. 102.6° F = _____ C   43. 0° F = _____ C

44. 10° C = _____ F   45. 10° F = _____ C   46. 95.6° F = _____ C

47. 32.2° C = _____ F   48. 92.5° F = _____ C   49. 212° F = _____ C

50. 100° C = _____ F

INTRODUCTION

It is important to be able to convert between time, temperature, and numerical systems when working in pharmacy. Many prescriptions include Roman numerals, medications must be stored at the correct temperatures, and the correct amount of medication must be prepared for the correct time. Pharmacy employees use both **Arabic numerals,** such as 1, 5, and 10, and **Roman numerals,** such as I, V, and X, when interpreting physicians' orders. Arabic numerals are commonly used in daily life, but Roman numerals are still occasionally used in the medical field and in literature. Similarly, we use the standard clock on a daily basis whereas institutional pharmacy settings use **military time** to prevent misinterpretation of order timing. Finally, temperature is read and recorded in **Fahrenheit** in daily lives in the United States, with 32° as the freezing point and 212° as the boiling point of water. The **Celsius** scale is the basic unit of temperature in the metric system and is used in most other parts of the world, with 0° as the freezing point and 100° as the boiling point of water. The Celsius scale is used in most clinical settings.

ARABIC AND ROMAN NUMERALS

Medication orders or prescriptions are written in both Arabic and Roman numerals, depending on the prescriber's preference. Arabic numerals, such as 2 for whole numbers, ½ for fractional numbers with the household system, and 0.5 for decimal numbers in the metric system, are used most often.

Roman numerals, which date back to the ancient Roman Empire, use letters to represent numerical amounts. The following equates Arabic numerals to Roman numerals.

ROMAN NUMERALS

½	s̄s̄	10	X
1	I	50	L
2	II	100	C
3	III	500	D
4	IV	1,000	M
5	V		

Rules for Roman Numerals

1. When a numeral is repeated, its value is repeated.
   II = 2   XXX = 30

2. A numeral may not be repeated more than 3 times.
   40 = XL **not** XXXX

3. V, L, and D are *never* repeated.
   VV is **incorrect** because 10 = X
   LL is **incorrect** because 100 = C
   DD is **incorrect** because 1000 = M

4. When a smaller numeral is placed after a larger numeral, it is added to the larger numeral.
   DC = 600 (500 + 100)   LXVI = 66 (50 + 10 + 5 + 1)

5. When a smaller numeral is placed before a larger numeral, it is subtracted from the larger numeral.
   XL = 40 (50 – 10)   XC = 90 (100 – 10)

6. *Never* subtract more than one numeral.
   8 = VIII **not** IIX

7. V, D, and L are *never* subtracted.
   LC is **not** correct because 50 = L

8. When subtracting, only use a numeral before the next *two* higher-value numerals.
   Only use: I before V or X
   X before L or C
   C before D or M

> **TECH NOTE**
> Roman numerals are often used when writing prescriptions because alphabetic symbols indicating quantity are more difficult to alter than Arabic numerals.

The most commonly used Roman numerals in pharmacy are combinations of I, V, and X. Medical notations of Roman numerals are often written in lowercase with a line drawn over the numerals to prevent misinterpretation. Lowercase i's are frequently written with a line between the letter and the dot.

CHAPTER 3 Conversion of Clinical Measurements of Numbers, Time, and Temperature

Converting Arabic Numerals to Roman Numerals

EXAMPLE 3.1

Change 24 to Roman numerals:

  20 is 10 + 10, or xx

  4 is (5 − 1), or iv (subtract 1 from 5)

  So 24 is written as xxiv

Practice Problems A

Convert the following Arabic numerals to Roman numerals, using the correct medical notation to prevent misinterpretation.

1. 6 _____
2. 11 _____
3. 21 _____

4. 56 _____
5. $7\frac{1}{2}$ _____
6. 9 _____

7. $54\frac{1}{2}$ _____
8. $17\frac{1}{2}$ _____
9. 75 _____

10. 101 _____
11. 66 _____
12. 35 _____

13. $1\frac{1}{2}$ _____
14. 49 _____
15. $33\frac{1}{2}$ _____

Converting Roman Numerals to Arabic Numerals

To change Roman numerals into Arabic numerals, divide the entire Roman numeral into the groups of letters that indicate a number, such as XIV where X = 10 and IV = 4. So the Roman numeral XIV = 14.

EXAMPLE 3.2

Change XLVII to an Arabic numeral.

  Divide the numeral into XL and VII.

  XL means to subtract 10 (X) from 50 (L), which equals 40

  VII is 5 (V) + 1 (I) + 1 (I), or 7

  When the numerals are placed together, XLVII (XL + VII) equals 47

Copyright © 2019 by Elsevier, Inc. All rights reserved.

EXAMPLE 3.3

Change xix$\overline{ss}$ into an Arabic numeral.

    Divide the Roman numeral into separate parts.

    x = 10   ix = (10 − 1) = 9 $\overline{ss}$ = ½

    10 + 9 + ½ = 19½

Practice Problems B

Convert the following Roman numerals to Arabic numerals.

1. viii _____
2. ix _____
3. xix _____

4. xxxix _____
5. xliv _____
6. lxvi _____

7. CXXV _____
8. xxv$\overline{ss}$ _____
9. xcv _____

10. vii$\overline{ss}$ _____
11. ix$\overline{ss}$ _____
12. xxxvii$\overline{ss}$ _____

13. xxv _____
14. LXIII _____
15. xcix _____

CONVERSION BETWEEN 12-HOUR AND UNIVERSAL (MILITARY OR 24-HOUR) TIME

Because traditional time can be misinterpreted when using AM and PM with the same numbers to indicate the time of day for medication administration, most hospitals and other health care facilities use the 24-hour clock, also called military or universal time. The differentiation of time is not just dependent on the initials AM or PM but is actually a different number from 0001 to 2400. Orders are written 24 hours a day, and all medical-related caretakers must understand exactly when an order was written and when the medication or treatment is to take place. With this system, there is never any question as to when an order was written or which order supersedes another.

    In universal time, all time is expressed in four-digit numbers beginning at 1 minute past midnight, or 0001. There is no colon between hours and minutes. The time is stated in hundreds of hours with 1 AM being 0100, "zero one-hundred hours." Ten in the morning, 1000, is "ten hundred hours." Noon is 1200, or "twelve hundred hours." One o'clock in the afternoon becomes 1300, or "thirteen hundred hours." Midnight is 2400, "twenty-four hundred hours," or 0000, "zero hundred hours." Fig. 3.1 shows an example of a military time clock. The AM (antemeridian, or before noon) readings are found on the inside of the clock face, and the PM (postmeridian, or after noon) readings are found on the outside of the clock face.

CHAPTER 3 Conversion of Clinical Measurements of Numbers, Time, and Temperature

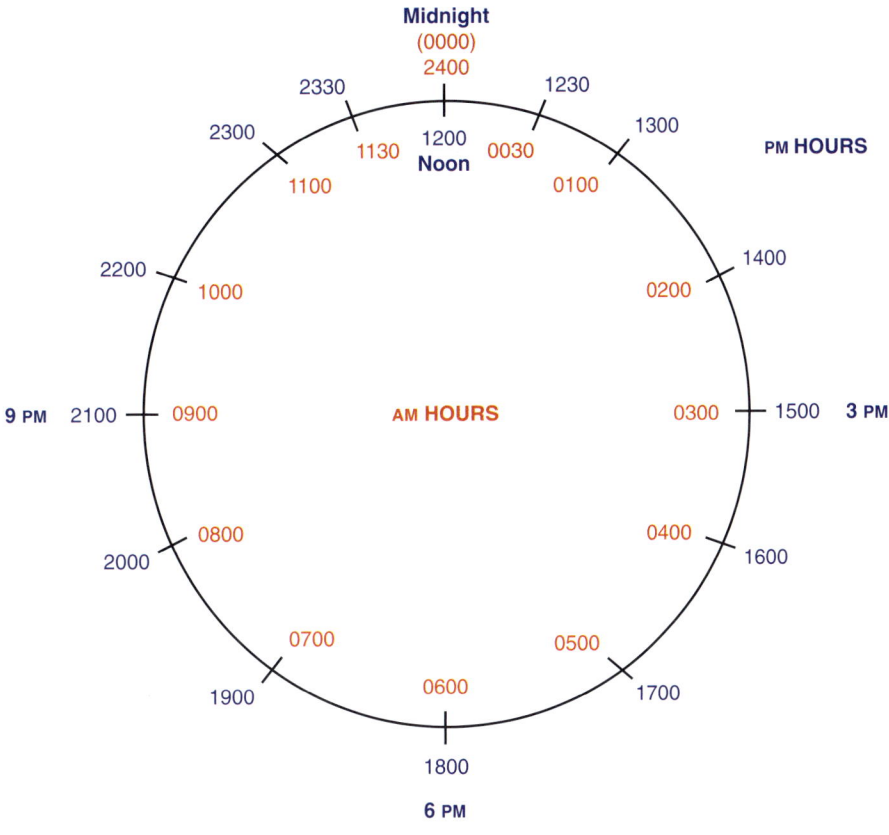

FIGURE 3.1 **Military Time Clock.** (Brown M, Mulholland JM: *Drug calculations: process and problems for clinical practice*, ed 8, St. Louis, Mosby, 2008.)

POINTS TO REMEMBER
CHANGING TO 24-HOUR, OR INTERNATIONAL, TIME
- Traditional and universal time use the same numbers from 1:00 AM (0100) to 12:59 PM (1259).
- Hours from 1:00 PM (1300) through 12:00 AM (2400 or 0000) are the 12-hour time plus 12; for instance, 5:00 PM would be 1700.
- Minutes are written in the third and fourth positions and are not separated by a colon, such as 1135 (11:35 AM). Minutes after midnight (0000) and before 1:00 AM (0100) are written as 00 with the number of minutes following, such as 0010 (12:10 AM).
- Midnight can be written as either 0000 or 2400 hours. In this text, we will use 0000 for midnight.

Practice Problems C

Convert the following 12-hour times to 24-hour times.

1. 12:35 AM _____
2. 2:45 PM _____
3. 6:15 AM _____

4. 6:20 PM _____
5. 12:05 AM _____
6. 3:45 AM _____

7. 12 AM _____   8. 12 PM _____   9. 6:55 AM _____

10. 7:25 PM _____   11. 2:15 PM _____   12. 8:20 PM _____

13. 9:05 AM _____   14. 11 AM _____   15. 11:59 PM _____

Convert the following 24-hour times to 12-hour times. Be sure to indicate morning and evening.

16. 1130 _____   17. 0354 _____   18. 1201 _____

19. 0030 _____   20. 1425 _____   21. 1615 _____

22. 0830 _____   23. 2345 _____   24. 0705 _____

25. 2145 _____   26. 0404 _____   27. 2020 _____

28. 1020 _____   29. 0330 _____   30. 0945 _____

CONVERSION BETWEEN FAHRENHEIT AND CELSIUS TEMPERATURE

In the United States, Fahrenheit (F) temperature is the measurement most commonly used. In countries where the metric system is used, Celsius (C) or centigrade temperature measurement is the most commonly used scale. In Fahrenheit, water boils at 212°, and in Celsius, water boils at 100°. Likewise, the freezing points are not the same; Fahrenheit is 32° and Celsius is 0°. Fig. 3.2 provides a comparison of the scales. As you can see, the Fahrenheit scale has 180° between the freezing and boiling points, whereas the Celsius scale contains only 100°. The formulas for conversion between the two scales have been developed with these differences as the basis. The following conversion formulas may be used to change from one temperature scale to the other.

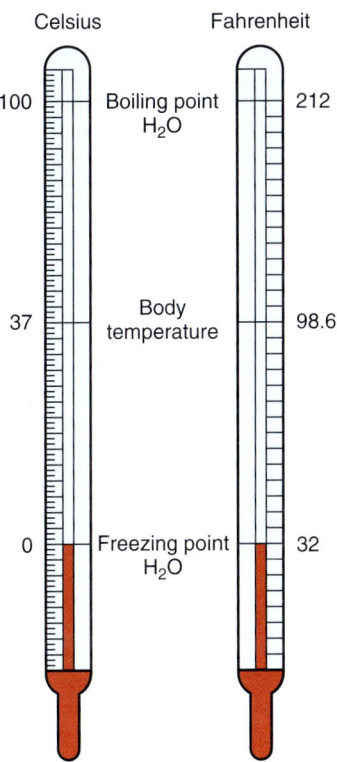

FIGURE 3.2 Comparison of Celsius and Fahrenheit Thermometers.

Converting Fahrenheit Temperature to Celsius Temperature

The equations can be written using decimals or fractions.

$$C = \frac{F - 32}{1.8} \quad \text{or} \quad C = (F - 32) \times \frac{5}{9}$$

In the first method, subtract 32 from the Fahrenheit temperature and then divide by 1.8. In the second method, subtract 32 from the Fahrenheit temperature, multiply that answer by 5, and then divide by 9. In either case, the remainder should be rounded to tenths.

Converting Celsius Temperature to Fahrenheit Temperature

To convert Celsius temperature to Fahrenheit temperature, you can also use two formulas:

$$F = 1.8\,C + 32 \quad \text{or} \quad F = \frac{9}{5}C + 32$$

In the first method, multiply the Celsius temperature by 1.8 and then add 32. In the second method, multiply the Celsius temperature by 9, divide that answer by 5, and then add 32 to that answer. In either case, the remainder should be rounded to tenths.

Alternate Formula for Converting Between Celsius and Fahrenheit

This one algebraic formula may be used for conversions for both systems: $9C = 5F - 160$
  Learn and use the formulas that are easiest for you.

EXAMPLE 3.4

Convert 96.5° F to C°.

$$C = (96.5° - 32) \div 1.8 = 35.833 \text{ or } 35.8°$$

OR

$$C = (96.5° - 32) \times 5 \div 9 = 35.8333 \text{ or } 35.8°$$

EXAMPLE 3.5

Convert 65° C to F°.

$$F = (65° \times 1.8) + 32 = 149° F$$

OR

$$F = (9 \times 65°) \div 5 + 32 = 149° F$$

EXAMPLE 3.6

Convert 65° C to F°.

$9 \times 65° = 5F - 160$ add 160 to both sides

$9 \times 65° + 160 = 5F$ solve left side

$745° = 5F$ divide each side by 5

$149° = F$

EXAMPLE 3.7

Convert 96.5° F to C°.

$9C = 96.5° \times 5 - 160$

$9C = 482.5° - 160$

$9C = 322.5°$ divide each side by 9

$C° = 322.5° \div 9$

$C° = 35.8°$

TECH NOTE

When checking conversions for accuracy, the Celsius temperature will always be a lower number than the corresponding Fahrenheit temperature.

Practice Problems D

Convert the following temperatures using the appropriate formulas. Round to tenths as appropriate.

1. 1° F = _____ C
2. 35° C = _____ F
3. 35° F = _____ C

4. 19° C = _____ F
5. 112° F = _____ C
6. 34° C = _____ F

7. 36.5° C = _____ F
8. 102.6° F = _____ C
9. 98.6° F = _____ C

10. 99.2° F = _____ C
11. 37.2° C = _____ F
12. 100.2° F = _____ C

13. 10.2° C = _____ F
14. 130.6° F = _____ C
15. 48.2° C = _____ F

16. If a serum is to be stored at a temperature cooler than 40° F, what is the temperature for storage in a refrigerator on a Celsius thermometer? _____

17. Mrs. Jones is to receive an antibiotic if her temperature is above 103.8° F. What is the Celsius conversion? _____

18. A parenteral medication arrives through the mail. The label on the box states that the medication cannot be exposed to temperatures higher than 47.8° C. The current outdoor temperature is 100.2° F. What is the temperature in C? _____ Can the medication be safely used? _____

19. If a bottle of medication must be stored at a temperature cooler than 45° F, what is the Celsius temperature at which the medication must be stored? _____

20. A bag of fluids must be given at body temperature of 98.6° F. What is that temperature in the Celsius measurement? _____

SECTION II Measurements and Conversions

REVIEW

This chapter covers the rules and equations used in time, temperature, and numerical system conversions, which will be important in your career as a pharmacy technician. Physicians use a combination of Arabic and Roman numerals when writing prescriptions and medication orders. Most clinical sites use the 24-hour clock, to avoid timing errors, as well as the Celsius temperature scale. Review these in the chapter and then proceed with the posttest to check your understanding.

Posttest

Complete the mathematical calculations as needed. Show your work.

Change the following to either Arabic or Roman numerals as appropriate.

1. xxviiss _____
2. xliv _____
3. xciiiss _____

4. ccl _____
5. 45 _____
6. $36\frac{1}{2}$ _____

7. 46 _____
8. 59 _____
9. 75 _____

10. viiiss _____
11. lxviii _____
12. cxxv _____

13. xii _____
14. 78 _____
15. 165 _____

Change the following to either 24-hour or 12-hour time as appropriate.

16. 0530 _____
17. 8:30 AM _____
18. 1625 _____

19. 2:30 PM _____
20. 1325 _____
21. 0045 _____

22. 12:05 AM _____
23. 9:30 PM _____
24. 12:10 PM _____

Posttest, cont.

25. 0010 _____   26. 1755 _____   27. 3:26 PM _____

28. 1455 _____   29. 5:30 PM _____   30. 0635 _____

Convert the following temperatures. If Fahrenheit is listed, change to Celsius; if Celsius is given, change to Fahrenheit. Round to tenths.

31. 38.6° C _____   32. 86° F _____   33. 180° F _____

34. 94.2° F _____   35. 103° F _____   36. 100° C _____

37. 32° F _____   38. 2° F _____   39. 2° C _____

Answer the following questions

40. A medication cannot be frozen. The refrigerator is set for 5° C. What is the temperature in Fahrenheit? _____ Will the medication freeze? _____

41. A patient has a temperature of 38.6° C. What is the temperature in Fahrenheit? _____ Should the medical professional be concerned about this body temperature? _____

42. A refrigerator in the pharmacy department shows a temperature of 35.2° C. What is the temperature in Fahrenheit? _____ Should the pharmacy technician be concerned about any medications that must be stored below 50° F? _____

43. A physician writes an order for xxiv tablets. How many tablets should be dispensed? _____

Posttest, cont.

44. An order shows to dispense xc tablets. How many tablets will be dispensed? _____

45. A physician wants medication to be given every 6 hours beginning at 6:00 AM. Write the universal time for every 6 hours. _____ _____ _____ _____

46. A chart reads that the patient had pain medication at 5:35 PM. The medication can be taken every 6 hours. At what time in universal time could the next dose of medicine be given? _____

47. A medication order is to dispense xlviii tablets. How many tablets is this in Arabic numerals? _____

48. You supply a medication to the floor at 4:30 PM. You must chart the supply in universal time. What is the time of delivery? _____

49. If a medication is to be stored below 45° F, what would be the temperature on a Celsius thermometer in a refrigerator? _____

50. If a medication must be frozen at all times and the label states that it should be stored below 27° F, what would the refrigerator temperature need to be in Celsius? _____

CHAPTER 4

Measurement Systems, Units, and Equivalencies

OBJECTIVES

1. Know the standard abbreviations, rules for expressing measurements, and basic equivalencies for the household system of measurement.
2. Know the standard abbreviations, rules for expressing measurements, and the basic equivalencies for the metric system of measurement.
3. Know the standard abbreviations, rules for expressing measurements, and the basic equivalencies for the apothecary system of measurement.

KEY WORDS

Apothecary system One of the oldest measurement systems used to calculate drug orders using measurements such as grains and minims

Biologicals Substances made from natural sources such as human, animal or microorganism that are used as drug treatments or to prevent or diagnose diseases; tested for potency in a biologic system

Electrolytes Elements such as sodium (Na), potassium (K), magnesium (Mg), and calcium (Ca) that are necessary for normal body functions

International System of Units (metric system) Internationally accepted system of measurement of mass, length, and time

International unit/Unit A specific unit of measurement used for biologicals; a measurement of a medication's action as opposed to its weight (as with the units mcg, mg, g); specific to each particular medication

Milliequivalents (mEq) A type of unit used to express the concentration of electrolytes

Specific gravity The ratio of the density of a substance to the density of water when dealing with liquids in pharmacy

Standards An exact quantity agreed on for use in comparing measurements

Unit A general term covering any quantity chosen as a standard; for a measurement to make sense, it must include a number and a unit; examples of units: mg, mL, teaspoon

U.S. customary system (household system) System of measurement based on common kitchen measuring devices

Viscosity Thickness of a substance

Pretest

If you are already comfortable with the material, answer the following to test your knowledge. If not, work your way through the chapter and return to them for extra practice.

Items marked with an asterisk (*) are apothecary symbols, which are included in the Institute for Safe Medication Practices (ISMP) List of Error Prone Abbreviations, Symbols, and Dose Designations. Technicians must still be familiar with them.

Continued

Pretest, cont.

Write the meaning of the following abbreviations or symbols.

1. mg _____
2. mcg _____
3. g _____
4. gr _____
5. kg _____
6. " _____
7. oz _____
8. *fl℥ _____
9. mEq _____
10. *fl℈ _____
11. gtt _____
12. tsp _____
13. Tbsp _____
14. *♏ _____
15. lb., # _____
16. mL _____
17. L _____

18. How should one and one-half teaspoons be written? _____

19. How should two and one-half milliliters be written? _____

20. How should nine and one-half grains be written? _____

21. How should one thousand units be written? _____

Pretest, cont.

22. *What is the symbol for twenty fluid drams? _____

23. How many teaspoons are in one tablespoon? _____

24. How many milliliters are in one liter? _____

25. How many ounces are in one cup? _____

26. How many micrograms are in one milligram? _____

27. How many drams are in one ounce (apothecary system)? _____

28. How many ounces are in a pound (household system)? _____

29. How many tablespoons are in one ounce? _____

30. How many quarts are in one gallon? _____

* On the Institute for Safe Medication Practices (ISMP) *List of Error-Prone Abbreviations, Symbols, and Dose Designations*

INTRODUCTION

Three measurement systems are presently used in the medical field to calculate length, volume, and weight, although length is not as commonly used in the pharmaceutical field as in other medical disciplines. Each system has a unique set of measurement units that have been chosen as standards. Numbers without units are meaningless. Consider telling someone that you will be gone for 3. Without the unit designating minutes, hours, days, months, or years, there is no meaning to the 3.

The U.S. customary system, or household system, uses measurements such as inches, teaspoons, and pounds. The International System of Units, or the metric system, which is used in most of the remaining world, uses meters, liters, and grams. The apothecary system, which uses grains and drams, is an older system used in pharmacy for many years, but less frequently today. All three systems—household, metric, and apothecary—have units of measure for weight and volume that are used in pharmacy, but only household and metric systems have commonly used units for length. Knowledge of the units for weight and volume in the three systems and length in the household and metric systems is necessary to interpret medication orders and prescriptions.

In pharmacy, length is used to measure medications that require application to the body that must be measured in inches, centimeters, or millimeters. In these instances, the means of application is usually premarked on a dispensing paper for ease in ensuring that the correct amount of medication is administered, such as with nitroglycerin ointment. Another pharmaceutical use of length is in finding body surface area (BSA) where height and weight are used for dosage calculations, which will be covered in Chapter 12.

Mass is the measurement of the amount of matter in an object and is commonly referred to as weight. Metric weight is the measurement used most often in pharmacy to express a dosage unit. Most medications are ordered and supplied by the weight of a drug in solid or liquid amounts. Most solid medications are supplied in micrograms, milligrams, or grams. A few older medications are still supplied in grains from the apothecary system. Household measurements of weight are not used in medication strengths.

Volume is the amount of space something occupies and is used to measure amounts of liquids. A derived unit that is used to describe liquid medication strengths is density, which is weight divided by volume. Most liquid medications are described in terms of mg/mL. Occasionally some products, such as Milk of Magnesia, are still labeled with the amount of active ingredient per tablespoon (15 mL).

Some other specific types of medications are dosed in **milliequivalents (mEq)** and **International units**, or **units** (not to be confused with the generic term *unit* that applies to a quantity chosen as a standard measurement). Milliequivalents are used to express concentrations of **electrolytes** that are needed for normal body functions. For example, K-Dur 20 tablets contain 20 mEq of potassium per tablet. Units, as a measurement, are assigned to various **biologicals**, which are substances made from living organisms that are used therapeutically as medications. The *unit* measurement is actually assigned according to a medication's *activity* in that system. Units are specific to each individual medication and do not relate to one another. For example, units of insulin cannot be compared with units of heparin. Measurements of these two medications are covered in detail in Chapter 11.

Most measurements need a unit to have meaning. The one exception to this is **specific gravity**, which is the density of a substance in g/mL, divided by the density of water, which is 1 g/mL. In this calculation, the units cancel, leaving specific gravity without a unit. If the density of a substance is x g/mL, once it is divided by the density of water or 1 g/mL, the units cancel and the specific gravity of the substance is x. Specific gravity is used occasionally in pharmacy to calculate the weight or volume of a solution.

> **TECH NOTE**
>
> The Joint Commission's Official "Do Not Use" List includes the use of the abbreviations u or U, which should be written "unit," and IU, which should be written "International unit."

Some of the previously mentioned measurements are used daily, whereas others may be foreign and need explanation. This chapter covers the basic measurements per system, which are essential for applying the conversion methods used in Chapters 5 and 6.

HOUSEHOLD OR U.S. CUSTOMARY SYSTEM

The household, or U.S. customary, system of measure is being introduced first because much of it is already familiar. Household measurements and abbreviations of weight can be found in Table 4.1, length in Table 4.2, and volume in Table 4.3. Learn the equivalents

TABLE 4.1 Household Measurements of Weight

MEASUREMENT UNIT	ABBREVIATION	EQUIVALENT
Ounce	oz	—
Pound	lb, #	16 oz
Ton	T	2,000 #

TABLE 4.2 Household Measurements of Length

MEASUREMENT UNIT	ABBREVIATION	EQUIVALENTS
Inch	in, "	—
Foot	ft, '	12 inches
Yard	yd	36 inches, 3 feet

TABLE 4.3 Household Measurements of Volume

MEASUREMENT UNIT	ABBREVIATION*	EQUIVALENTS
Drops	**gtt**	—
Teaspoon	**tsp**, Tsp, t	60 drops (depending on the size of the dropper and the viscosity of the medication)
Tablespoon	tbsp, **Tbsp**, tbs, T	3 teaspoons
Ounce	**oz**	2 Tbsp or 6 tsp
Cup	C, **c**	8 oz
Pint	**pt**	2 c, 16 oz
Quart	**qt**	2 pt, 4 c, 32 oz
Gallon	**gal**	4 qt, 8 pt, 16 c, 128 oz

*Preferred abbreviations used in this text are **bolded**.

presented, because an equivalency table may not be available when you need to make a conversion.

Household measurements are expressed in Arabic numerals with fractions for expressing parts of a whole, such as ½, ⅔, or ¾. The abbreviation for each measurement follows the number, such as 5 tsp or 2½ pt.

When looking the smallest measurement of volume, a drop, it is totally dependent on the size of the opening in the dropper and the **viscosity** (thickness) of the liquid; therefore the 60 drops per teaspoon often found in tables of household measurements is only an approximation. Drops should not be used for measuring drugs unless there is a specific dropper calibrated for the medication.

Household measurements are often used in the home setting for administration of medications, although they are not optimal and should be considered approximations. The use of a measurement device provided with the medication by the pharmacy increases the accuracy of dosing and therefore patient safety. The household system is *not* used in hospital settings.

TECH NOTE

Pharmacy technicians should commit the following basic household equivalencies to memory and can use methods presented in Chapter 5 to calculate any of the others.

Volume		Weight	
	3 tsp = 1 Tbsp		16 oz = 1 lb
	2 Tbsp = 1 oz		
	8 oz = 1 c		
	2 c = 1 pt		
	2 pt = 1 qt		
	4 qt = 1 gal		

POINTS TO REMEMBER
THE HOUSEHOLD SYSTEM
- The household system uses fractions and Arabic numerals.
- Teaspoon and tablespoon are common household measurements.
- For patient safety, household utensils should not be used except when absolutely necessary.
- Household utensils are only approximations.
- For correct dosing, use the measuring device provided with the medication.

Practice Problems A

1. 1 c = _____ oz
2. 1 Tbsp = _____ tsp
3. 1 qt = _____ pt
4. 1 gal = _____ qt
5. 1 pt = _____ c
6. 1 lb = _____ oz

Write the meaning of the following abbreviations.

7. c _____
8. Tbsp _____
9. tsp _____
10. oz _____
11. gal _____
12. pt _____

METRIC SYSTEM OF MEASUREMENT

The metric system of measurement is the most widely used throughout the world and is the most commonly used system for measuring medications and dosages because of its accuracy. Most prescriptions are written in the metric system, and most liquid drugs are administered using this system. The *U.S. Pharmacopeia* considers the metric system the appropriate system for use on drug labels.

Medication labels should be written in the appropriate metric units. Some medication labels include household measurements as well as metric measurements, as seen with the label for zidovudine (Retrovir) in Fig. 4.1. Additionally, some labels still contain nonrecommended abbreviations, such as µg (microgram) found on the labels for digoxin (Lanoxin), Fig. 4.2, and cc (cubic centimeter), which is equivalent to mL (milliliter).

The metric system is based on units of 10. The basic measurements are the gram for weight, liter for volume, and meter for length. Prefixes for the base measurements are used to indicate the multiple or submultiple of the base that is being described. Fig. 4.3 illustrates the following prefixes: Deka (10 base units), hecto (100 base units), and kilo (1,000 base units) indicate multiples. Deci (one-tenth of the base), centi (one-hundredth of the base), milli (one-thousandth of the base), and micro (one-millionth of the base) are submultiples. Table 4.4 applies these prefixes to weight, volume, and length. Table 4.5 lists the equivalents between the measurements.

TECH NOTE
The prefixes most commonly used in pharmacy are micro, milli, and kilo.

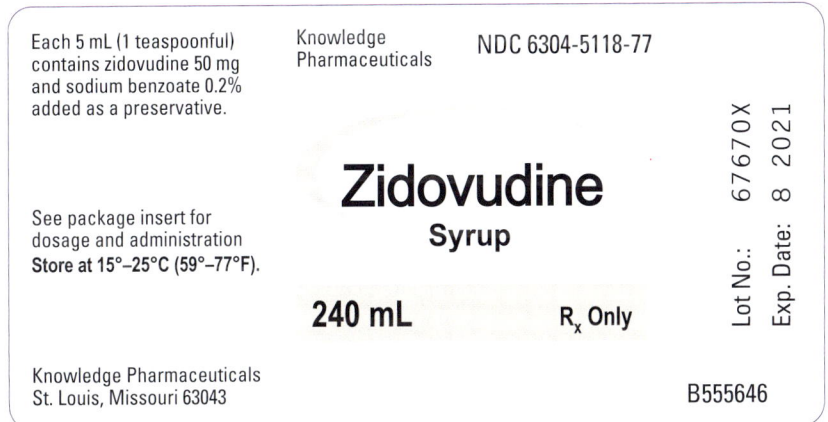

FIGURE 4.1 Label for zidovudine syrup.

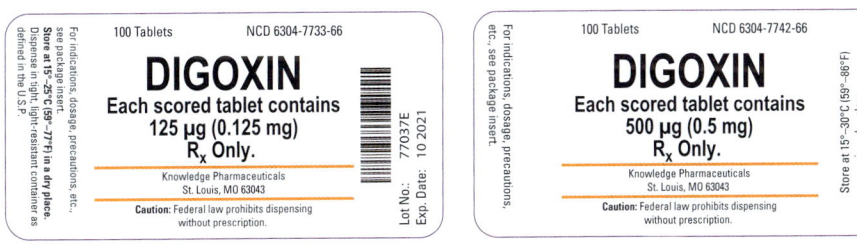

FIGURE 4.2 Labels for digoxin tablets.

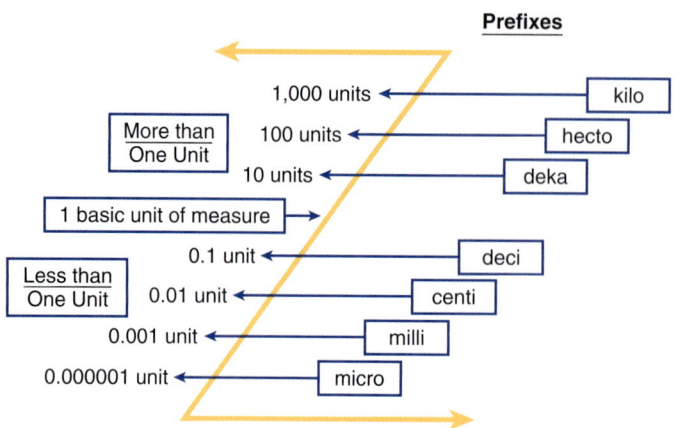

FIGURE 4.3 The Basic Units of Measure—Gram, Liter, and Meter—With Prefixes Indicating Larger or Smaller Measures. (Modified from Fulcher EM, Soto CD, Fulcher RM: *Pharmacology: principles and applications*, ed 3, St. Louis, Saunders, 2012.)

TABLE 4.4 Metric System of Measurements*

UNIT	WEIGHT	VOLUME	LENGTH
1,000 units	**kilogram**	kiloliter	kilometer
100 units	hectogram	hectoliter	hectometer
10 units	dekagram	dekaliter	dekameter
Base Unit	**gram**	**liter**	**meter**
1/10th unit	decigram	deciliter	decimeter
1/100th unit	centigram	centiliter	centimeter
1/1,000th unit	**milligram**	**milliliter**	millimeter
1/1,000,000th unit	**microgram**	microliter	micrometer

*****Bolded** measurements are commonly used in pharmacy.

TABLE 4.5 Metric Equivalents Used in Pharmacy*

TYPE OF SUBSTANCE	ABBREVIATION	UNIT OF MEASURE	COMMON EQUIVALENTS
Volume/liquid	**L**, l	liter	1,000 mL, 1,000 cc**
	mL, cc**	milliliter, cubic centimeter*	0.001 L
Weight	**g**	gram	1,000 mg, 0.001 kg
	kg	kilogram	1,000 g
	mg	milligram	0.001 g, 1,000 mcg
	mcg, µg**	microgram	0.000001 g, 0.001 mg
Length	**m**	meter	100 cm, 1,000 mm

*Prefered abbreviations used in this text are **bolded**.
**On the *ISMP List of Error-Prone Abbreviations, Symbols, and Dose Designations*.

A cubic centimeter is another way to express a milliliter. One cubic centimeter is the amount of space that is required to hold one milliliter of liquid. The abbreviation "cc" is *not recommended* because of the danger of misreading it as "00" (double zeros), but it is occasionally still found on prescriptions and medication orders. The preferred abbreviation is **mL**. The abbreviation "µg" for microgram may be misinterpreted as mg, causing a 1,000-fold error. The preferred abbreviation is **mcg**.

It is important to have a general idea of the weight, volume, or length of a unit. Most people in the United States are familiar with household but not metric units. The following comparisons may be helpful.

A gram is about the weight of two large-sized paper clips.

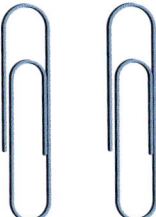

A liter is about the size of a quart container.

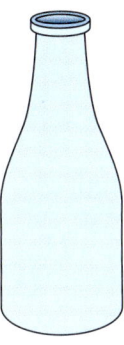

A meter is a little longer than a yardstick.

Fractional parts of numbers in the metric system are indicated with decimals. A zero, called *leading zero*, should always be placed before a decimal when the number is less than 1 to prevent confusion and a possible error in interpretation. For instance, .25 mg might be misread as 25 mg if the measurement was not written as 0.25 mg. The potential error would be 100 times too much medication being administered to a patient. Also *no* zeros, called *trailing zeros*, should be added at the end of a fractional portion after a decimal point. For instance, to prevent errors, 2.50 mg should be written 2.5 mg, and 1.500 L should be written 1.5 L. Zeros found at the *end* of a number to the right of the decimal point may be removed without changing the value of the number.

The following depicts the weight measurements used in pharmacy from largest to smallest. There is a 1,000-unit difference between each of the following measurements of mass.

Metric Measurements of Mass in Pharmacy

kg _____ g _____ mg _____ mcg
 (1 kg = 1,000 g)   (1 g = 1,000 mg)   (1 mg = 1,000 mcg)

Metric Measurements of Volume in Pharmacy

L _____ mL
   1 L = 1,000 mL

TECH NOTE

Pharmacy technicians should commit the following basic metric equivalencies to memory and can use methods presented in Chapter 5 to calculate any of the others needed.

Weight: 1,000 mcg = 1 mg   1,000 mg = 1 g   1,000 g = 1 kg
Volume: 1,000 mL = 1 L

POINTS TO REMEMBER
THE METRIC SYSTEM

- The metric system is a system of "place values" with the *base* being the unit from which all place values are measured. The gram, meter, and liter are at place 1, or the base site; kilo is at place 10^3 (the thousands place); milli is 10^{-3} (the one-thousandths place); and micro is 10^{-6} (the one-millionths place).
- When using the metric system of measurement, the numeral is written before the abbreviation for the quantity, with a full space between the number and abbreviation (e.g., 10 mg, 2.5 mm, 1.5 L).
- All fraction parts are written as a *decimal* number (e.g., 1.5 mL, 2.5 g, or 2.75 m).
- Be sure that any number with a value less than zero has a "0" preceding the decimal point, a leading zero.
- Any unnecessary, or trailing, zeros should be eliminated.
- Avoid using a decimal number if a whole number can be used.

Practice Problems B

1. 1 mg = 1,000 _____   2. 1 kg = 1,000 _____

3. 1 L = 1,000 _____   4. 1 g = 1,000 _____

Write the meanings of the following abbreviations:

5. kg _____   6. g _____

7. mg _____   8. L _____

9. mL _____   10. mcg _____

APOTHECARY SYSTEM OF MEASUREMENT

The apothecary system is one of the oldest systems of measurement. First used by an apothecary (early pharmacist), this system is gradually being replaced with the metric system. In ancient times, a minim (drop) of water was considered to weigh the same as a grain of wheat. Therefore the basic unit of liquid in the apothecary system is a minim (♏) and the basic unit of weight is a grain (gr). Apothecary measurements of volume such as minims (♏), fluid drams (fl℥), and fluid ounces (fl℥) are still found on some pharmacy bottles and medication-dispensing cups even though the use of these measurements is discouraged. These apothecary symbols are found on the *ISMP List of Error-Prone Abbreviations, Symbols, and Dose Designations*. Although the metric system is preferred, the apothecary grain is still used with some older medications, such as nitroglycerin sublingual tablets (Nitrostat) (Fig. 4.4).

In the apothecary system, lowercase Roman numerals are used for expression of numbers 10 and below, rather than Arabic numerals as found in the metric and household systems. The Roman numerals should be expressed with lines placed over them to tie them together, such as ī, īī, īīī, īv̄, v̄ and x̄, and lowercase i's are often expressed with the dots above that line. Arabic numerals may be used for numbers higher than 10, except for 20 ($\overline{xx}$) and 30 ($\overline{xxx}$), for which Roman numerals are required. Over the years the use of the line over the Roman numeral has gradually diminished, but using it is correct. Fractions other than ½, which is $\overline{ss}$, are expressed using Arabic numerals. Roman numerals and Arabic numerals are never used together in one measurement, so when using a fraction other than $\overline{ss}$, use Arabic numerals for the whole number as well. Therefore seven and three-fourths would be 7¾, not vii ¾. Decimals are *not* used with the apothecary system. The unit abbreviation is written first with Roman numerals placed to the right of the unit of measure. For example, 5 ounces is written ℥ v and 10 drams is ℨ x. See Table 4.6 for equivalents in the apothecary system.

TECH NOTE

The household pound (#) is 16 ounces; the apothecary pound is 12 ounces. The household pound (16 oz) will be used for conversions with body weight in pharmacy.

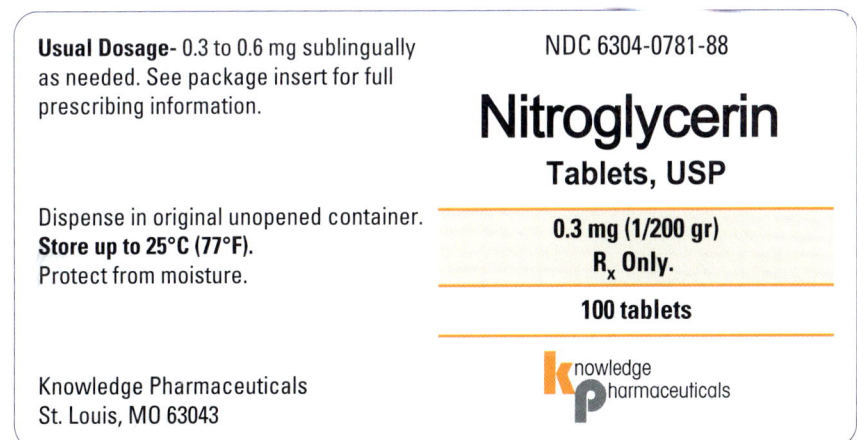

FIGURE 4.4 Label for nitroglycerin sublingual tablets.

TABLE 4.6 Equivalents in the Apothecary System

TYPE OF SUBSTANCE	ABBREVIATION	UNIT OF MEASURE	COMMON EQUIVALENTS
Volume/liquid	♏	minim	—
	fl ʒ*	fluid dram	♏ lx (60)
	fl ℥*	fluid ounce	ʒ viii (8)
Mass/weight	gr	grain	—
	ʒ	dram	gr lx (60)
	℥	ounce	ʒ viii (8)
	#	pound	℥ xii (12)

*On the *ISMP List of Error-Prone Abbreviations, Symbols, and Dose Designations*. An ounce is larger than a dram; the ounce symbol has one more loop than the dram symbol.

TECH NOTE
Although they are not used often, pharmacy technicians should be familiar with the following apothecary equivalencies.

Weight: ℥ i = ʒ viii   Volume: fl ℥ i = fl ʒ viii

POINTS TO REMEMBER
THE APOTHECARY SYSTEM
- The quantity should be expressed in lowercase Roman numerals, frequently with a line placed over the entire numeral and a dot above the line with the numeral i, although this line is not used as often as it used to be.
- An amount greater than 10, other than 20 and 30, *may* be written in Arabic numerals.
- Numbers less than 1 are written as fractions, except ½, which is written s̄s̄.
- Do not combine Roman and Arabic numerals in the same measurement.
- The symbol or abbreviation is written before the quantity.

Practice Problems C
Identify the following symbols and abbreviations.

1. fl ℥ _____
2. ♏ _____
3. # _____
4. fl ʒ _____
5. gr _____

REVIEW

Three measurement systems are used in the field of medicine in the United States. The household system is the most commonly used on a daily basis in homes in the United States. However, using the household system provides only approximate measurements because of the differences in utensils; it may lead to inaccurate dosing when used for administering medication. The use of actual measuring spoons as opposed to individual flatware can help decrease the variation. The metric system is used as the standard unit of measure throughout the rest of the world and is structured on multiples of 10. Most medications are designated in the metric system today. The final system, rarely used today but found with some medications, is the apothecary system, which is based on grains for weight and minims, fluid drams, and fluid ounces for volume. Although this system is not popular and its use is being discouraged, these measurements are still seen occasionally with some medications. The measurements for length, weight, and volume must be learned for conversions within and between the systems, which will be discussed in the next two chapters.

Posttest

Rewrite the following using the appropriate numerals and abbreviations (or numerals and symbols with the apothecary system).

1. 36 kilograms = _____
2. 5.4 grams = _____
3. 3 teaspoons = _____
4. 9 tablespoons = _____
5. 5 grains = _____
6. 10 fluid drams = _____
7. 6 pints = _____
8. 125 micrograms = _____
9. twelve and one-half milligrams = _____
10. one-half milliliter = _____
11. one and three-fourths liters = _____
12. two and one-half quarts = _____
13. 3 drops = _____
14. 2 ounces = _____

Continued

Posttest, cont

15. 4 cups = _____

16. 6 apothecary fluid ounces = _____

17. 4 minims = _____

18. 110 pounds = _____

19. 65 grains = _____

20. three and one-half fluid drams = ____

21. forty milliequivalents = _____

22. one thousand units = _____

Complete the following equivalencies.

23. one fluid ounce = _____ fluid drams

24. 1 c = _____ oz

25. 1 kg = 1,000 _____

26. 1 L = 1,000 _____

27. 3 tsp = 1 _____

28. 2 pt = 1 _____

29. 1 gal = _____ qt

30. 1,000 mcg = 1 _____

REVIEW OF RULES

Household System

- The household system uses fractions and Arabic numerals.

Metric System

- The metric system uses decimals and Arabic numerals.

Apothecary System

- The quantity should be expressed in lowercase Roman numerals, frequently with a line placed over the entire numeral and a dot above the line for the numeral i.
- An amount greater than 10, other than 20 and 30, *may* be written in Arabic numerals.
- Numbers less than 1 are written as fractions, except ½, which is written $\overline{ss}$.
- Do not combine Roman and Arabic numerals in the same measurement.
- The symbol or abbreviation is written before the quantity.

CHAPTER 5

Conversions Within Measurement Systems

OBJECTIVES

1. Identify, convert, and calculate among household system measurements of weight and volume used in the medical field using both the ratio and proportion method and dimensional analysis.
2. Identify, convert, and calculate among metric system measurements of weight and volume used in the medical field using both the ratio and proportion method and dimensional analysis.
3. Identify, convert, and calculate among apothecary system measurements of weight and volume used in the medical field.

KEY WORDS

Conversion factor A ratio equal to 1 that is used to change one *unit* to another without changing the value of the answer

Dimensional analysis (DA) A method used for converting between units and calculating medication doses and dosages that involves multiplying a series of fractions in an order whereby all unnecessary units are sequentially canceled until the desired unit is reached

Ratio and proportion (R&P) A method used for *single-step* conversions between units and for calculating medication doses and dosages; involves solving for two equivalent fractions using cross-multiplication and division

Pretest

If you are comfortable with the subject matter, answer the following to test your knowledge. If not, work your way through the chapter and return to them for extra practice. Show your calculations. Perform ounce and pound weight conversions in the household system. Do not round your answers.

1. 15 gtt = _____ tsp
2. 6 Tbsp = _____ oz
3. 15 tsp = _____ Tbsp
4. 2 mcg = _____ mg
5. 6 kg = _____ mg
6. ℥ viii = ʒ _____
7. 4 c = _____ oz
8. 6 pt = _____ qt

Pretest, cont.

9. 3 Tbsp = _____ oz

10. 250 mg = _____ g

11. 0.125 mg = _____ mcg

12. 1.56 g = _____ mg

13. 5.6 kg = _____ g

14. ℨ ii = ℥ _____

15. 2.5 g = _____ mg

16. 60″ = _____ ′

17. 2′ = _____ ″

18. 5 kg = _____ mcg

19. 44# = _____ oz

20. ℨ $\frac{3}{4}$ = ℥ _____

21. 6 Tbsp = _____ tsp

22. 2.5 g = _____ kg

23. 60 gtt = _____ tsp

24. ℥ iv = ℨ _____

25. 6 c = _____ oz

INTRODUCTION

Now that we are familiar with the standard units of measurement in the household, metric, and apothecary systems, we will focus on converting from one unit to another within each system. All conversions, and most pharmaceutical calculations, can be completed using one of two basic calculation methods: **dimensional analysis (DA)** or **ratio and proportion (R&P)**.

HOUSEHOLD OR U.S. CUSTOMARY SYSTEM

How many inches are in 2 feet? That is fairly simple for people in United States because it is used in everyday life. We know that 1 foot equals 12 inches, so 2 feet will equal 24 inches. This is actually an example of the R&P method of solving a conversion.

Copyright © 2019 by Elsevier, Inc. All rights reserved.

Ratio and Proportion

This method is also known as cross-multiply and divide.

1. Identify the unknown unit of measurement.
2. Find the known equivalent for the problem to be solved.
3. Write the known equivalents in a fraction on the left side of the equation.
4. Write the unknown desired equivalent in a fraction on the right side of the equation, using *x* for the unknown value.
5. Cross-multiply the numerators and denominators.
6. Divide to solve for the value of *x*.

EXAMPLE 5.1

How many inches are in 2 feet? We know that there are 12 inches in 1 foot.

$$\frac{12''}{1'} = \frac{x}{2'}$$
$$1 \cdot x = 2 \cdot 12$$
$$x = 24''$$

> **! TECH ALERT**
>
> The units in the numerators of equivalent fractions must be the same and the units in the denominators of equivalent fractions must be the same!

EXAMPLE 5.2

How many tablespoons are equivalent to 7 tsp?

Once you know all of the basic equivalencies from Chapter 4, this becomes much easier. We can see from Table 4.3 that 3 tsp equals 1 Tbsp; therefore:

$$\frac{1 \text{ Tbsp}}{3 \text{ tsp}} = \frac{x}{7 \text{ tsp}} \quad 3x = 7$$

Divide each side by 3.

$$x = \frac{7}{3} \text{ Tbsp}$$

Reduce the answer to $2\frac{1}{3}$ Tbsp.

> **TECH NOTE**
>
> Leave your answer as a whole number and a fraction when using the household measurement system.

Using dimensional analysis is another choice for converting between units. Some students prefer using this method to keep track of units. We will use DA exclusively when dealing with multistep calculations specifically for this reason.

A **conversion factor** is a ratio that is equal to 1 and is used to change one unit to another. Because it is equivalent to 1, it does not change the value of the answer, only the unit. $\frac{12''}{1'}$ is a conversion factor; 12″ divided by 1′ has a value of one because they are equivalent amounts.

Dimensional Analysis

1. Identify the unit of the *answer* needed and follow it with an equal sign.
2. Set up a fraction such that the unit of the *desired* answer is in the numerator of the first fraction of the DA equation—this unit will *never* be cancelled.
3. Set up the next fraction in the equation so the unit of its numerator is the same as the unit of the denominator of the first fraction (so they will cancel when the fractions are multiplied).
4. These steps are continued when dealing with multistep problems but are sufficient for the single-step conversions in the following examples.

EXAMPLE 5.3

How many inches are in 2 feet?

The conversion factor is $\frac{12''}{1'}$, which equals the *value* of 1.

$$'' = \frac{12''}{1'} \cdot \frac{2'}{1} = 24''$$

The unit of feet cancels, and inches is left.

! TECH ALERT

DA involves multiplication of fractions—NOT cross-multiplication as with R&P!

EXAMPLE 5.4

How many Tbsp are equivalent to 7 tsp?

The conversion factor is $\frac{1\,\text{Tbsp}}{3\,\text{tsp}}$, which equals the value of 1.

$$\text{Tbsp} = \frac{1\,\text{Tbsp}}{3\,\text{tsp}} \times \frac{7\,\text{tsp}}{1} = \frac{7\,\text{Tbsp}}{3} = 2\frac{1}{3}\,\text{Tbsp}$$

The unit *tsp* cancels, leaving *Tbsp*.

EXAMPLE 5.5

24 Tbsp is equivalent to how many cups?

If you do not remember exactly how many tablespoons are in one cup, you can go to what you know and use DA. For instance, if you remember that there are 2 Tbsp in 1 oz and 8 oz in 1 cup, set up a DA equation as follows:

$$\text{cups} = \frac{1\,\text{c}}{8\,\text{oz}} \times \frac{1\,\text{oz}}{2\,\text{Tbsp}} \times \frac{24\,\text{Tbsp}}{1} = \frac{24\,\text{c}}{16} = 1\frac{1}{2}\,\text{c}$$

As long as you learn the sequence in Table 5.1, you can solve any conversion within the household system.

TECH NOTE

The use of R&P is only appropriate with single-step conversions. DA can be used for single-step or multistep conversions.

TABLE 5.1 Household Equivalencies/Conversions

LIQUID MEASUREMENTS (VOLUME)

Measurement	Abbreviation	Equivalent
1 drop	gtt	1 mL
1 teaspoon	tsp	60 gtt (varies with viscosity and dropper size)
1 tablespoon	Tbsp	3 tsp
1 ounce	oz	2 Tbsp
1 cup	c	8 oz
1 pint	pt	2 c
1 quart	qt	2 pt
1 gallon	gal	4 qt

DRY WEIGHT MEASUREMENT

Measurement	Abbreviation	Equivalent
1 pound	lb or #	16 oz

Practice Problems A

Calculate the following conversions using your preferred method. Show your calculations.

1. 9 tsp = _____ Tbsp
2. 2 qt = _____ gal
3. 3 Tbsp = _____ oz
4. 6 oz = _____ c
5. 5 c = _____ oz
6. 15 tsp = _____ Tbsp
7. 4½ oz = _____ tsp
8. 4 c = _____ pt
9. 20 oz = _____ #
10. 4′ 6″ = _____ ″ (Hint: convert 4′ to inches and then add 6″)
11. 3½ # = _____ oz
12. ½ Tbsp = _____ tsp
13. 3 pt = _____ qt
14. 6 qt = _____ gal

15. 3 tsp = _____ gtt

16. 45 gtt = _____ tsp

17. 24 oz = _____ c

18. 10 c = _____ oz

19. 32 oz = _____ #

20. 8 Tbsp = _____ oz

Patients often use calibrated medication cups or oral syringes at home to take medications; however, these utensils may not be provided or may be misplaced, so the pharmacy technician must have an understanding of conversions within household measurements. Convert the following problems to easier-to-use household measurements.

21. The physician orders 4½ tsp of amoxicillin.

How many tablespoons would the patient take? _____

22. The physician orders 1 oz of milk of magnesia.

How many tablespoons are ordered? _____

23. The physician orders 120 gtt of Rondec DM for a child.

How many teaspoons would you give the child? _____

24. A patient is to take 1 quart of Go-Lytely in preparation for x-rays.

How many cups of the medication should the patient drink? _____

25. The physician tells the patient to drink at least 24 additional ounces of water a day.

How many additional cups of water would the patient need to drink to follow the physician's order? _____

METRIC SYSTEM CONVERSIONS

Because the metric system is based on units of 10, conversions can be made within the system by moving decimal places. This is a quick method, but a thorough understanding of the relationship between units is needed to master it. DA and R&P can always be used as well.

Metric Measurements of Mass Used in Pharmacy

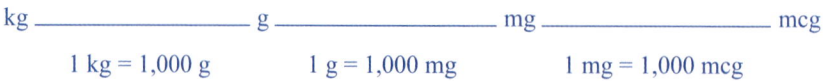

1 kg = 1,000 g　　1 g = 1,000 mg　　1 mg = 1,000 mcg

There is a 1,000-fold (3 decimal place) difference between (*kg & g*), (*g & mg*), & (*mg & mcg*)
There is a 1,000,000-fold (6 decimal place) difference between (kg & mg) & (g & mcg)
There is a 1,000,000,000-fold (9 decimal place) difference between (kg & mcg)

FIGURE 5.1 Metric system conversions.

TABLE 5.2　Metric Conversions Used in Pharmacy

WEIGHT
1 kg = 1,000 g
1 g = 1,000 mg
1 mg = 1,000 mcg

VOLUME
1 L = 1,000 mL

The units used for weight in pharmacy are, from largest to smallest, kilogram, gram, milligram, and microgram, with a 1,000-fold or 3-decimal-place-factor difference between each closest measurement. Fig. 5.1 is helpful for remembering this.

The units used for volume in pharmacy are, from largest to smallest, liter and milliliter, with a 1,000-fold or 3-decimal-place difference between each. The only conversion factor that is used in pharmacy for volume is 1 L = 1,000 mL. See Table 5.2.

! TECH ALERT
Be careful to distinguish between mcg, mg, g, and kg (weight) and mL and L (volume) to prevent medication errors. The abbreviation μg (mcg) is on the "Do Not Use" list but is still found on some medications labels.

TECH NOTE
When numbers in an answer are 1,000 or more, add commas to avoid mistakes.

CONVERTING FROM LARGER METRIC NUMBERS TO SMALLER METRIC NUMBERS

The placement of the decimal point is based on moving through powers of 10 by moving the decimal point. First, determine the number of the decimal place difference between the two numbers. When converting from a larger metric unit to a smaller one, move the decimal point to the right by the number of the decimal place difference between the two *or* multiply by 1 plus the number of zeros in the equivalent (large unit to smaller unit → multiply). This method can be verified or checked by using R&P or DA as well. The following examples depict moving the decimal point, multiplying by 1 plus the number of zeros difference, R&P, and DA.

EXAMPLE 5.6

Moving the decimal or multiplying

1.2 L = _____ mL

A liter is larger than a milliliter by three place values, so move the decimal three places to the right or multiply by 1,000.

1.2 L becomes 1.2 0 0. or 1,200 mL

$$1.2 \times 1{,}000 = 1{,}200.0$$

1.2 L = 1,200 mL

Ratio and Proportion

$$\frac{1\,L}{1{,}000\,mL} = \frac{1.2\,L}{x}$$

$$x = 1{,}200\,mL$$

Dimensional Analysis

$$mL = \frac{1{,}000\,mL}{1\,L} \cdot \frac{1.2\,L}{1} = 1{,}200\,mL$$

EXAMPLE 5.7

Moving the decimal or multiplying

5.4 kg = _____ mg

A kilogram is larger than a milligram by six place values, so move the decimal six places to the right or multiply by 1,000,000.

5.4 kg becomes 5.4 0 0 0 0 0.

$$5.4 \times 1{,}000{,}000 = 5{,}400{,}000.0$$

5.4 kg = 5,400,000 mg

Ratio and Proportion

$$\frac{1\,kg}{1{,}000{,}000\,mg} = \frac{5.4\,kg}{x} \qquad x = 5{,}400{,}000\,mg$$

Dimensional Analysis

If you are more comfortable moving from the closest unit in steps, DA analysis can be used.

$$mg = \frac{1{,}000\,mg}{1\,g} \cdot \frac{1{,}000\,g}{1\,kg} \cdot \frac{5.4\,kg}{1} = 5{,}400{,}000\,mg$$

> **TECH NOTE**
> To convert a **L**arger unit to a **S**maller unit, move the decimal to the **R**ight: **"L to S go R."**

CONVERTING FROM A SMALLER METRIC NUMBER TO A LARGER METRIC NUMBER

First, determine the number of the decimal place difference between the two numbers. When converting from a smaller metric unit to a larger one, move the decimal point to the left by the number of the decimal place difference between the two *or* divide by 1 plus the number of zeros in the equivalent (small unit to large unit → divide).

EXAMPLE 5.8

Moving the decimal or dividing

$$5 \text{ mg} = \underline{\hspace{2cm}} \text{ g}$$

A milligram is smaller than a gram by three place values, so move the decimal three places to the left or divide by 1,000.

5 mg is the same as 0.005 g or 5 ÷ 1,000

$$5 \text{ mg} = 0.005 \text{ g}$$

Ratio and Proportion

$$\frac{1{,}000 \text{ mg}}{1 \text{ g}} = \frac{5 \text{ mg}}{x}$$

$$1{,}000x = 5 \text{ g}$$

Divide both sides by 1,000.

$$x = 0.005 \text{ g}$$

Dimensional Analysis

$$g = \frac{1 \text{ g}}{1{,}000 \text{ mg}} \cdot \frac{5 \text{ mg}}{1} = 0.005 \text{ g}$$

> **TECH NOTE**
> Always place a leading zero before the decimal point if the number is less than 1.

EXAMPLE 5.9

$$500 \text{ g} = \underline{\hspace{2cm}} \text{ kg}$$

A gram is smaller than a kilogram by three place values, so move the decimal three places to the left or divide by 1,000.

500 g is the same as 0.500 kg or 500 ÷ 1,000

Because zeros at the end of a decimal (trailing zeros) can be dropped, the answer is 0.5 kg.

TECH NOTE
To convert from a **S**maller unit to a **L**arger unit, move the decimal to the **L**eft: **"S to L go L."**

Practice Problems B

Complete the following problems

1. 2 L = _____ mL
2. 2.5 mg = _____ mcg
3. 4 kg = _____ g
4. 450 g = _____ kg
5. 0.5 L = _____ mL
6. 0.5 mg = _____ mcg
7. 0.5 mg = _____ g
8. 2.5 mL = _____ L
9. 50 mL = _____ L
10. 5.5 L = _____ mL
11. 1.5 g = _____ mg
12. 6.54 kg = _____ mg
13. 450 mg = _____ g
14. 25 mcg = _____ mg
15. 50.6 kg = _____ g
16. 10 L = _____ mL
17. 500 mL = _____ L
18. 3,500 mL = _____ L
19. 0.0045 kg = _____ g
20. 0.3 mg = _____ mcg
21. 5 mL = _____ L
22. 58,400 mL = _____ L
23. 510 mL = _____ L
24. 300 mg = _____ mcg

25. A container of IV fluids contains 0.5 L.

    How many milliliters is this? _____

26. Amoxicillin is available as 250 mg/capsule.

    How many grams of amoxicillin does each capsule contain? _____

27. A tablet of digoxin contains 250 mcg.

    How would this be written in mg? _____

28. A physician orders 1 g of Cipro.

    How many mg should be administered to the patient? _____

29. A physician orders a thyroid replacement, Synthroid 0.175 mg.

    How many micrograms would be given to the patient? _____

30. A physician orders 1,500 mg of cephalexin.

    How many grams of cephalexin are in a 1,500 mg dose? _____

! **TECH ALERT**

The abbreviation "cc" is on the ISMP List of Error Prone Abbreviations, Symbols, and Dose Designations because of the danger of reading the abbreviation as "00" (zeros); the unit mL should be used instead.

APOTHECARY SYSTEM OF MEASUREMENT

The measurement of grains is still found on labels of nitroglycerin, codeine, phenobarbital, aspirin, and ferrous sulfate (iron). Some physicians will order these medications, as well as acetaminophen, in grains, which is the apothecary unit used most in pharmacy. Apothecary symbols are found on the ISMP List of Error Prone Abbreviations, Symbols, and Dose Designations. They will be used in Chapters 5 and 6 only. Apothecary equivalents that will be used as conversion factors in Practice Problems C are found in Table 5.3.

! TECH ALERT

Care should be taken that gr (grain) and g or gm (which is sometimes still used for gram) are not confused. These measurements have different weights and are in two separate measurement systems.

TABLE 5.3 Apothecary System Symbols and Equivalencies

Volume

1 minim	♏	
1 fluid dram	fl ʒ	♏ 60
1 fluid ounce	fl ʒ	fl ʒ viii (8)

Weight

1 grain*	gr	
1 dram	ʒ	gr 60
1 ounce	ʒ	ʒ viii (8)
1 pound	#	ʒ xii (12)

*The only weight measurement frequently used in pharmacy is the grain.

TECH NOTE

Although symbols used for the apothecary system may be unfamiliar, they cancel just like units for the metric and household systems. Set these problems up the same as with those systems.

EXAMPLE 5.10

How many fluid drams are in 2 apothecary fluid ounces?

Ratio and Proportion

Known   Unknown

$$\frac{ʒ\ i}{ʒ\ viii} \bowtie \frac{ʒ\ ii}{x}$$

$x = viii \cdot ʒii$ (The math may be easier to perform if it is changed to $x = 8 \cdot ʒ\ 2$)

$x = ʒ\ 16$, so $\frac{ʒ\ i}{ʒ\ viii} = \frac{ʒ\ ii}{ʒ\ xvi}$ or $ʒ\ ii = ʒ\ xvi$

Single-step and multistep conversions can be solved using DA.

TECH NOTE

It may be easier to change your numbers to Arabic numerals while performing calculations. Just be sure to change your answer back into Roman numerals if necessary. This is especially helpful with multistep conversions using DA. Remember that apothecary symbols cancel the same as metric and household units.

Practice Problems C

Practice your skills in the apothecary system, using Roman numerals in your answers when required. Show your calculations.

1. fl℈ vi = fl℥ _____

2. fl℈ xii = fl℥ _____

3. gr iv = ℈ _____

4. gr xxx = ℈ _____

5. gr x = ℈ _____

6. fl℥ v = fl℈ _____

7. fl℥ ii = fl℈ _____

8. fl℈ iii = fl℥ _____

REVIEW

Three measurement systems are used in practicing pharmacology. The household system is used most commonly on a daily basis in the United States and is also used for administration of liquid medications at home if the appropriate dispenser is not provided. However, using the household system for volume provides only approximate measurements because of the difference in utensils; it may cause an inaccurate dose when used for administering medication. The metric system is used as a standard unit of measure throughout the world and is structured on multiples of 10. Most medications are designated in the metric system. The final system, rarely used today but still found with some medications, is the apothecary system. Although this system is not popular and its use is being discouraged, these measurements are still seen occasionally with some medications.

R&P and DA may be used for the calculation of conversions within a system. With the metric system, the decimal may be moved as a shortcut to make the necessary conversion. Use the method that is best for you and use it consistently.

Posttest

Using the appropriate system of measurement, figure the equivalents found in this posttest. Show your calculations.

1. 36 kg = _____ g

2. 5.4 g = _____ mg

3. 2 tsp = _____ gtt

4. 4 Tbsp = _____ tsp

5. gr v = ℈ _____

6. fl℈ x = fl℥ _____

Posttest, cont

7. 6 pt = _____ qt

8. 125 mcg = _____ mg

9. 12.5 mg = _____ g

10. 0.5 mL = _____ cc (on ISMP List of Error Prone Abbreviations)

11. 1.75 L = _____ mL

12. 2 qt = _____ gal

13. 2 Tbsp = _____ oz

14. 4 oz = _____ c

15. 4 c = _____ pt

16. 0.4 mg = _____ mcg

17. 1.3 kg = _____ mg

18. 1 Tbsp = _____ oz

19. 4 oz = _____ tsp

20. fl℥ xvi = fl℥ _____

21. 40.5 mg = _____ g

22. 40.5 mg = _____ mcg

23. 3.75 L = _____ mL

24. 12 c = _____ qt

25. 250 mg = _____ g

26. 0.25 g = _____ mg

27. 75 mL = _____ L

28. 250 mL = _____ L

29. 2 tsp = _____ Tbsp

30. 8 Tbsp = _____ oz

31. 32 oz = _____ c

32. 64 oz = _____ pt

Continued

Posttest, cont

33. 24 tsp = _____ oz

34. 1.2 mg = _____ mcg

35. ʒ xxiv = ℥ _____

36. 4 c = _____ oz

37. 9 tsp = _____ Tbsp

38. 55 mg = _____ g

39. 600 mg = _____ g

40. 650 mcg = _____ mg

41. 15 Tbsp = _____ oz

42. 15 tsp = _____ oz

43. 0.05 g = _____ mg

44. 0.0025 g = _____ mg

45. 2.5 kg = _____ g

46. A physician orders digoxin 0.125 mg tablet.
    How many micrograms of medication is this?

47. An order is given for amoxicillin 250 mg.
    How many grams is this?

48. A physician writes a prescription for Benadryl fl℥ viii.
    How many fluid drams is this?

49. An order is written for ranitidine 0.075 g.
    How many milligrams is this?

Posttest, cont

50. A patient is given a prescription for sulfamethoxazole 2,000 mg.
How many grams is this?

51. An order is written for a patient with hypertension for hydralazine 25 mg tablets.
How many grams are in each tablet?

52. A physician asks a patient to take an ounce of Mylanta every 4 hours.
How many tablespoons need to be taken per dose?

53. A child is to take ½ Tbsp of amoxicillin suspension.
How many teaspoons should the parent give the child?

54. A physician orders Carafate Suspension 2 Tbsp to be taken 30 minutes before meals.
How many teaspoons is this per dose?

55. Because of hyperlipidemia, a patient is given a prescription for Zetia 0.01 g.
How many milligrams is this?

CHAPTER 6

Conversions Between Measurement Systems

OBJECTIVES

1. Discuss conversions and conversion factors, including the rules for using ratio and proportion and dimensional analysis.
2. Describe how to perform conversions among household, apothecary, and metric systems of measurement.

KEY WORDS

Measurable amount The quantity of medication that can be most accurately measured with the device available

! TECH ALERT

When converting between two measurement systems, the answers will not be exact due to the differences between the measurement systems. Other factors include the viscosity of the medication and the size of the devices used to provide the medication.

Pretest

If you are already comfortable with the subject matter, answer the following to test your knowledge. If not, work your way through the chapter and return to them for extra practice. Show your calculations and round to the nearest tenth.

1. 1 oz = _____ mL
2. 1 gal = _____ mL
3. 2 kg = _____ #
4. 1 Tbsp = _____ mL
5. 1# = _____ g
6. 2 tsp = _____ mL
7. 2 pt = _____ mL
8. 4 oz = _____ mL
9. 4 tsp = ℨ _____
10. gr $\frac{1}{4}$ = _____ mg

Pretest, cont.

11. 88# = _____ kg

12. 120 mg = gr _____

13. 180 mL = _____ oz

14. 15 mL = _____ tsp

15. 325 mg aspirin = gr _____

16. 1½ tsp = _____ mL

17. 15 tsp = ℨ _____

18. nitroglycerin gr 1/150 = _____ mg

19. nitroglycerin 0.6 mg = gr _____

20. 60 g = _____ oz

21. 2.5 mL = _____ tsp

22. 3.84 L = _____ gal

23. 4 Tbsp = ℨ _____

24. 6″ = _____ cm

25. 1 c = _____ mL

26. 2 Tbsp = _____ mL

27. codeine gr i = _____ mg

28. 5 kg = _____ #

29. 44# = _____ kg

30. flℨ vi = _____ Tbsp

INTRODUCTION

The previous chapter covered conversions within the household, metric, and apothecary systems of measurement. Each of these is used today in prescribing and administering medications, although the metric system is the most common. Because all three systems are used, conversions between the systems must be covered in detail. The two other units used in dosage calculations—milliequivalents and units—are rarely converted because they are unique to individual medications.

If a physician writes an order in the apothecary system and the medication is available in a metric dose, you need to convert the apothecary dose to an approximate metric equivalent to ensure that the patient receives the correct amount of medication. Conversions from the apothecary system are approximations and may incur dosing variability. As the metric system becomes more widely accepted, the need for conversion will decrease, although the need to calculate a dose in household measurements will remain as long as the United States continues measuring in household equivalents. Household measurements use common measuring tools found in most homes. Therefore, for the person taking medication to be able to use readily available utensils, you may need to convert orders written in apothecary or metric systems to household measurements for ease of drug administration. Household measurements are more accurate when using actual measuring spoons as opposed to flatware; however, it is appropriate to dispense a measuring device to ensure accurate dosing in the home environment because people may use their own flatware, which varies greatly in measurements.

CONVERSION FACTORS

Conversion factors are equivalents between two measurements, whether within the same system or between different systems. Each part of a conversion factor includes a value (number) and a label (unit of measurement).

> **TECH NOTE**
> The **value** of a conversion factor is always 1. It is used to change one unit to another **without** changing the value of the original measurement. For example, 5 mL = 1 tsp has a numerical value of 1.

Table 6.1 lists necessary equivalents between the three systems of measurement that are used as conversion factors. The **bolded** conversion factors used most often in pharmaceutical calculations should be learned and committed to memory.

TABLE 6.1 Common Conversions: Metric, Apothecary, and Household Systems of Measurement

PARAMETER	APOTHECARY UNITS	HOUSEHOLD UNITS	METRIC UNITS
VOLUME	♏ i	1 gtt	
		20 gtt	1 mL
	fl ʒ i	1 tsp	5 mL
	fl ʒ ss	1 Tbsp	15 mL
	fl ℥ i	1 oz	30 mL
	fl ℥ viii	1 c	240 mL
	1 pt	**1 pt**	473.2 mL/**480 mL***
	1 qt	1 qt	960 mL
	1 gal	**1 gal**	3,840 mL
MASS/WEIGHT	gr i	N/A	60–65 mg
	ʒ i	1 oz	30 g
	**	1# or **1 lb**	454 g
		2.2#	1 kg
LENGTH		1″	2.54 cm

*The exact conversion is 1 pt = 473.2 mL. The approximate value of 1 pt = 480 mL is often used in conversions because 1 pt = 16 oz and 1 oz = 30 mL. **1 pt = 480 mL** will be used in this text.

**An apothecary pound contains only 12 oz, whereas a household pound contains 16 oz, which is considered to be equivalent to 454 g. The apothecary pound is not used in this text.

TECH NOTE

Remember that the equivalents are approximate and not exact; therefore, when converting between two measurement systems, the conversion is approximate. The final answer should always be one that is measurable in the system; 1.7 tsp would be 1¾ tsp in household measurements, because 0.7 tsp cannot be measured.

As you can see from Table 6.1, the apothecary grain has a range of equivalencies. The conversion between grains and milligrams actually varies between different medications. Table 6.2 illustrates some of the more common medications that are still dosed in both grains and milligrams. This illustrates the degree of approximation between these two systems. Because the measurement systems are not identical, *any* conversions between them are approximations. Another example is that a dram is often used as a symbol for a teaspoon when a dram is actually about 4 mL and a teaspoon may measure either 4 or 5 mL depending on the device.

The conversion of 20 drops per 1 mL is based on a viscosity close to that of water. Remember that the number of drops varies according to drop size and thickness of the liquid. This conversion is not used in dosing because medications dosed in drops come with a specific dropper for administration. It is mostly used for determining day's supply with eyedrops or eardrops for submission to insurance companies.

! TECH ALERT

Medicine droppers provided by the manufacturer with specific medications are the only ones that are guaranteed to deliver the correct dose. Random droppers may not deliver the correct amount.

TABLE 6.2 Commmon Medications Dosed in Grains and Milligrams

MEDICATION	CONVERSION FACTOR
codeine NTG SL—sublingual nitroglycerin phenobarbital*	60 mg/gr
ASA—aspirin APAP—acetaminophen ferrous sulfate—iron	65 mg/gr

*Phenobarbital also comes in strengths based on 64.8 mg/gr.

Practice Problems A

After reviewing Tables 6.1 and 6.2, complete the following equivalents. These are some of the most important conversion factors used in pharmaceutical calculations.

1. 1 oz = _____ g

2. gr i aspirin = _____ mg

3. 1 tsp = _____ mL

4. 1 pt = _____ mL

5. 1 gal = _____ mL

6. 1 Tbsp = _____ mL

7. fl℥ i = _____ tsp

8. 1# = _____ g

9. 1 kg = _____ #

10. 1 oz = _____ mL

11. gr i codeine = _____ mg

12. 1 mL = _____ gtt

CONVERSIONS

If one factor is in one system, such as the metric system, and the other factor is in another system, such as the household system, either ratio and proportion (R&P) or dimensional analysis (DA) may be used for conversion. *Always* use DA with multistep problems to keep track of units.

POINTS TO REMEMBER
RULES FOR USING RATIO AND PROPORTION
- Set up the conversion ratio with the known conversion units on the left of the equation.
- Set up the second ratio of the proportion with the conversion units for the unknowns.
- Label the units so that the like unit is placed in the same position within each R&P. This sets the ratios so that they are equivalent to each other.
- Cross-multiply and divide to solve for the unknown.

EXAMPLE 6.1

A physician orders a 10-mL dose of antibiotic tid. How many teaspoons constitute one dose? This is a single-step conversion, so it is performed easily with R&P.

R & P $\dfrac{1 \text{ tsp}}{5 \text{ mL}} = \dfrac{x}{10 \text{ mL}}$

$5x = 10$ tsp   divide both sides by 5

$x = 2$ tsp

POINTS TO REMEMBER
RULES FOR USING DIMENSIONAL ANALYSIS
- Identify the unit of the *answer* needed followed by an equal sign.
- Set up a fraction such that the unit of the *desired* answer is in the numerator of the first fraction of the DA equation—this unit will *never* be canceled.
- Set up the next fraction in the equation so the unit in its numerator is the same as the unit in the denominator of the first fraction (so these units will cancel when the fractions are multiplied).
- Continue this process when dealing with multistep problems.
- Cancel units to ensure proper setup of the fractions.
- Multiply the numerators and denominators.
- Complete the problem by reducing if necessary.

EXAMPLE 6.2

A physician orders a 10-mL dose of antibiotic tid. How many teaspoons constitute one dose?

$$\text{DA} \quad \text{tsp} = \frac{1 \text{ tsp}}{5 \text{ mL}} \times \frac{10 \text{ mL}}{1} = 2 \text{ tsp}$$

> **! TECH ALERT**
>
> When using DA, be sure to place the unit desired for the answer in the numerator of the first fraction and follow with the additional information in the sequence needed to cancel all unnecessary units.

CONVERSIONS BETWEEN HOUSEHOLD AND APOTHECARY SYSTEMS

The apothecary system has only a few significant measurements that, although not commonly used, do convert into household measurements. Of importance are minims to drops, drams to teaspoons, and ounces to tablespoons (Fig. 6.1). Cups, pints, quarts, and gallons are used by both systems. Length is not measured in the apothecary system.

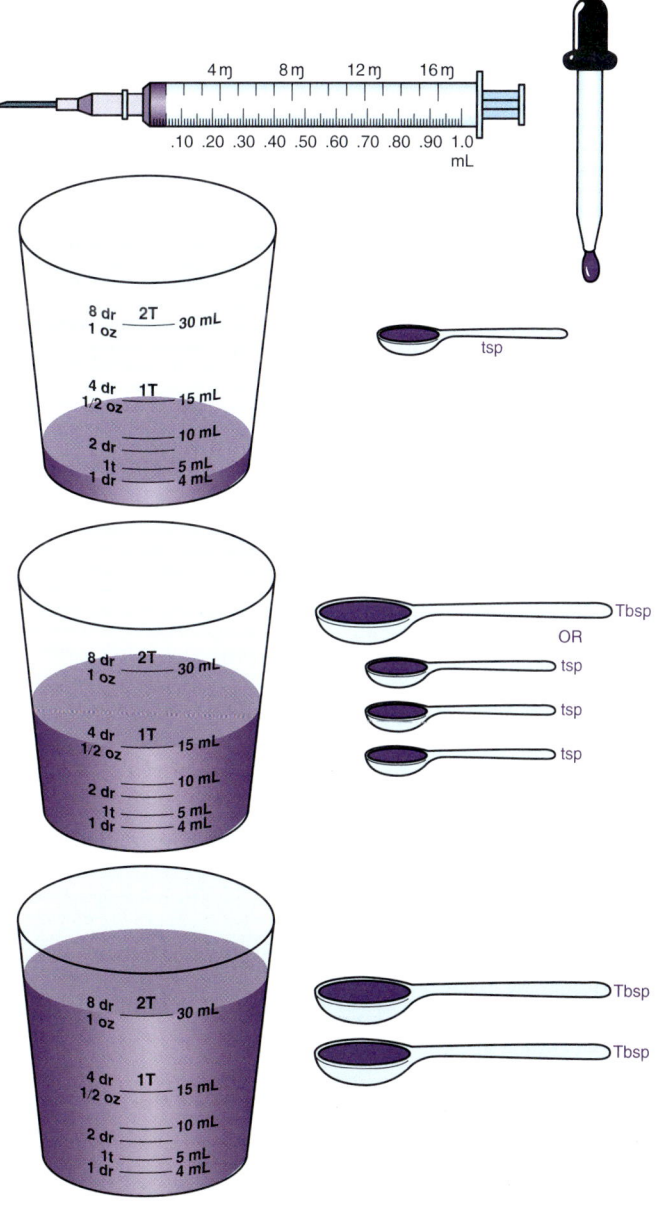

FIGURE 6.1 Equivalents between apothecary and household measurements.

! **TECH ALERT**
Do not confuse the symbols for ʒ (dram) and ʒ (ounce). If it is difficult to work with the symbols, use the words in your R&P or DA setup. Just remember to change the answer back to symbols if it is an apothecary measurement.

EXAMPLE 6.3

fl ʒ iii = _____ tsp

R & P

$$\frac{1 \text{ tsp}}{1 \text{ fluid dram}} = \frac{x}{3 \text{ fluid dram}} \quad x = 3 \text{ tsp}$$

DA

Start with tsp =
Use the conversion factor 1 tsp = fl ʒ i

$$\text{tsp} = \frac{1 \text{ tsp}}{1 \text{ fluid dram}} \times \frac{3 \text{ fluid dram}}{1} = 3 \text{ tsp}$$

Practice Problems B

Calculate the following problems using either R&P or DA. Show your calculations. Be sure to use the correct numeral form (Roman or Arabic) for the measurement system. Remember that these answers are approximate.

1. 6 tsp = fl ʒ _____

2. 2 tsp = fl ʒ _____

3. 16 gtt = ♏ _____

4. 4 Tbsp = fl ʒ _____

5. fl ʒ s̄s̄ = _____ tsp

6. 24 gtts = ♏ _____

7. fl ʒ v = _____ tsp

8. 3 Tbsp = fl ʒ _____

9. 8 c = fl ʒ _____

10. fl ʒ xxiv = _____ c

11. 4 tsp = fl ʒ _____

12. 30 tsp = fl ʒ _____

13. fl ʒ xxx = _____ Tbsp

14. A physician writes a prescription for ℥ ii of Robitussin cough medication q4h.

    How much is this in household measurements?

    How often will the person take the medication? _____

15. The directions on the bottle of Maalox read fl℥ iss q3–4h prn indigestion.

    How many tablespoons are equivalent to one dose?

    How often can a dose be taken? _____

16. A physician writes a prescription for MiraLax one capful in H₂O fl℥ viii.

    How could you tell the patient to easily measure the water? *(Hint: convert to household measurement.)*

CONVERSIONS BETWEEN HOUSEHOLD AND METRIC UNITS

Most conversions from metric to household, such as milliliters to teaspoons or ounces, are volume conversions, although length from inches to centimeters is sometimes used in the medical field. Fig. 6.2 illustrates some of the conversions from Table 6.1.

EXAMPLE 6.4

60 mL = _____ oz

$$\frac{1\ oz}{30\ mL} = \frac{x}{60\ mL}$$

$30x = 60$ oz   Divide both sides by 30.

$x = 2$ oz

EXAMPLE 6.5

4′ = _____ cm

Because most of us do not know how many centimeters are in 1 foot, this is calculated more easily as a multistep DA equation using two familiar conversion factors.

$$cm = \frac{2.54\ cm}{1\ in} \times \frac{12\ in}{1\ ft} \times \frac{4\ ft}{1} = 121.92\ cm$$

TECH NOTE

When converting between systems, make sure the answer is a **measurable amount**. For example, an answer of 0.9 tsp should be rounded to 1 tsp.

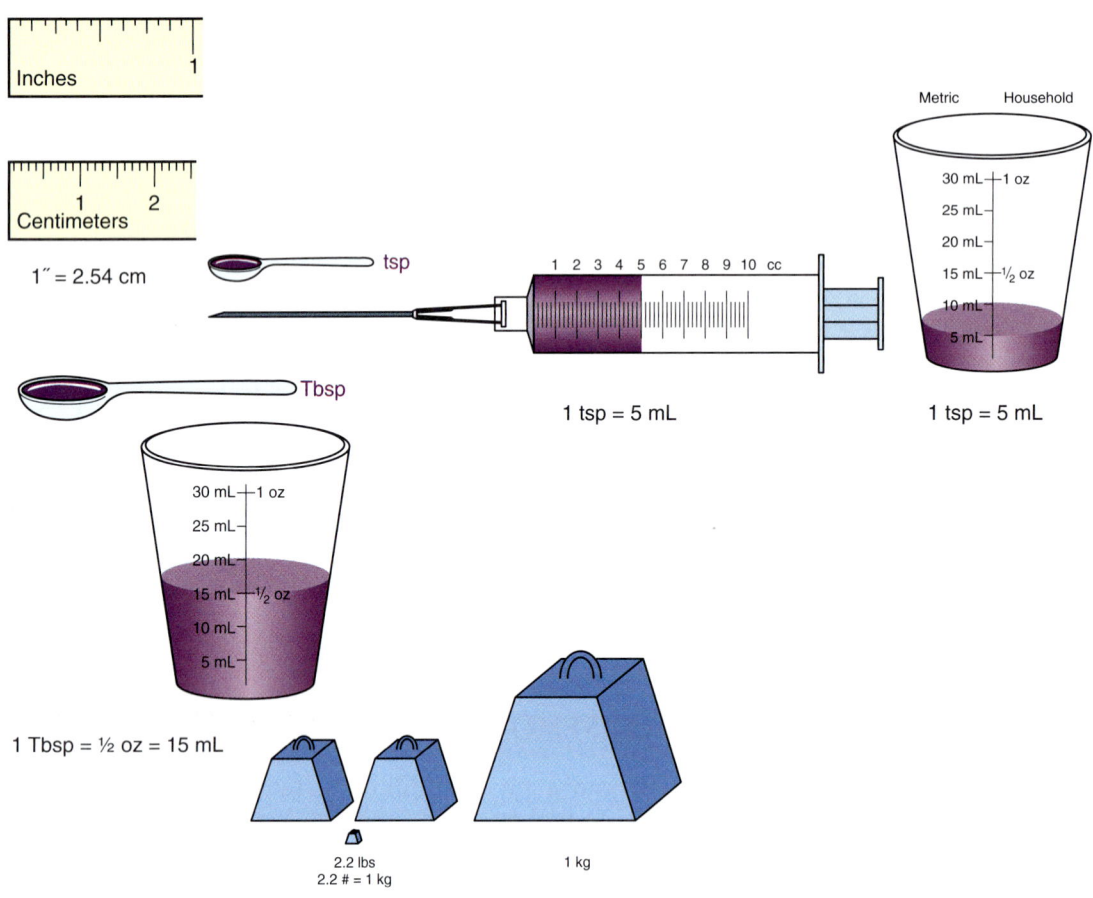

FIGURE 6.2 Equivalents between household and metric measurements.

Practice Problems C

Calculate the following conversions. Use fractions with the household system and decimals with the metric system. Use DA with multistep problems. Round to the nearest tenth. Show your calculations.

1. 16 oz = _____ mL

2. 8 kg = _____ #

3. 3 tsp = _____ mL

4. 2 pt = _____ mL

5. 5″ = _____ cm

6. 3 c = _____ mL

7. 90 mL = _____ oz

8. 10.2 cm = _____"

9. 75 mL = _____ oz

10. 10 kg = _____#

11. 720 mL = _____ pt

12. 720 mL = _____ qt

13. 10 tsp = _____ mL

14. 500 mL = _____ qt

15. 6 tsp = _____ mL

16. 1.5 L = _____ pt

17. 10 c = _____ L

18. 5 ft = _____ cm

19. A physician writes an order for an antihelmintic for a child weighing 35#. The dosage must be calculated in mg/kg body weight.

    How many kilograms does the child weigh?

20. A physician writes a prescription for 5 mL of azithromycin liquid for a child.

    How many teaspoons would you tell the parent to give the child?

CONVERSIONS BETWEEN METRIC AND APOTHECARY SYSTEMS

The metric system uses grams, liters, and meters, whereas the apothecary system uses grains, minims, drams, and ounces. When converting between two systems of measurement, the equivalents are approximate. R&P or DA may be used, depending on the method that is most comfortable for you.

The important conversions to remember are as follows and these are approximations as stated earlier in the chapter:

MASS	VOLUME
gr i = 60–65 mg	fl ʒ i = 5 mL
1 g = gr xv	fl ℥ i = 30 mL

TECH NOTE

The numbers are approximations, NOT EXACT NUMBERS, so you need to use the conversion that will give you a measurable answer.

An interesting way to remember the strengths of medications based on the conversion gr i = 60 mg is to think of a clock. There are 60 minutes in 1 hour, just as there are 60 mg in 1 grain. Therefore, if you think of ¼ of an hour as being 15 minutes, gr ¼ = 15 mg. Likewise, if you think of ½ hour as being 30 minutes, gr ½ = 30 mg, and if you think of ¾ of an hour as being 45 minutes, gr ¾ = 45 mg.

R&P or DA may be used for conversions as desired.

EXAMPLE 6.6

codeine 15 mg = gr _____

R & P

$$\frac{\text{gr i}}{60 \text{ mg}} = \frac{x}{15 \text{ mg}}$$

$60x = \text{gr } 15$ Divide both sides by 60.

$x = \frac{1}{4} = \text{gr } \frac{1}{4}$

DA

$$\text{gr} = \frac{\text{gr i}}{60 \text{ mg}} \times \frac{15 \text{ mg}}{1} = \frac{\text{gr } 15}{60} = \text{gr } \frac{1}{4}$$

EXAMPLE 6.7

NTG SL gr 1/100 = _____ mg

R & P

$$\frac{\text{gr i}}{60 \text{ mg}} = \frac{\text{gr } \frac{1}{100}}{x}$$

$$x = 60 \text{ mg} \cdot \frac{1}{100} = \frac{60}{100} \text{ mg} = \frac{6}{10} \text{ mg} = 0.6 \text{ mg}$$

DA

$$\text{mg} = \frac{60 \text{ mg}}{\text{gr i}} \times \frac{\text{gr } \frac{1}{100}}{1} = 60 \text{ mg} \times \frac{1}{100} = \frac{60}{100} \text{ mg} = \frac{6}{10} \text{ mg} = 0.6 \text{ mg}$$

Practice Problems D

Calculate the following practice problems. **If no medication is specified**, *use gr i = 60 mg. Show all of your calculations.*

1. acetaminophen gr v = _____ mg

2. 45 mL = fl℥ _____

3. 15 mg = gr _____

4. 60 mL = fl℥ _____

5. 1.5 mL = ♏ _____ Use 1 mL = ♏ xvi   6. gr viiss = _____ g

7. 750 mL = fl℥ _____   8. NTG SL gr $\frac{1}{150}$ = _____ mg

9. codeine gr s̄s̄ = _____ mg   10. 15 mL = fl℥ _____

11. NTG SL 0.3 mg = gr _____   12. gr $\frac{3}{4}$ = _____ mcg

13. 4 mL = ♏ _____ Use 1 mL = ♏ xv

14. A physician writes a medication order for phenobarbital gr iss. The available medication is phenobarbital 30 mg tablets.

    How many tablets should be administered?

15. A prescription is written for phenobarbital gr ¼. The medication stock bottle reads phenobarbital 30 mg per unscored tablet.

    What strength in mg should be used for the dose?

    Is this the correct medication stock bottle for the prescription? _____

TECH NOTE

Nitroglycerin sublingual (NTG SL) tablets are available in three strengths, which are ordered in either milligrams or grains. It is a good idea to learn the strength conversions to verify that your conversion calculations are correct.

NTG SL   gr 1/200   0.3 mg $\left(60 \text{ mg} \times \frac{1}{200}\right)$

NTG SL   gr 1/150   0.4 mg $\left(60 \text{ mg} \times \frac{1}{150}\right)$

NTG SL   gr 1/100   0.6 mg $\left(60 \text{ mg} \times \frac{1}{100}\right)$

REVIEW

The methods of conversion between metric, apothecary, and household systems have been presented. Conversions between measurement systems are approximations, and some will vary depending on the conversion factor used, such as the number of milliliters in a dram. The metric system is the most accurate method of measurement and therefore is used exclusively when compounding prescriptions and making intravenous preparations.

Conversions within and between measurement systems may be accomplished using either R&P or DA. Once you learn the basic equivalencies listed in Table 6.3, you should be able to accomplish almost any conversion needed in the pharmacy setting.

TABLE 6.3 Common Measurements and Conversions

HOUSEHOLD LIQUID MEASUREMENTS (VOLUME)

1 drop	gtt	
1 teaspoon	tsp	60 drops (varies with viscosity and dropper size)
1 tablespoon	Tbsp	3 teaspoons
1 ounce	oz	2 Tbsp
1 cup	c	8 oz
1 pint	pt	2 c
1 quart	qt	2 pt
1 gallon	gal	4 qt

HOUSEHOLD DRY WEIGHT MEASUREMENT

1 pound	lb or #	16 oz

METRIC WEIGHT MEASUREMENTS

1 kg = 1,000 g
1 g = 1,000 mg
1 mg = 1,000 mcg

METRIC VOLUME MEASUREMENTS

1 L = 1,000 mL

HOUSEHOLD TO METRIC CONVERSIONS

Volume
1 tsp = 5 mL
1 Tbsp = 15 mL
1 fl oz = 30 mL
1 pt = 480 mL
1 gal = 3,840 mL

Dry Weight
1# = 454 g
2.2# = 1 kg
1 oz = 30 g

APOTHECARY SYSTEM VOLUME

1 minim	♏	
1 fluid dram	fl ʒ	♏ 60
1 fluid ounce	fl ʒ	fl ʒ viii (8)

TABLE 6.3 Common Measurements and Conversions—cont'd

APOTHECARY SYSTEM WEIGHT

1 grain	gr	
1 dram	ʒ	gr 60
1 ounce	℥	ʒ viii (8)

APPROXIMATE CONVERSIONS

gr i = 60–65 mg
    60 mg with codeine, phenobarbital,* and NTG SL
    65 mg with ASA, APAP, and iron
fl ʒ i = 1 tsp = 5 mL
fl ℥ i = 2 Tbsp = 30 mL

MISCELLANEOUS

Drops: 20 gtt = 1 mL (mostly used for day's supply calculations for insurance companies)

*Some phenobarbital doses are based on gr i = 64.8 mg.

Posttest

Use the correct numeral form (Roman or Arabic) for each system. Be sure the answers are measurable doses. Use either R&P or DA. Round all answers to the nearest tenth. If no medication is specified, use gr i = 60 mg

1. 3 tsp = fl ʒ _____
2. 6 tsp = _____ mL
3. codeine gr ¾ = _____ mg
4. fl ʒ v = _____ mL
5. 88# = _____ kg
6. 0.6 mg = _____ gr
7. 1,250 mL = _____ pt
8. 2.5 mL = _____ gtt
9. 4 qt = _____ L
10. 45 mg = gr _____
11. fl ℥ 24 = _____ c
12. 16 Tbsp = fl ℥ _____
13. 17″ = _____ cm
14. 46# = _____ kg

Continued

Posttest, cont.

15. 0.1 mg = gr _____

16. 2,500 g = _____#

17. 12 mL = _____ gtt

18. 45 mL = flʒ _____

19. 45 mL = _____ tsp

20. gr $\frac{1}{200}$ = _____ mg

21. 5 Tbsp = flʒ _____

22. 10 kg = _____#

23. 328 cm = _____ ″

24. 35 mL = _____ tsp

25. gr 45 = _____ g (use 1 g = gr xv)

26. aspirin gr x = _____ mg

27. 2,500 mL = _____ pt

28. A physician orders acetylsalicylic acid 325 mg. Available are gr v tablets.

    Should this medication be used for the order? _____ Why or why not?

29. A child is to receive Benadryl elixir 7.5 mL. The parent needs to give this with a teaspoon.

    How many teaspoons should the parent give per dose?

30. A physician orders atropine sulfate 0.4 mg as a preoperative order.

    How many grains will the patient receive?

IN SECTION III

7 Interpretation of Medication Labels and Orders
8 Calculation of Oral Solid Doses
9 Calculation of Oral Liquid Doses
10 Calculation of Parenteral Doses
11 Unit Calculations With Anticoagulants and Insulin
12 Calculation of Medications by Age, Body Weight, and Body Surface Area
13 Interpreting Physicians' Orders for Dosages and Days' Supply

SECTION III
Calculations With Prescriptions and Medication Orders

CHAPTER 7

Interpretation of Medication Labels and Orders

OBJECTIVES

1. Discuss what a prescription indicates, and describe the components of a prescription.
2. Describe what a medication order is, and list the parts of a medication order.
3. Interpret stock medication labels.

KEY WORDS

Auxiliary label Label added to prescriptions to provide important supplementary instructions

Dosage strength Weight of medication in a dose

Generic name Official nonproprietary name approved for a drug by the U.S. Food and Drug Administration (FDA)

Indication Reason to prescribe a medication

Inscription Part of prescription indicating medication name, dosage form, strength, and quantity

Medication order Physician's written or verbal direction for administration of medication in an inpatient health care setting

National Drug Code (NDC) Unique number on a drug product label that identifies the manufacturer, product, and size of container

Pharmacokinetics Movement of drugs through the body; absorption, distribution, metabolism, and excretion

Pharmacotherapeutics Uses and effects of drugs in treatment of conditions and diseases in the body

Prescription Written order by a licensed health care professional for dispensing medications

Scheduled medications Classification of medications with potential for abuse and misuse: CII, CIII, CIV, and CV

Signa (Sig) Part of prescription; directions for the patient—how, how much, when, how long

Subscription Part of a prescription that contains instructions for the pharmacist on how to compound if necessary

Superscription Part of a prescription designated with the symbol ℞, meaning, "Take this drug"

Toxicology Study of adverse toxic reactions or toxic levels of chemicals and drugs

Trade/Brand name Proprietary name given to a medication by the manufacturer

Pretest

If you are already comfortable with the subject matter, complete the Pretest to test your knowledge. If not, work your way through the chapter and return to it for extra practice. For the prescriptions, write the directions in lay terms as they should be written on a prescription label for the patient. Inpatient medication orders just need to be interpreted.

1. Prescription: penicillin 250 mg po qid × 10 days
   In stock: penicillin 250 mg tablets
   Label directions: _____
   _____

2. Prescription: nitroglycerin 0.4 mg SL q5min × 3 doses prn; if no relief, call 9-1-1
   In stock: NTG 0.4 mg SL tablets
   Label directions: _____
   _____

3. Prescription: hydrochlorothiazide 25 mg i tab po qam prn swelling
   In stock: HCTZ 25 mg tablets
   Label directions: _____
   _____

4. Prescription: Synthroid 0.025 mg po daily @ 8 am
   In stock: Synthroid 25 mcg tablets
   Label directions: _____
   _____

5. Prescription: Premarin 1.25 mg tab po daily × 21d
   In stock: Premarin 1.25 mg tablets
   Label directions: _____
   _____

6. Prescription: Zithromax 250 mg tab ii po stat, then tab i po daily on days 2 to 5
   In stock: Zithromax 250 mg tablets:
   Label directions: _____
   _____

Pretest, cont.

7. Prescription: Lanoxin 0.25 mg tab po qam if P 60 or ↑

In stock: Lanoxin 250 mcg tablets

Label directions: _____

_____

8.

```
           Lawrence Merry, M.D.
         4th Street and Jones Ave.
              Holly, GA 00111
          phone# - 001-555-2176

Patient Name_____     Date _____
Address_____     Age _____

   ℞      Pen-V 250 mg
          #40
          Sig: i tab po q6h

    _____    Refill _____
    DEA#_____
```

Label directions: _____

_____

9.

```
           Lawrence Merry, M.D.
         4th Street and Jones Ave.
              Holly, GA 00111
          phone# - 001-555-2176

Patient Name_____     Date _____
Address_____     Age _____

   ℞      Thorazine 100 mg
          #100
          Sig: tab i po tid

    _____    Refill _____
    DEA#_____
```

Label directions: _____

_____

Continued

Pretest, cont.

10.

Lawrence Merry, M.D.
4th Street and Jones Ave.
Holly, GA 00111
phone# - 001-555-2176

Patient Name_____ Date_____
Address_____ Age_____

℞ tetracycline 250 mg
   #120
   Sig: ii cap po qid x 2wk; i cap po bid x 2wk;
   then i cap po daily

_____ Refill _____
DEA#_____

Label directions: _____
_____

11.

Lawrence Merry, M.D.
4th Street and Jones Ave.
Holly, GA 00111
phone# - 001-555-2176

Patient Name_____ Date_____
Address_____ Age_____

℞ furosemide 40 mg
   #30
   Sig: i tab po daily @ 10am

_____ Refill _____
DEA#_____

Label directions: _____
_____

Pretest, cont.

12.

Lawrence Merry, M.D.
4th Street and Jones Ave.
Holly, GA 00111
phone# - 001-555-2176

Patient Name_____ Date _____
Address_____ Age _____

℞ lovastatin 10 mg
#30
Sig: i tab po daily c̄ evening meal or at bedtime c̄ snack for hyperlipidemia

_____ Refill _____
DEA#_____

Label directions: _____
_____

13.

Lawrence Merry, M.D.
4th Street and Jones Ave.
Holly, GA 00111
phone# - 001-555-2176

Patient Name_____ Date _____
Address_____ Age _____

℞ Humulin 70/30
10 mL vial
Sig: 22 units subcutaneously qam

_____ Refill _____
DEA#_____

Label directions: _____
_____

Continued

Pretest, cont.

14.

Lawrence Merry, M.D.
4th Street and Jones Ave.
Holly, GA 00111
phone# - 001-555-2176

Patient Name_____ Date _____
Address_____ Age _____

℞ Reg Insulin
10 mL vial
Sig: 16 units subcutaneously qam and 20 units subcutaneously 30 min ac evening meal

_____ Refill _____
DEA#_____

Label directions: _____
_____

15.

Lawrence Merry, M.D.
4th Street and Jones Ave.
Holly, GA 00111
phone# - 001-555-2176

Patient Name_____ Date _____
Address_____ Age _____

℞ diazepam 10 mg
#30
Sig: ss̄ – i tab po q4-6h prn anxiety or muscle spasms

_____ Refill _____
DEA#_____

Label directions: _____
_____

Pretest, cont.

16. *

```
            Lawrence Merry, M.D.
           4th Street and Jones Ave.
                Holly, GA 00111
             phone# - 001-555-2176

  Patient Name_____   Date _____
  Address_____   Age _____

     ℞      Robitussin DM syrup ʒviii
            Sig: ʒ ii po q4-6h prn cough


  _____   Refill _____
  DEA#_____
```

*Apothecary symbols for drams and ounces are on the ISMP List of Error Prone Abbreviations, Symbols, and Dose Designations.

Prescription interpretation: _____

_____

Label directions: _____

_____

17. Medication Order: meperidine 50 mg and promethazine 25 mg IM q4–6h prn pain

Interpretation: _____

_____

18. Medication Order: metoprolol 50 mg po bid

Interpretation: _____

_____

19. Medication Order: temazepam 7.5 mg i-ii po at bedtime prn sleep

Interpretation: _____

_____

Continued

Pretest, cont.

20.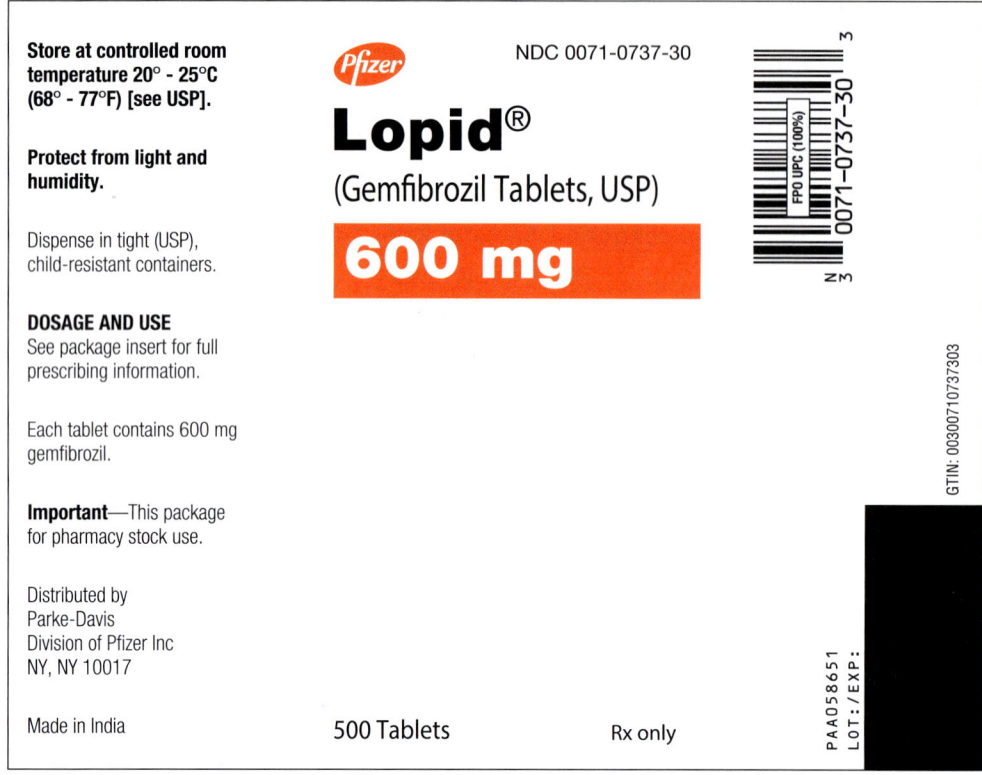

(© Pfizer. Used with permission.)

What is the trade name for this medication? _____

What is the generic name for this medication? _____

What is the NDC number for this medication container? _____

What is the total number of tablets in the container? _____

INTRODUCTION

Prescriptions are medications ordered by prescribers in outpatient settings, and **medication orders** are medications ordered by prescribers in inpatient settings. Whatever the setting, it is important for the pharmacy technician to be able to read and interpret these orders accurately. This is why it is important to learn the abbreviations from Chapter 1. Every order must be reduced to writing as soon as possible, and the pharmacist must transcribe any verbal orders. Also, a pharmacist is required to handle any clarification of orders with the prescriber. The ability to interpret a medication order or prescription is an essential skill for professionals who work with medications.

The pharmacist is ultimately responsible for dispensing the medication as ordered. As a pharmacy technician, you have the training to perform most functions in the pharmacy. Because the field of medicine is always changing, stay current with new medications and new **indications** for older medications. Patient safety is the most important aspect of dispensing medications.

Knowledge of pharmacy includes **pharmacokinetics**, the movement of the drugs through the body, and **pharmacotherapeutics**, the therapeutic uses and effects of drugs, whether beneficial or harmful. The field of **toxicology** includes the study of the adverse effects of chemical substances on the human body. It is important to learn the normal dosage range for medications so that you can check your calculations to see if your answers make sense. It is easier to check your answers for accuracy when you have an idea of what doses should be. The differences between therapeutic (desired) and toxic (harmful) levels of medications must be considered, as well as possible drug-drug interactions, drug-food interactions, and drug-disease state interactions.

WHAT DOES A PRESCRIPTION INDICATE?

A prescription is a means for a physician or other health professional to provide the information needed by the pharmacist to dispense the desired medication for a patient in an outpatient setting. It is an order written for a specific person by a medical professional licensed to prescribe for a specific condition. The rules about who may prescribe vary from state to state, so the statutes of the state of practice determine the legalities of prescription writing. As a legal document, the prescription indicates the medication desired and the directions for its use. The components of a prescription are included in Fig. 7.1.

TECH NOTE
Legally, the physician's Drug Enforcement Agency (DEA) number must be on a prescription if it is written for a controlled substance!

TECH NOTE
As you work through prescriptions, an understood meaning is that if a tablet or capsule is ordered, the route of administration is by mouth (po) unless otherwise indicated.

When typing prescription labels for the public, make sure that the instructions are clear and easy to understand. Begin oral prescriptions with "Take" and always state the number of tablets, capsules, or milliliters as opposed to the strength. For example, if the prescription is for 500 mg and the medication comes in 250 mg tablets, type "Take 2 tablets," not "Take 500 mg." Other direction words used include "Instill" for eye or ear medications, "Insert" for suppositories, "Apply" for topical preparations and patches, and "Inhale" for nasal and oral inhalers. A few medications, including insulin preparations, are prescribed for subcutaneous use, in which case you could use, "Inject subcutaneously" or "Inject under the skin." Special training should be provided before a patient self administers subcutaneous medication.

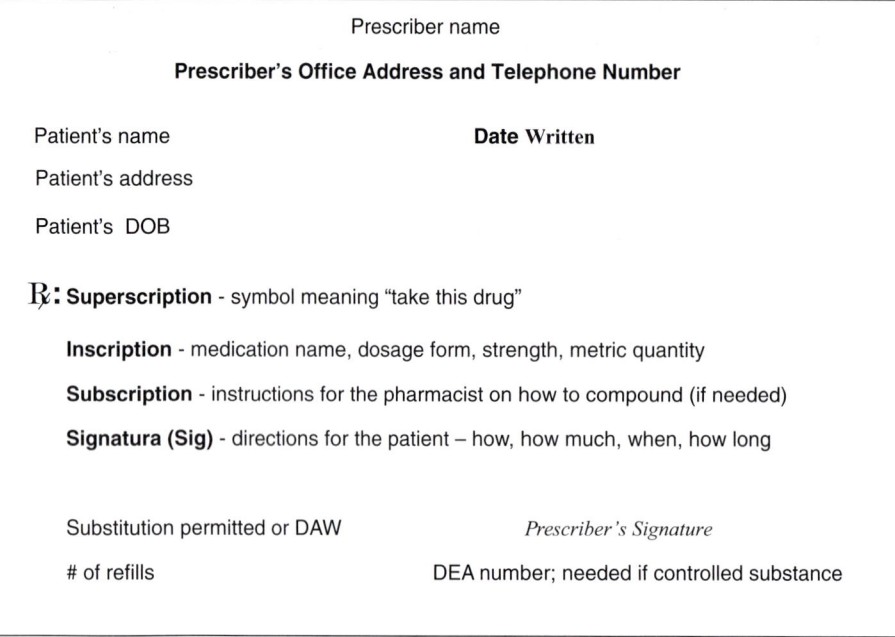

FIGURE 7.1 Elements of a prescription.

FIGURE 7.2 Elements of a label.

The Institute for Safe Medication Practices (ISMP) recommends the use of numeric rather than alphabetic characters on prescription labels. Therefore, in this text, use numbers such as 1, 2, and 3 on prescription labels as opposed to one, two, and three. In its quest to reduce medication errors, the ISMP also recommends the use of numbers over ambiguous terms such as twice daily (https://www.ismp.org). This should be written, "Take 2 times a day."

> **TECH NOTE**
>
> If a prescription is written for a brand name and substituted with a generic, you must put "generic for (Brand name)," with the specific brand name entered, on the label.

As seen in Figs. 7.1 and 7.2, a prescription must include the *prescriber's* address and phone number and the date it was *written*, whereas a prescription label includes the *pharmacy's* name, address, and phone number and the date it was *filled*. These concepts are bolded in Figs. 7.1 and 7.2 to emphasize this important difference.

The prescription interpretation is how one would read the prescription without the use of abbreviations. The label directions are written for the patient in language that is easily understood.

EXAMPLE 7.1

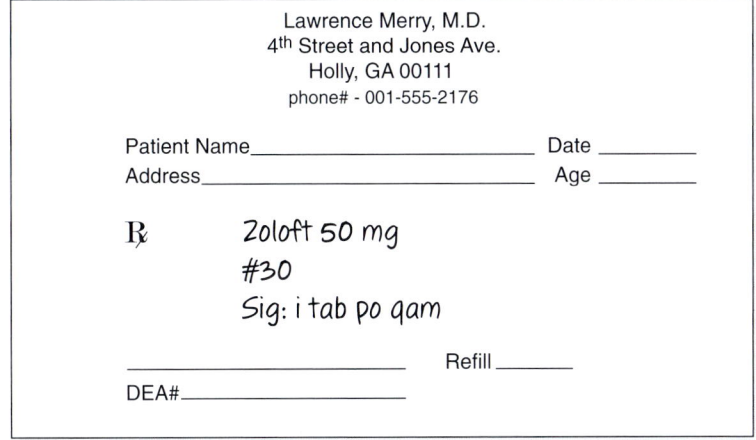

```
            Lawrence Merry, M.D.
          4th Street and Jones Ave.
               Holly, GA 00111
             phone# - 001-555-2176

Patient Name_____   Date _____
Address_____   Age _____

  R    Zoloft 50 mg
       #30
       Sig: i tab po qam

  _____   Refill _____
  DEA#_____
```

Prescription interpretation: *Zoloft 50 mg, 30 tablets, one tablet by mouth every morning*

Label directions: *Take 1 tablet by mouth every morning.*

EXAMPLE 7.2

```
            Lawrence Merry, M.D.
          4th Street and Jones Ave.
               Holly, GA 00111
             phone# - 001-555-2176

Patient Name_____   Date _____
Address_____   Age _____

  R    Mycostatin Oral Suspension
       60 mL
       Sig: Agit then swish and swallow 5 mL
       q4-6h

  _____   Refill _____
  DEA#_____
```

Prescription interpretation:

Mycostatin Oral Suspension, 60 mL, agitate, then swish and swallow 5 mL every 4 to 6 hours.

Label directions:

Shake medication, and then swish and swallow 5 mL every 4 to 6 hours.

This prescription should be dispensed with a measuring device appropriate for 5 mL.

Practice Problems A

Interpret the following prescriptions and then write the instructions, as they should appear on a prescription label.

1.
```
            Lawrence Merry, M.D.
           4th Street and Jones Ave.
                Holly, GA 00111
             phone# - 001-555-2176

   Patient Name_____    Date _____
   Address_____     Age _____

       ℞       atorvastatin 10 mg
               #30
               Sig: i tab po nightly at bedtime

       _____           Refill _____
       DEA#_____
```

Prescription interpretation: _____

_____

Label directions: _____

2.
```
            Lawrence Merry, M.D.
           4th Street and Jones Ave.
                Holly, GA 00111
             phone# - 001-555-2176

   Patient Name_____    Date _____
   Address_____     Age _____

       ℞       Premarin 0.625 mg
               #30
               Sig: i tab po daily at approximately
               same hour

       _____           Refill _____
       DEA#_____
```

Prescription interpretation: _____

_____

Label directions: _____

3.

```
                    Lawrence Merry, M.D.
                   4th Street and Jones Ave.
                        Holly, GA 00111
                     phone# - 001-555-2176

   Patient Name_____   Date _____
   Address_____    Age _____

   ℞      Zoloft 50 mg
          #30
          Sig: i tab po daily c̄ morning meal

          _____        Refill _____
   DEA#_____
```

Prescription interpretation: _____
_____

Label directions: _____

4.

```
                    Lawrence Merry, M.D.
                   4th Street and Jones Ave.
                        Holly, GA 00111
                     phone# - 001-555-2176

   Patient Name_____   Date _____
   Address_____    Age _____

   ℞      Prednisone 10 mg
          #40
          Sig: i tab po qid x 4 d ; i tab po tid x 4 d ; i tab
          po bid x 4 d ; i tab po daily x 4
          _____        Refill _____
   DEA#_____
```

Prescription interpretation: _____
_____
_____

Label directions: _____
_____
_____

5.

Lawrence Merry, M.D.
4th Street and Jones Ave.
Holly, GA 00111
phone# - 001-555-2176

Patient Name_____ Date _____
Address_____ Age _____

℞   Allegra 180 mg
       #30
       Sig: i tab po daily

_____   Refill _____
DEA#_____

Prescription interpretation: _____

_____

Label directions: _____

6.

Lawrence Merry, M.D.
4th Street and Jones Ave.
Holly, GA 00111
phone# - 001-555-2176

Patient Name_____ Date _____
Address_____ Age _____

℞   ibuprofen 800 mg
       #100
       Sig: i tab po q8h

_____   Refill _____
DEA#_____

Prescription interpretation: _____

_____

Label directions: _____

7.

```
              Lawrence Merry, M.D.
             4th Street and Jones Ave.
                   Holly, GA 00111
                phone# - 001-555-2176

Patient Name_____  Date _____
Address_____  Age _____

    ℞      Norvasc 5 mg
           #30
           Sig: i tab po qam for ↑ B/P

    _____  Refill _____
    DEA#_____
```

Prescription interpretation: _____

_____

Label directions: _____

8.

```
              Lawrence Merry, M.D.
             4th Street and Jones Ave.
                   Holly, GA 00111
                phone# - 001-555-2176

Patient Name_____  Date _____
Address_____  Age _____

    ℞      furosemide 40 mg
           #30
           Sig: i tab po daily @ 10am

    _____  Refill _____
    DEA#_____
```

Prescription interpretation: _____

_____

Label directions: _____

9.

```
          Lawrence Merry, M.D.
         4th Street and Jones Ave.
              Holly, GA 00111
           phone# - 001-555-2176

Patient Name_____   Date_____
Address_____    Age_____

  ℞      Fosamax 70 mg
         #4
         Sig: i po on same d qwk

  _____       Refill_____
  DEA#_____
```

Prescription interpretation: _____

_____

Label directions: _____

10.

```
          Lawrence Merry, M.D.
         4th Street and Jones Ave.
              Holly, GA 00111
           phone# - 001-555-2176

Patient Name_____   Date_____
Address_____    Age_____

  ℞      diazepam 5 mg
         #100
         Sig: i po tid prn anxiety

  _____       Refill_____
  DEA# AM123321
```

Prescription interpretation: _____

_____

Label directions: _____

11.

Lawrence Merry, M.D.
4th Street and Jones Ave.
Holly, GA 00111
phone# - 001-555-2176

Patient Name_____ Date _____
Address_____ Age _____

℞ Neurontin 600 mg
   #50
   Sig: i po daily x 5 d ; i po bid x 5 d ;
   then i po tid

_____ Refill _____
DEA#_____

Prescription interpretation: _____

_____

Label directions: _____

_____

12.

Lawrence Merry, M.D.
4th Street and Jones Ave.
Holly, GA 00111
phone# - 001-555-2176

Patient Name_____ Date _____
Address_____ Age _____

℞ Glucotrol XL 10 mg
   #30
   Sig: i tab po c̄ am meal

_____ Refill _____
DEA#_____

Prescription interpretation: _____

_____

Label directions: _____

What Is a Medication Order?

A medication order is a method of providing the same information as is found on an outpatient prescription, but it is used in an inpatient environment (Fig. 7.3). Whereas a prescription is written for either the number of doses or length of time of therapy, a medication order tells a health care professional what drug or drugs should be administered, how

PHYSICIAN'S ORDERS

Patient, James A.

DATE	ORDERS			TRANS BY
	Diagnosis:	Weight:	Height:	
	Sensitivities/Drug Allergies:			
1/12/17	0900 Lasix 80 mg. p.o. b.i.d.			
	Digoxin 0.125 mg. p.o. q.d.			
	Slow-K 10 mEq. p.o. b.i.d.			
	A. Physician, M.D.			

MEDICAL RECORDS COPY **PHYSICIAN'S ORDERS** **T-5**

B-CLIN. NOTES	E-LAB	G-X-RAY	K-DIAGNOSTIC	M-SURGERY	Q-THERAPY	T-ORDERS	W-NURSING	Y-MISC.

A

Transcription of Med Sheet by: ____________

Reviewed by: ____________ Page ____ of ____

Patient, James A.

Initials	Signature
NJ	N. Jones R.N.
AN	A. Nurse R.N.

Allergies: ☑ NKDA

Injection Sites: A = RUE, B = LUE, C = RLE, D = LLE, E = Abdomen, F = R Glut, G = L Glut

Special Notes:

See Legend on Back

☐ Inpatient ☐ Outpatient

#	DATE	DRUG	dose	route	interval	08 09 10 11	12 13 14 15	16 17 18 19	20 21 22 23	24 01 02 03	04 05 06 07	1/12/17	1/13/17	1/14/17	1/15/17	1/16/17
1	1/12	Lasix	80 mg	p.o.	b.i.d.	09			21			09 AN, 21 NJ	09 AN, 21 NJ			
2	1/12	Digoxin	0.125 mg	p.o.	q.d.	09						09 AN	09 AN			
3	1/12	Slow-K	10 mEq	p.o.	b.i.d.	09			21			09 AN, 21 NJ	09 AN, 21 NJ			
4			dose	route	interval											
5			dose	route	interval											

MEDICATION PROFILE

B-CLIN. NOTES	E-LAB	G-X-RAY	K-DIAGNOSTIC	M-SURGERY	Q-THERAPY	T-ORDERS	W-NURSING	Y-MISC.

B

FIGURE 7.3 Examples of physician's orders: **(A)** a patient's medication administration record **(B)** with appropriate drug interpretations. (Forms courtesy Clarian Health, Indianapolis, IN.)

to administer them, the strength of the medication, and the frequency with which they should be given in an inpatient setting. The medication order contains the date, patient name, medication name, dose, route of administration, time and frequency of administration, and the signature of the prescribing professional. Although only recommended in emergency situations, medication orders may be verbally communicated. However, for legal purposes, each order should be transcribed into writing by the health care professional who accepts the order, and the order must be countersigned by the health care professional who communicates the order and is licensed to prescribe medications in the state of practice.

> ! **TECH ALERT**
>
> Even though, in most inpatient pharmacies, a pharmacist enters medication orders into the computer, the pharmacy technician still has a responsibility to check as he or she is filling orders and report any concerns to the pharmacist.

When interpreting medication orders, simply restate the order without the use of abbreviations. Include the name of the drug ordered and strength because these are orders that will only be seen by other health care professionals, not patients.

EXAMPLE 7.3

[PAIN] Discontinue naproxen 375 mg; start naproxen 500 mg po bid

Discontinue naproxen 375 mg; start naproxen 500 mg by mouth twice daily

Practice Problems B

Interpret the following as medication orders.

1. Discontinue Zocor; add Lipitor 10 mg tab i po at bedtime

   _____

   _____

2. amoxicillin suspension 250 mg po tid until discontinued

   _____

3. cephalexin 500 mg po q8h × 3 d

   _____

4. [ENDO] metformin-XR 500 mg po qd c̄ pm meal

   _____

5. Discontinue Septra; start Cipro 500 mg po bid × 2 d

6. albuterol sulfate 2 puffs q4h SOB

7. Levaquin 500 mg IV q24h

8. Coumadin 5 mg po q even day; 7.5 mg po q odd day

9. Levothroid 100 mcg po daily c̄ am meal

10. Advair Diskus 250/50 i puff bid

11. diazepam 5 mg po tid prn anxiety

12. hydrocodone/APAP 7.5/325 po q6h prn pain

13. Flonase i spray each nostril bid

14. Ambien 10 mg po at bedtime prn sleep

_____

15. furosemide 40 mg po qam prn swelling

_____

INTERPRETING STOCK MEDICATION LABELS

The label on the stock medication bottle identifies the drug within the container. It also indicates the important information needed (**in bold**) to dispense the drug as follows:

- **Generic name**—the official name that is assigned to a medication after approval by the FDA; found in the *U.S. Pharmacopeia–National Formulary* (USP-NF)
- **Trade/Brand name**—the name assigned by the manufacturer
- **National Drug Code (NDC)** number—a 10-digit, 3-segment number that identifies the manufacturer (labeler), the product, and the size of the container in which the medication is packaged; a universal product identifier in the United States
- **Dosage strength**—the amount of active ingredient found in the medication, such as micrograms (mcg), milligrams (mg), grams (g), grains (gr), units, or milliequivalents (mEq), per dosage form
- **Total quantity of medication**—amount in the container as packed by the manufacturer
- **Dosage form**
- **Name of the manufacturer**
- **Special instructions** for mixing or compounding if indicated by the manufacturer
- **Storage requirements** of the medication
- **Lot and batch numbers or control number** of the medication that can be used for identification if the medication is recalled
- **Expiration date**
- **Controlled substance indicators** as appropriate—indicated by a large "C" with the schedule number in Roman numerals within the "C"

TECH NOTE

The generic name should be expressed with a lowercase letter, such as diazepam. The brand name is expressed with a capital letter, such as Valium. If the medication is a generic form of the drug, a trade name will not be found on the manufacturer's label.

One of the most important aspects of patient safety is the careful interpretation of the medication label. To ensure that the proper medication has been provided for dispensing, the label (drug name, drug strength, drug form, expiration date, and NDC number) should be read when taking the medication from the shelf, before preparing the medication for dispensing, and when returning the medication container to the shelf for storage. By reading medication labels carefully, you can reduce errors and avoid confusion, and the therapeutic potential of the drug is maximized. The pharmacy technician must be fully aware of the information on the label, including the expiration date, to ensure that the medicine dispensed is of the highest quality and exactly as ordered.

SECTION III Calculations with Prescriptions and Medication Orders

> **! TECH ALERT**
> Always read medication labels at least three times. Read before removing from the storage place; before counting when preparing the prescription; and before passing it to the pharmacist for the final check.

EXAMPLE 7.4

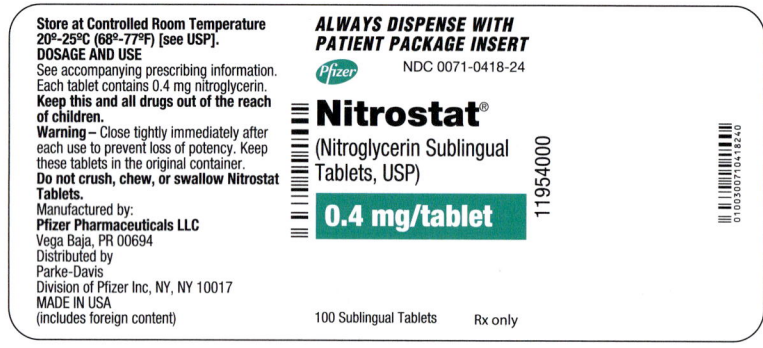

(© Pfizer. Used with permission.)

What is the NDC number for this medication? *0071-0418-24*

    0071—manufacturer (labeler)   0418—product identification   24—package size

How many tablets are in a full container? *100*

What is the strength of this medication? *0.4 mg/tablet*

Who manufactures this medication? *Pfizer Pharmaceuticals LLC*

Where is it manufactured? *Vega Baja, Puerto Rico*

What is the trade name of this medication? *Nitrostat*

What is the generic name of this medication? *nitroglycerin*

What are the warnings that must accompany a prescription for Nitrostat?

    Close tightly immediately after use to prevent loss of potency. Keep these tablets in the original container. Do not crush, chew, or swallow.

Practice Problems C

Using the following labels, answer the questions that follow.

1.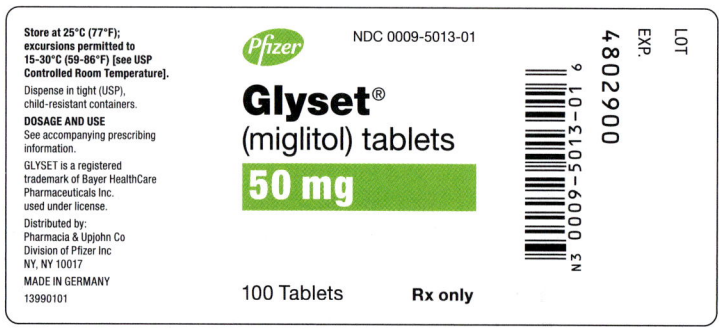

(© Pfizer. Used with permission.)

Who is the manufacturer of this medication? _____

What is the NDC number on this container? _____

What is the trade name for this medication? _____

What is the generic name for this medication? _____

What is the strength of this medication? _____

How many tablets are in an unopened container? _____

2.

ALWAYS DISPENSE WITH MEDICATION GUIDE

NDC 0071-2214-20

Pfizer

Dilantin-125®
(Phenytoin
Oral Suspension, USP)

125 mg per 5 mL

**IMPORTANT–SHAKE WELL
BEFORE EACH USE**

NOT FOR PARENTERAL USE

8 fl oz (237 mL)   Rx only

THIS PRODUCT MUST BE SHAKEN WELL ESPECIALLY PRIOR TO INITIAL USE.

Each 5 mL contains 125 mg phenytoin, with a maximum alcohol content not greater than 0.6 percent.

DOSAGE AND USE
Adults, 1 teaspoonful (5 mL) three times daily; pediatric patients, see package insert.

Advice to Pharmacist and Patient–Patient must be advised to use an accurate measuring device when using this product.

See package insert for complete prescribing information.

Store at Controlled Room Temperature 20°-25°C (68°-77°F) [see USP].

Protect from freezing and light.

Keep this and all drugs out of the reach of children.

Distributed by
Parke-Davis
Division of Pfizer Inc
NY, NY 10017

(© Pfizer. Used with permission.)

Who manufactures the medication? _____

What is the dosage form of this medication? _____

What are the specific directions (capitalized information) accompanying this medication? _____
_____

What is the dosage strength? _____

What is the total volume in metric measurements? _____

What is the trade name? _____

What is the generic name? _____

REVIEW

It is absolutely necessary that you interpret medication orders and prescriptions correctly. There must be checks and balances among the prescriber, the pharmacist, and the person responsible for obtaining the medications for dispensing, such as the pharmacy technician, as well as the person administering the medication. Any break in this checking process could result in the patient getting the wrong medication or strength, which could have dire consequences.

SECTION III Calculations with Prescriptions and Medication Orders

TECH NOTE
As a pharmacy technician, you have the responsibility to be sure you understand any order or prescription. Ask for verification if you have any concerns. Never make assumptions! As part of the medical team, you must assist in continuous quality control for patient safety.

Posttest

Interpret the following prescriptions or medication orders and show the directions as they should appear on a prescription label. If the prescription calls for the liquid form of a medication, use the metric system and assume that a dispensing utensil is provided.

1.
```
Lawrence Merry, M.D.
4th Street and Jones Ave.
Holly, GA 00111
phone# - 001-555-2176

Patient Name_____    Date _____
Address_____    Age _____

Rx      Xanax 500 mcg
        #30
        Sig: i tab po at bedtime

   _____   Refill _____
   DEA#_____
```

Label directions: _____

_____

 2.
```
Lawrence Merry, M.D.
4th Street and Jones Ave.
Holly, GA 00111
phone# - 001-555-2176

Patient Name_____    Date _____
Address_____    Age _____

Rx      K-Clor 20 mEq ℥xvi
        Sig: ʒ ss̄ po qam p̄ breakfast

   _____   Refill _____
   DEA#_____
```

Prescription interpretation: _____

Label directions: _____

Posttest, cont.

3.

```
              Lawrence Merry, M.D.
            4th Street and Jones Ave.
                  Holly, GA 00111
              phone# - 001-555-2176

Patient Name_____   Date _____
Address_____   Age _____

  ℞        Dilantin 100 mg caps
           #120
           Sig: cap iv po stat then cap ī po qid

    _____   Refill _____
    DEA#_____
```

Prescription interpretation: _____
_____

Label directions: _____
_____

4.

```
              Lawrence Merry, M.D.
            4th Street and Jones Ave.
                  Holly, GA 00111
              phone# - 001-555-2176

Patient Name_____   Date _____
Address_____   Age _____

  ℞        amlodipine 5 mg
           #30
           Sig: tab ī po daily @ 10 am

    _____   Refill _____
    DEA#_____
```

Label directions: _____
_____

Continued

Posttest, cont.

5.

```
            Lawrence Merry, M.D.
           4th Street and Jones Ave.
               Holly, GA 00111
             phone# - 001-555-2176

Patient Name_____   Date _____
Address_____    Age _____

    ℞    Vasotec 10 mg
         #30
         Sig: tab ss̄ po x 1 wk then ī tab po daily.
         Check B/P and record daily.

    _____         Refill _____
    DEA#_____
```

Prescription interpretation: _____

_____

Label directions: _____

_____

6.

```
            Lawrence Merry, M.D.
           4th Street and Jones Ave.
               Holly, GA 00111
             phone# - 001-555-2176

Patient Name_____   Date _____
Address_____    Age _____

    ℞    Antivert 12.5 mg
         #60
         Sig: tab ī po q4-6h prn

    _____         Refill _____
    DEA#_____
```

Label directions: _____

_____

Posttest, cont.

7.

Lawrence Merry, M.D.
4th Street and Jones Ave.
Holly, GA 00111
phone# - 001-555-2176

Patient Name_____ Date_____
Address_____ Age_____

℞   Ocuflox Ophthalmic Solution
    5 mL
    Sig: i gtt each eye qid x 5 d

_____ Refill _____
DEA#_____

Prescription interpretation: _____
_____

Label directions: _____

8.

Lawrence Merry, M.D.
4th Street and Jones Ave.
Holly, GA 00111
phone# - 001-555-2176

Patient Name_____ Date_____
Address_____ Age_____

℞   Actos 30 mg
    #30
    Sig: i tab po qam ac breakfast

_____ Refill _____
DEA#_____

Label directions: _____
_____

Continued

Posttest, cont.

Interpret the following medication orders.

9. meperidine 75 mg and Phenergan 25 mg IM q4–6h prn extreme pain

10. Nafcillin i g q6h added to IV fluids

11. Humulin 70/30 25 units subcut qam ac breakfast and ac supper

12. Tagamet 300 mg IM stat

13. ampicillin 250 mg po qid c̄ meals and hs c̄ snack

14. warfarin sodium 5 mg po on even days and 2.5 mg po on odd days

15. digoxin 250 mcg po qam c̄ pulse ↑60

16. Sudafed 60 mg po q4–6h prn nasal congestion

Posttest, cont.

Interpret these labels by answering the following questions.

 17.

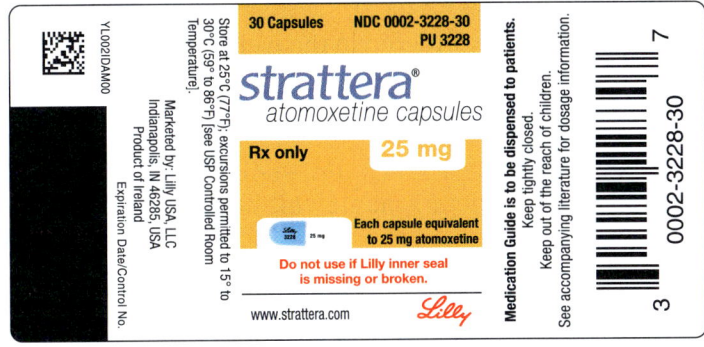

(© Eli Lilly and Company. All Rights Reserved. Used with Permission.)

What is the brand name of this medication? _____

What is the generic name? _____

Who manufactures this medication? _____

How many capsules are in a full stock container? _____

What is the strength per capsule? _____

What are the corresponding number codes for the following segments of the NDC number?

labeler: _____; product: _____; package size: _____

18.

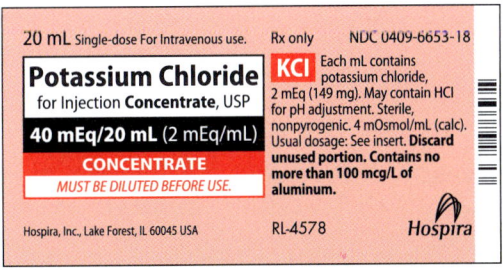

(© Pfizer. Used with permission.)

What is the total strength of medication in the vial? _____

What is the total volume of medication in the vial? _____

Who manufactures the medication? _____

What is the dosage form? _____

What is the major warning on this label? _____

REVIEW OF RULES

Interpreting Medication Labels and Orders

- Always read the entire label/prescription/medication order before making decisions concerning the medication to be dispensed.

- Solid medications are usually ordered in the weight of medication per tablet or capsule.

- Liquid medications will be found as weight per volume of medication, such as mg/mL.

- The generic name for the medication should be written in lowercase letters, whereas the trade or proprietary name will begin with a capital letter and may be followed by ®.

- If there is a question about the medication ordered, always ask the pharmacist to verify before beginning the process of preparing it for dispensing.

- Always read medication labels three times to ensure correctness of the dispensed medication to the medication order/prescription (1) when removing stock medication from the storage shelf; (2) before preparing medication; and (3) before returning stock medication back to the shelf, if applicable.

CHAPTER 8

Calculation of Oral Solid Doses

OBJECTIVES

1. Calculate solid oral medication doses using both ratio and proportion and dimensional analysis, following the rules that should be considered when calculating medication doses.
2. Convert equivalent measurements of oral solid doses between different units or measurement systems.
3. Maintain patient safety.

KEY WORDS

Buccal Between gum and cheek
Dosage Size, frequency, and number of doses of medication prescribed *over a period of time*
Dosage form Physical structure of a dose; for example: capsule, tablet, solution
Dose Amount of a medication to be administered *at one time*
Enteric-coated tablet Dosage form that allows medication to pass through stomach unchanged; to prevent stomach irritation or prevent degradation of the active ingredient by stomach acid
Oral medications Medications taken by mouth (po)
Stock strength Strength or weight of medication available for doses
Sublingual medications Medications placed under the tongue to dissolve (SL)

Pretest

If you are already comfortable with the subject matter, perform the following calculations to test your knowledge. If not, work your way through the chapter and return to them for extra practice. Determine how many capsules or tablets must be given per dose of the stock available. Any labels included represent the stock strength available. Show your calculations.

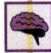
1. Dose ordered: phenobarbital 30 mg

   Stock strength: phenobarbital 60 mg tablets _____

2. Dose ordered: AcipHex 60 mg

   Stock strength: AcipHex (rabeprazole) 20 mg tablets _____

3. Dose ordered: digoxin 0.25 mg

   Stock strength: digoxin 250 mcg tablets _____

Continued

Pretest, cont.

4. Dose ordered: Mobic 7.5–15 mg
   Stock strength: meloxicam 7.5 mg tablets _____

5. Dose ordered: theophylline 0.4 g
   Stock strength: theophylline 200 mg capsules _____

6. Dose ordered: potassium chloride 10 mEq
   Stock strength: potassium chloride 20 mEq scored tablets _____

7. Dose ordered: aspirin gr x
   Stock strength: aspirin gr v tablets _____

8. Dose ordered: Pepcid 40 mg
   Stock strength: famotidine 20 mg tablets _____

9. Dose ordered: amoxicillin 1 g
   Stock strength: amoxicillin 500 mg capsules _____

10. Dose ordered: Haldol 2 mg
    Stock strength: haloperidol 1 mg tablets _____

11. Dose ordered: Synthroid 350 mcg
    Stock strength: levothyroxine 0.175 mg tablets _____

12. Dose ordered: ferrous sulfate 324 mg
    Stock available: ferrous sulfate 5 grain tablets _____

Pretest, cont.

13. Dose ordered: Glyset 50 mg

Number of tablets needed: _____

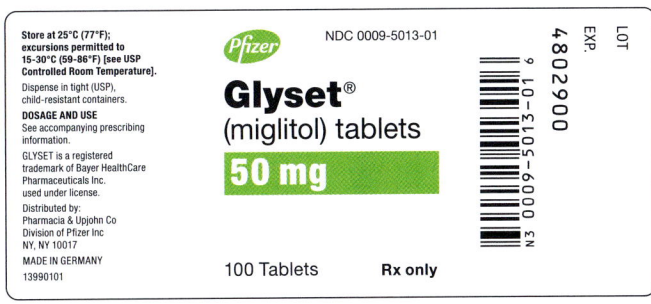

(© Pfizer. Used with permission.)

14. Dose ordered: Cogentin 1.5 mg

Stock available: benztropine 0.5 mg tablets _____

15. Dose ordered: Synthroid 50 mcg

Stock available: levothyroxine 0.05 mg tablets _____

INTRODUCTION

Oral medications come in solid forms, such as tablets and capsules, and liquid forms, such as solutions and suspensions. Variations of solid forms, such as powders and granules, may be dissolved in liquid for administration. The oral route is the most frequently used due to convenience for the patient, safety, and reduced cost of administration and manufacturing.

Oral medications are absorbed in the gastrointestinal tract, primarily in the small intestine. A prescription or medication order is written to accommodate individual differences due to age, weight, and concurrent medical conditions, among others. These differences must be considered by the physician and further checked and verified by the pharmacy professional as a means of checks and balances. Drug manufacturers often provide drugs in different strengths to meet the needs of most patients. The pharmacy technician must be aware of the various strengths of medications and choose the correct drug strength to dispense.

Calculation of exact doses and dosages is a critical factor in both dispensing and administering medications. Many drugs are prescribed in the exact amount found in stock, whereas others must be calculated. When the dose ordered is available in the ordered strength and form, no calculations are needed and fewer errors occur.

Some tablets are scored to allow breaking them in half or even thirds. Medications that are not scored are generally not to be divided into smaller doses. Some tablets are enteric-coated to delay release until they pass through the stomach to either prevent irritation of the stomach or avoid the inactivation of the medication by stomach acid. Enteric-coated medications should *never* be divided, crushed, or chewed. This rule also applies to most extended-release (over time) formulations and delayed-release formulations. Capsules should not be crushed, chewed, or divided, although a few can be opened and sprinkled on food for ease of administration. Be certain of these restrictions when calculating solid doses.

CALCULATING SOLID ORAL MEDICATION DOSES

The pharmacy technician must be sure to calculate the correct amount of medicine to be given to the patient both for an individual dose and the entire course of therapy. A **dose** is the amount of medicine to be given at one specific time, whereas **dosage** indicates the size, frequency, and number of doses of medication prescribed over a period of time. Also, be sure that the medication name is correct because many medications have sound-alike or look-alike names. If there is ever a doubt about the medicine to be used or if the answer calculated is not what you expect, obtain clarification from the pharmacist, a practice that is always safe, important, and acceptable. The pharmacist is the person ultimately responsible for dispensing the medication and would prefer to answer questions before medication preparation rather than make a medication error by dispensing incorrect doses, dosages, or medications.

> **TECH NOTE**
> Remember that dose refers to the amount of medication given at a single time; dosage refers to the amount of medication to fill the physician's entire order.

Rules that should be considered when calculating medication doses follow:
- Most capsules are not meant to be opened or divided.
- Scored tablets may be divided, but unscored tablets are not typically meant to be divided.
- **Enteric-coated**, **buccal**, and **sublingual** tablets, as well as most extended- and delayed-release capsules, are not intended for crushing, dividing, or chewing.
- Buccal and sublingual tablets should not be swallowed whole but should be dissolved within the oral cavity in the designated location.
- If a part of a tablet (usually ½) is the answer to a dose problem, be sure dividing the tablet will not alter the pharmaceutical action, the calculations are correct, and the correct medication and strength have been chosen.

> **! TECH ALERT**
> Always double-check your calculations! If your answer seems incorrect, recalculate. If the answer still does not seem correct, ALWAYS ask for help from a pharmacist. Never fill an order or prescription if you have a question regarding the accuracy of your calculations.

Single-step calculations are easily performed with the ratio and proportion (R&P) method, using cross-multiplication and division. Any of these calculations can also be performed with dimensional analysis (DA). Choose which method is best for you.

Calculating Medications Using Ratio and Proportion

First, write the relationships as fractional units. Note that the ***known*** dosage and the **dosage form** are on the left side of the proportion.

For example, if you have 250 mg capsules available and you need a 500 mg dose:

$$\frac{250 \text{ mg}}{1 \text{ cap}} = \frac{500 \text{ mg}}{x} \quad \text{1 times 500 divided by 250 equals 2 capsules}$$

This is read as follows: If there are 250 mg in one capsule, there are 500 mg in *x* capsules.

> **! TECH ALERT**
> ONLY cross-multiply and divide with the R&P method!

Remember that the units of the numerators must be the same and the units of the denominators must be the same, since these are equivalent fractions. If the units of measurement differ, a conversion must be performed to bring these components into the same system. This then becomes a multistep problem, which is performed more easily with DA using a conversion factor.

EXAMPLE 8.1

 A medication order is written for fluoxetine (Prozac) 80 mg and the stock medication available is Prozac 40 mg capsules. What is the dose to be given to the patient?

$$\frac{40 \text{ mg}}{1 \text{ cap}} = \frac{80 \text{ mg}}{x} \quad \text{Cross-multiply.}$$

Drop the mg because it appears on both sides so it can be canceled.

$40x = 80$ caps   Divide both sides by 40.

$x = 2$ caps

EXAMPLE 8.2

 A medication order is written for gr $\frac{3}{4}$ codeine.

Stock strength available is codeine gr $\frac{1}{4}$ tablet. What is the dose to be given to the patient?

$$\frac{\text{gr } 1/4}{1 \text{ tab}} = \frac{\text{gr } 3/4}{x} \quad \text{Cross-multiply.}$$

Drop the "gr" because this appears on both sides of the equation.

$\frac{1}{4}x = \frac{3}{4}$ tabs   Multiply both sides by 4. $x = 3$ tabs

Calculating Medications Using Dimensional Analysis

Although DA is most useful when performing calculations with more than one step, to keep track of units, it can be used for single-step calculations. To use DA, fractional units must allow for the cancellation of measurements from one fraction to the next. When orders are written in different measurement systems or units, DA is used to incorporate a conversion factor.

> **TECH NOTE**
> Remember to always start with whatever unit you want for your answer, follow it with an equal sign, and place the known quantity with that unit in the numerator of the first fraction to the right of the equal sign. Continue with this process until you cancel all but your desired unit.

If you have 250 mg capsules available and you need a 500 mg dose, start with the unit needed for the answer, capsules, and follow with an equal sign. Then use the known quantity with that unit as the numerator first. Follow with the fraction that will cancel the unit of the previous denominator, and solve.

$$\text{caps} = \frac{1 \text{ cap}}{250 \text{ mg}} \cdot \frac{500 \text{ mg}}{1} = 2 \text{ caps}$$

> **! TECH ALERT**
> DA is multiplication of fractions. NEVER cross-multiply unless using R&P!

As we have seen previously, this one-step problem was solved more simply with R&P. The following examples show Examples 8.1 and 8.2 performed with DA.

EXAMPLE 8.3

A medication order is written for Prozac (fluoxetine) 80 mg, and the stock medication available is Prozac 40 mg capsules. What is the dose to be given to the patient?

$$\text{caps} = \frac{1 \text{ cap}}{40 \text{ mg}} \cdot \frac{80 \text{ mg}}{1} \quad \text{Milligrams are canceled because this is a fraction multiplication.}$$

$$\text{caps} = \frac{80 \text{ caps}}{40} = 2 \text{ caps}$$

EXAMPLE 8.4

A medication order is written for gr ¾ codeine to be given, and stock strength available is codeine gr ¼/tablet. What is the dose to be given to the patient?

$$\text{tabs} = \frac{1 \text{ tab}}{\text{gr } 1/4} \cdot \frac{\text{gr } 3/4}{1} \quad \text{gr cancel because this is a fraction multiplication}$$

$$\text{tabs} = \frac{3}{4} \text{ tabs} \Big/ \frac{1}{4} \quad \text{Invert the second fraction and multiply.}$$

$$\text{tabs} = \frac{3}{4} \text{ tabs} \cdot \frac{4}{1} = 3 \text{ tabs}$$

Either method can be used for Practice Problems A, but DA should be used for Practice Problems B, which are multistep problems.

Practice Problems A

Calculate the number of tablets or capsules to be given per dose in the following orders. Show your calculations.

1. Order: Dilantin (phenytoin) 200 mg po

   Number of capsules needed: _____

   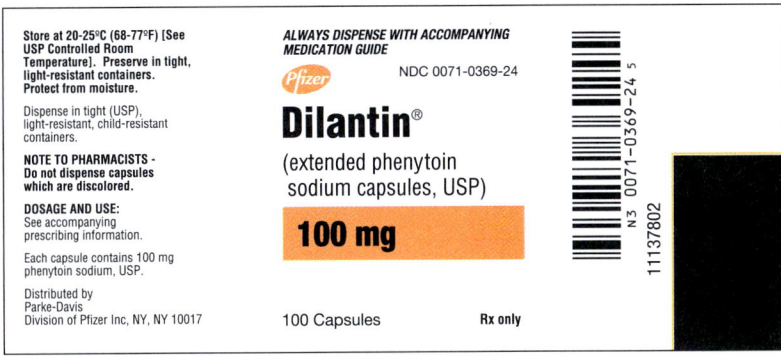

   (© Pfizer. Used with permission.)

2. Order: ferrous sulfate gr x po qam

   Stock strength: ferrous sulfate gr v tablets _____

3. Order: digoxin cap 0.1 mg po qam c̄ P ↑ 60 until changed by MD

   Stock strength: Lanoxicaps 0.05 mg (50 mcg) capsules _____

4. Order: Biaxin 500 mg po bid c̄ food

   Stock strength: clarithromycin 250 mg tablets _____

5. Order: Pravachol 20 mg po daily

   Stock strength: pravastatin 10 mg tablets _____

6. Order: Ativan 0.5 mg po q6–8h prn anxiety

   Stock strength: lorazepam 1 mg tablets _____

7. Order: Retrovir 200 mg po qpm

   Stock strength: Retrovir (zidovudine) 100 mg capsules _____

8. **PAIN** Order: ASA gr x po q4–6h prn aching; do not exceed 8 tab q24h

   Stock strength: aspirin gr v tablets _____

9. **ENDO** Order: Decadron 0.75 mg daily @ same time

   Stock strength: dexamethasone 0.25 mg tablets _____

10. Order: isoniazid 250 mg tid c̄ meals

    Stock strength: isoniazid 100 mg tablets _____

Some medications are combination products that will need to be looked at individually, such as Lotrel 2.5/10. Each tablet contains 2.5 mg of amlodipine and 10 mg of benazapril. If a different dosage of Lotrel is ordered, such as *Lotrel 5/20 daily in am*, it must be ordered in equal multiples of each component. This order is for two times the amount of amlodipine (2 × 2.5 = 5) and two times the amount of benazapril (2 × 10 = 20); therefore the dose can be obtained with two tablets of Lotrel 2.5/10. If it were not ordered in equal multiples, the order could not be filled with this medication.

CALCULATIONS INVOLVING DIFFERENT UNITS OR MEASUREMENT SYSTEMS

These conversions involve multiple steps and are most easily solved using DA to keep track of units. DA allows you to make the entire conversion in one equation. Using DA, the step of changing from one metric unit to another is done as part of the equation.

EXAMPLE 8.5

A physician orders metformin 1 g qam. Available stock is 500 mg tablets. How many tablets are needed for one dose?

This requires the use of a conversion factor between g and mg.

$$\frac{\text{tabs}}{\text{dose}} = \frac{1 \text{ tab}}{500 \text{ mg}} \cdot \frac{1{,}000 \text{ mg}}{1 \text{ g}} \cdot \frac{1 \text{ g}}{\text{dose}} = 2 \text{ tabs/dose}$$

Frequently this type of problem is set up without using per dose each time, as that is understood from the question:

$$\text{tabs} = \frac{1 \text{ tab}}{500 \text{ mg}} \cdot \frac{1{,}000 \text{ mg}}{1 \text{ g}} \cdot \frac{1 \text{ g}}{1} = 2 \text{ tabs}$$

TECH NOTE

Using DA is especially helpful when conversions between measurement systems are necessary to arrive at the answer.

EXAMPLE 8.6

A physician orders phenobarbital gr ½ tid. Available stock is phenobarbital 15 mg tablets. How many tablets are needed for one dose?

This requires the use of a conversion factor between gr and mg.

$$\frac{\text{tabs}}{\text{dose}} = \frac{1 \text{ tab}}{15 \text{ mg}} \cdot \frac{60 \text{ mg}}{\text{gr i}} \cdot \frac{\text{gr } 1/2}{\text{dose}} = 2 \text{ tabs/dose}$$

How many tablets are needed per day?

$$\frac{\text{tabs}}{\text{day}} = \frac{1 \text{ tab}}{15 \text{ mg}} \cdot \frac{60 \text{ mg}}{\text{gr i}} \cdot \frac{\text{gr } 1/2}{\text{dose}} \cdot \frac{3 \text{ doses}}{\text{day}} = 6 \text{ tabs/day}$$

TECH NOTE
When converting, the answer may be approximate rather than exact. Close answers may be rounded to the nearest whole number of capsules or tablets. An answer such as 1.9 tablets would be rounded to 2. If tablets are scored, they can be rounded to the nearest half tablet.

Practice Problems B

Calculate number of tablets or capsules to be given per dose with each of the following orders using DA. Show calculations.

1. Order: ciprofloxacin 1.5 g po qam

   Stock available: ciprofloxacin 750 mg tablets _____

2. Order: Lopid 1.2 g qam c̄ am meal _____

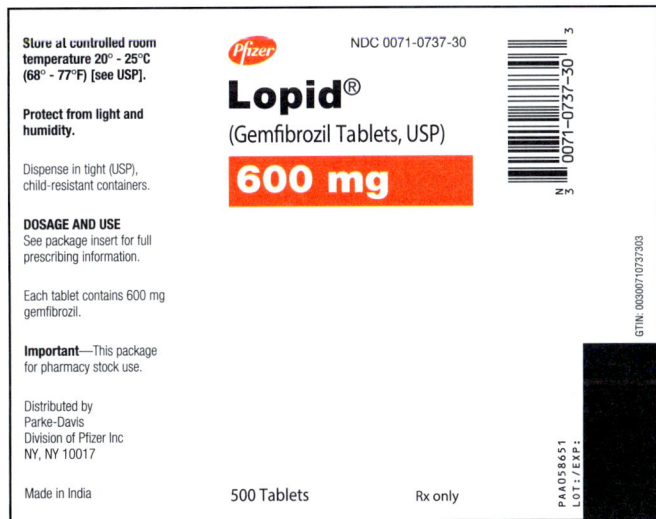

(© Pfizer. Used with permission.)

3. Order: Dilantin 0.3 g bid c̄ breakfast and evening meal _____

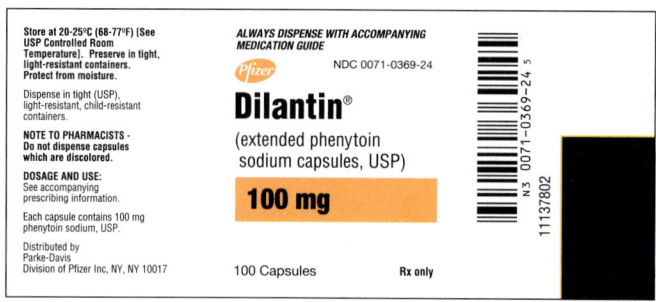

(© Pfizer. Used with permission.)

4. Order: Glucophage 1 g po bid c̄ meals
Stock strength: metformin 500 mg tablets _____

5. Order: cephalexin 0.75 g po bid
Stock strength: cephalexin 250 mg capsules _____

6. Order: Evista 0.12 g po daily _____

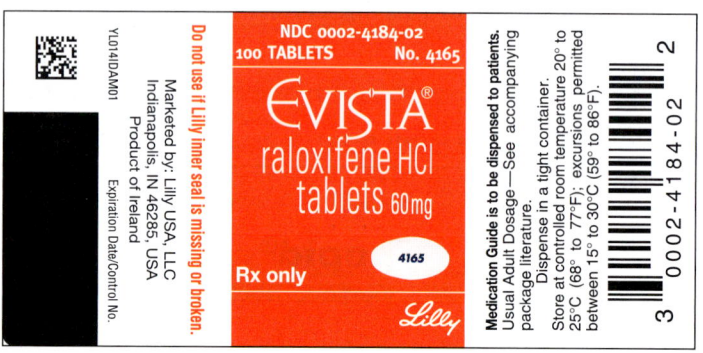

(© Eli Lilly and Company. All Rights Reserved. Used with Permission.)

7. A physician orders ferrous sulfate gr v po bid. The available stock medication is ferrous sulfate 325 mg tabs. _____

8. A physician orders phenobarbital gr s̄s̄ tab po qpm. The available stock medication is phenobarbital 60 mg tabs. _____

9. 🟪 A physician orders codeine sulfate 60 mg q4–6h prn pain. The available stock is codeine sulfate gr ¼ tab. _____

10. ♥ A physician orders Nitrostat gr 1/150 SL q5min up to 3 doses prn angina. The available stock medication is Nitrostat 0.4 mg tab. _____

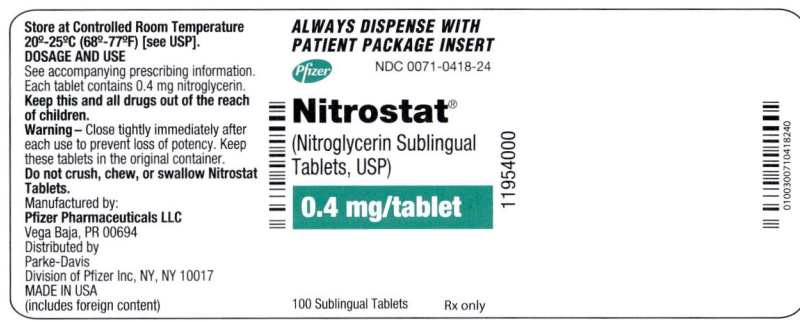

(© Pfizer. Used with permission.)

PATIENT SAFETY WHEN CALCULATING DOSES AND DOSAGES

Accurate calculations are essential for patient safety. Medication orders or prescriptions are the physician's determination of what medication and dosage should be safe for the patient. The physician, pharmacist, pharmacy technician, nurse, and other health care team members work together to ensure this safety. The patient is dependent on health care professionals to provide medications that are as risk-free as possible.

To be certain that the medication is correct and in the correct dosage, you should follow certain safety rules:

- Always recheck calculations after the dose has been figured. Learn and practice calculations until you are confident using them.
- If you have any calculation questions, check with the pharmacist. Remember that he or she is ultimately responsible.
- As you work from either a medication order or a prescription, verify that what you have on hand is the medication ordered and that it is in the dosage form required.
- Check labels three times before presenting the prescription to the pharmacist for verification—before taking the medication from the shelf, before preparing the medication, and before passing it to the pharmacist.
- Compare the label on the medication with the order from the physician. Be sure these are the same, being careful of look-alike and sound-alike medications. Do not allow yourself to be distracted; keep your full attention on the task at hand.
- Know your medication and the average dose that is required for a patient of the age, gender, and weight of the person for whom the prescription or medication order is written. If in doubt, read the drug insert or other reference materials related to the specific medication before preparing it so that you are aware of the usual dose.
- Finally, remember that the pharmacist would rather have you ask a question than have the incorrect medication dispensed to the patient.

REVIEW

When calculating solid oral medication doses, the amount of medication should be calculated to that of the physician's order. If the medication order and the available medications are in different measurement systems, use a conversion factor to be sure the medications are converted to the same system.

Single-step medication doses can be calculated using R&P or DA. As a pharmacy technician, find the method that is most comfortable for you. Multistep problems involving one or more conversion factors should be performed using DA.

Posttest

Determine the number of capsules or tablets to be given per dose. Show all calculations.

1. Order: Tagamet 0.8 g bid
   Stock available: cimetidine 400 mg tablets _____

2. Order: HydroDIURIL 100 mg qam pc am meal
   Stock strength available: hydrochlorothiazide 50 mg tablets _____

3. Order: Tylenol gr x q4–6h prn fever
   Stock available: acetaminophen 325 mg tablets _____

4. Order: ciprofloxacin HCl 0.5 g tid c̄ meals × 7 days
   Stock strength available: ciprofloxacin 250 mg capsules _____

5. Order: cefaclor 0.75 g daily *in 3 divided doses*
   Stock strength: cefaclor 250 mg capsules _____

6. Order: codeine phosphate gr s̄s̄ po stat and q4–6h prn pain
   Stock strength: codeine phosphate 30 mg tablets _____

Posttest, cont.

7. Order: Urecholine 20 mg po bid c̄ meals × 10 d
Stock available: bethanechol 10 mg tablets _____

8. Order: Benadryl 50 mg po tid prn itching
Stock strength: diphenhydramine 50 mg capsules _____

9. Order: Cipro 0.75 g po bid × 10 days
Stock available: ciprofloxacin 750 mg tablets _____

10. Order: ampicillin 1 g po stat, then 500 mg po qid × 12 d
Stock strength available: ampicillin 500 mg capsules
Number of capsules to be given stat: _____
Number of capsules to be given qid: _____

11. Order: Restoril 0.015 g po at bedtime prn sleep
Stock strength available: temazepam 15 mg capsules _____

12. Order: Lopressor 100 mg po bid today, then 50 mg po bid
Stock strength: metoprolol 50 mg tablets

What is the total dosage to be given today (mg)? _____
How many tablets are needed per dose today? _____
What is the total *daily* dosage to be given starting tomorrow (mg)? _____
How many tablets are needed per dose starting tomorrow? _____

Continued

Posttest, cont.

13. Order: tetracycline 500 mg qid × 5 d; then 500 mg bid × 5 d; then 500 mg daily × 5 d for acne

Stock available: tetracycline 500 mg capsules

How many capsules are needed per dose? _____

What is the total number of capsules that will be given over the first 5 days?

What is the total number of capsules that will be given over days 6 through 10?

What is the total number of capsules that will be given over the last 5 days?

What is the total number of capsules necessary to fill the prescription?

What is the total dosage per day in the first 5 days (g)?

What is the total dosage per day for days 6 to 10 (g)?

What is the total dosage per day for the last 5 days (mg)?

Continued

Posttest, cont.

14. Order: Strattera 0.05 g po daily c̄ breakfast

How many capsules are needed for one dose? _____

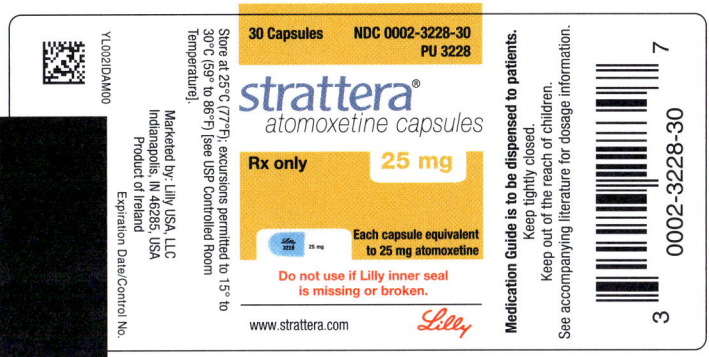

(© Eli Lilly and Company. All Rights Reserved. Used with Permission.)

REVIEW OF RULES

Calculating Solid Oral Medications

- Calculations for oral solid medications may be accomplished by using R&P or DA.
- Use DA if the problem requires a conversion factor.
- Solid medications usually have a quantity of a single solid form such as per tablet, per capsule, or per package of powder.
- Scored tablets may be broken at scores or on indented marks.
- To solve using R&P, place the known measurements on the left side of the equation and the unknowns on the right. Remember to place the values in each ratio so that the units are in the same position to make the proportion equal. Cross multiply and divide.
- To solve using DA, always start with the unit of the numerator of your desired answer as the numerator of the first fraction and add the remaining known information as fractions in the order that will cancel unwanted units by multiplication of the fractions.

CHAPTER 9

Calculation of Oral Liquid Doses

OBJECTIVES

1. Interpret orders and calculate the volume of oral liquid medication necessary to administer ordered doses using either ratio and proportion or dimensional analysis.
2. Discuss the process of reconstitution of powders into oral liquid medications.

KEY WORDS

Beyond use date (BUD) Date assigned by the pharmacy to a reconstituted or repackaged medication beyond which the preparation is no longer considered usable

Diluent Agent that dilutes a substance; in pharmacy, the liquid added to a powder to change the powder to a liquid or the liquid used to dilute another liquid; also known as **solvent**

Elixir Sweetened, flavored medication dissolved in a mixture of alcohol and water

Expiration date Date assigned by the manufacturer of a medication beyond which it is not considered usable (no longer valid once a medication is repackaged or reconstituted)

Graduates Containers, calibrated in the metric system, that are used to measure liquid

Lyophilized Freeze-dried

Meniscus Curved line that develops on the upper surface of a liquid when poured into a container; always read at the bottom of the curve at eye level

Powder volume Space occupied by the powdered active ingredient relative to the total volume of medication after reconstitution; also known as **displacement value;** a measurement of the amount of active substance that displaces (takes the place of) some of the liquid diluent

Reconstitution Process of adding fluid, such as distilled water, to a powdered or crystalline form of medication to make a specific liquid dosage strength

Solution Dosage form in which the medication is completely dissolved in the liquid

Solute Substance that is being dissolved; in this chapter, the powdered medication

Suspension Dosage form in which small particles of medication are dispersed throughout the liquid; most require shaking before dispensing and administering

Syrup Aqueous solution sweetened with sugar or a sugar substitute to disguise taste

Pretest

If you are already comfortable with the subject matter, perform the following calculations to test your knowledge. If not, work your way through the chapter and return to them for extra practice. Show all calculations. Answer in milliliters unless otherwise specified. Round answers to nearest tenth.

1. A physician orders Ceclor 250 mg po tid for a child with otitis media.

   Stock strength: cefaclor 125 mg/5 mL

   What volume of medication is needed for one dose?

   What is one dose in household measurements?

Pretest, cont.

2. A physician orders hydroxyzine hydrochloride syrup 15 mg po qid for itching.

   Stock strength: hydroxyzine HCl syrup 10 mg/5 mL

   What volume of medication is needed per dose?

3. A physician orders Tylenol gr v q4h prn fever and aches for a child who has a high fever.

   The drug available is acetaminophen suspension 160 mg/5 mL

   What volume of medication is needed per dose? (Round to nearest whole number)

4. A physician orders Amoxil 62.5 mg po tid for an infant.

   The drug available is amoxicillin suspension 125 mg/5 mL

   What volume of medication is needed per dose?

5. A physician orders Benadryl 25 mg tid prn for severe itching.

   The strength available is diphenhydramine 12.5 mg/5 mL

   What volume of medication is needed per dose?

   What volume is needed in household measurements?

6. Ordered medication: amoxicillin 375 mg po tid

   Stock available: amoxicillin oral suspension 250 mg/5 mL

   What volume of medication is needed per dose?

   What is the equivalent household measurement in teaspoons?

Continued

Pretest, cont.

7. Ordered medication: erythromycin 0.3 g po tid

   Stock available: erythromycin ethylsuccinate oral suspension 200 mg/5 mL

   What volume of medication is needed per dose?

8. Ordered medication: phenobarbital 30 mg po at bedtime

   Stock strength: phenobarbital elixir 20 mg/5 mL

   What volume of medication is needed per dose?

9. Ordered medication: Prozac 10 mg po qam

   Stock available: fluoxetine 20 mg/5 mL oral solution

   What volume of medication is needed per dose?

   What is this volume in household measurements?

10. A bottle of ampicillin suspension is marked 125 mg/5 mL. The 200-mL bottle instructs that 158 mL of water be added for an oral suspension. The physician wants the child to receive ampicillin 250 mg qid.

    What volume of water should be added to the powder?

    What is the powder volume?

    What is the volume per dose that the child should receive?

    What is this dose in household measurements?

INTRODUCTION

Oral liquid formulations include **solutions**, tinctures, **elixirs**, **suspensions**, and **syrups**. Oral medications given in liquid form are absorbed more quickly than solids that have to dissolve before absorption. Most oral medications are absorbed in the small intestine, although some are absorbed beginning in the mouth or stomach. For some patients, solid medications such as tablets and capsules are difficult to swallow, and the physician will order oral liquid formulations. This is most common with children and elderly patients. These preparations are stated in weight per unit of volume such as milligrams per milliliter. Most liquid medications are dosed in household or metric units, with metric being preferred. As with solid medications, conversions may be accomplished by either ratio and proportion (R&P) or dimensional analysis (DA). Some medications for oral administration are supplied in a powder form for reconstitution to a liquid form before dispensing.

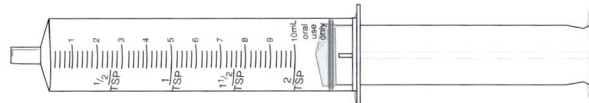

FIGURE 9.1 Typical oral syringe. (Fulcher EM, Soto CD, Fulcher RM: *Pharmacology: Principles and Applications*, ed 3, St. Louis, Saunders, 2012.)

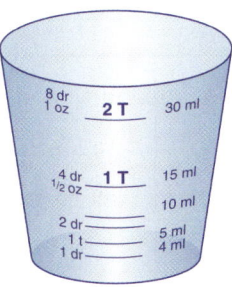

FIGURE 9.2 Typical medication cup. (Kee J, Hayes E, McCuistion LE: *Pharmacology: A nursing Process Approach*, ed 7, St. Louis, Saunders, 2012.)

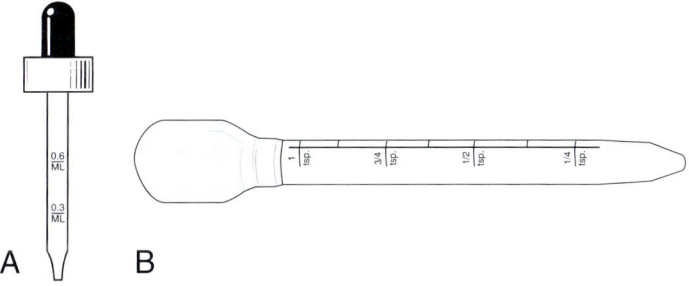

FIGURE 9.3 Typical medicine droppers. (*A*, From Brown M, Mulholland JM: *Drug Calculations: Process and Problems for Clinical Practice*, ed 8, St. Louis, Mosby, 2008. *B*, From Fulcher EM, Soto CD, Fulcher RM: *Pharmacology: Principles and Applications*, ed 3, St. Louis, Saunders, 2012.)

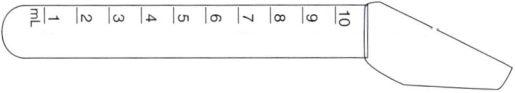

FIGURE 9.4 Typical dosespoon found with oral liquid pediatric medications. (Fulcher EM, Soto CD, Fulcher RM: *Pharmacology: Principles and Applications*, ed 3, St. Louis, Saunders, 2012.)

ADMINISTRATION OF ORAL LIQUID MEDICATIONS

Liquid medications may be administered with oral syringes that are available in 1-mL, 3-mL, 5-mL, 6-mL, and 10-mL sizes (Fig. 9.1), a medication cup (Fig. 9.2), a dropper that is available in different measurements and is usually tailored by the manufacturer for a specific drug (Fig. 9.3), dosespoons (Fig. 9.4), or by using household devices such as teaspoons and tablespoons (not recommended). A newer form of administration of oral medications is a pacifier that will hold a measured amount of medication (Fig. 9.5). The choice of administration device depends on the volume of medication to be administered and the availability of supplies. Teaspoons and tablespoons are the measurements occasionally used for doses in the home setting or when calibrated devises are not available. The use of kitchen utensils is discouraged because of inaccuracy.

When measuring oral liquid medications using a medicine cup, read the line of the medication to the **meniscus** at eye level. The meniscus is the curved line that develops when

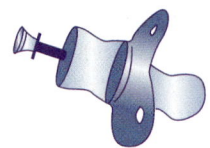

FIGURE 9.5 Pacifier used to administer oral liquid medication to infant. (Modified from Kee J, Hayes E, McCuistion LE: *Pharmacology: A Nursing Process Approach*, ed 7, St. Louis, Saunders, 2012.)

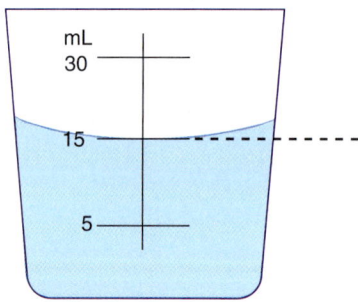

FIGURE 9.6 Reading the meniscus or curved line to 15 mL. (Clayton BD, Stock, YN, Cooper S: *Basic Pharmacology for Nurses*, ed 15, St. Louis, Mosby, 2010.)

> **TECH NOTE**
> When a medication dropper is provided by the manufacturer, it should be used for administration of that particular medication.

a liquid is poured into a container (Fig. 9.6) and should be measured at the lowest point. For medications that must be more accurately measured, an oral syringe should be used. With the 1-mL and 3-mL oral syringes, the dose is measured using 0.1-mL increments. With the 5-mL, 6-mL, and 10-mL oral syringes, the calibrations are in 0.2-mL increments.

> **! TECH ALERT**
> Household utensils are sources of potential errors and are not the ideal means of measuring doses. The abbreviations for teaspoon (tsp) and tablespoon (Tbsp) can be easily confused, leading to errors in administration. Also, when people use their own flatware to measure, there is too much variation. Patient safety is better ensured if calibrated medication administration utensils are used. However, household utensils are used in some necessary instances, and understanding these conversions is needed to assist people with proper dosing.

Calculation of Oral Liquid Medication

Liquid drug preparations are labeled with the weight of the drug per unit of volume. Most are expressed in metric units as mg/mL. Occasionally you will still see per teaspoon or per tablespoon on a manufacturer's label. Even more rare is the use of the apothecary system. Most labels using grains will include the metric measurement as well.

> **TECH NOTE**
> Volume is usually the unknown value when calculating oral liquid medication doses and dosages.

Remember, the *dose* is the amount of medication to be administered at a specific given time, whereas *dosage* is the total amount of medication that will be dispensed and administered over a particular length of time. A physician may order amoxicillin 500 mg tid for

7 days for a patient who requests a liquid dosage form. If the medication on hand is amoxicillin 250 mg (weight) per 5 mL (volume), the known amounts can be placed into an R&P or a DA equation to determine the correct dose of medication. The total dosage to dispense is found by multiplying the amount for one dose by the number of doses per day by 7 days, which will be discussed in detail in Chapter 13.

Calculating Oral Liquid Medications Using Ratio and Proportion

EXAMPLE 9.1

A physician orders amoxicillin oral suspension 500 mg tid for 7 days. The medication available is amoxicillin 250 mg/5 mL. How many mL are needed for one dose?

$$\frac{250 \text{ mg}}{5 \text{ mL}} = \frac{500 \text{ mg}}{x} \quad 250x = 2{,}500 \text{ mL} \quad x = 10 \text{ mL}$$

EXAMPLE 9.2

A physician orders Ceftin oral suspension 200 mg every 12 hours for 10 days. The medication on hand is cefuroxime 125 mg/5 mL. What volume should be given per dose?

$$\frac{125 \text{ mg}}{5 \text{ mL}} = \frac{200 \text{ mg}}{x} \quad 125x = 1{,}000 \text{ mL} \quad x = 8 \text{ mL}$$

This prescription should be dispensed with an administration device such as an oral syringe to accurately measure the 8 mL dose.

Calculating Oral Liquid Medications Using Dimensional Analysis

The problems in Examples 9.1 and 9.2 would appear as follows if calculated using DA.

EXAMPLE 9.3

A physician orders amoxicillin oral suspension 500 mg tid for 7 days. The medication available is amoxicillin 250 mg/5 mL. How many mL are needed for one dose?

$$\text{mL} = \frac{5 \text{ mL}}{250 \text{ mg}} \cdot \frac{500 \text{ mg}}{1} = 10 \text{ mL}$$

Because "mg" is found in both the numerator and denominator, "mg" may be canceled.

The amount needed for a 10-day supply is 10 mL/dose × 3 doses/day × 7 days = 210 mL

EXAMPLE 9.4

A physician orders Ceftin oral suspension 200 mg every 12 hours for 10 days. The medication on hand is cefuroxime 125 mg/5 mL. What volume should be given for one dose?

$$\text{mL} = \frac{5 \text{ mL}}{125 \text{ mg}} \cdot \frac{200 \text{ mg}}{1} = 8 \text{ mL}$$

To obtain the answer in teaspoons, one more step of fractional components needs to be added to the calculation.

$$\text{tsp} = \frac{1\ \text{tsp}}{5\ \text{mL}} \cdot \frac{5\ \text{mL}}{125\ \text{mg}} \cdot \frac{200\ \text{mg}}{1} = 1\frac{6}{10}\ \text{tsp or } 1\frac{3}{5}\ \text{tsp}$$

This is not a measureable amount and would need to be rounded to 1½ tsp. As mentioned earlier, this leads to variation in the actual dose and is not the recommended system to use. 8 mL is much more accurate than rounding to 1½ tsp, which is equivalent to only 7.5 mL.

TECH NOTE

An apothecary dram is approximately 4 to 5 mL and is considered a teaspoon in the household measurement system. Neither the apothecary nor the household measurement system is extremely accurate.

! TECH ALERT

When it is necessary to compute medication doses and equivalencies, the equivalent should be no more than 10% above or below the amount of the prescribed dose. Some doses will require rounding to a measureable quantity; however, the dose, once rounded, should be within the 10% margin. Be aware that some medications require that rounding be within a much lower percentage of variation. This is due to the narrow range between effectiveness and toxicity. If you have questions regarding acceptable rounding techniques, ask your pharmacist for assistance.

Practice Problems A

Calculate the following medication orders, and answer the questions listed. If there is a dispensing device shown, mark the correct dose. Show your calculations.

Remember to use the method of calculation and conversion that is most comfortable for you.

1. Medication order: phenobarbital elixir 60 mg po qid

   Stock strength: phenobarbital elixir 20 mg/5 mL
   What volume of medication is needed per dose?

2. Prescribed: Diflucan suspension 60 mg po stat, then 30 mg po qd × 20 d

   Stock strength available: fluconazole oral suspension 10 mg/mL (35 mL after reconstitution)
   What volume of medication is needed for the stat dose?

   What volume of medication is needed per dose thereafter?

3. Prescribed: cephalexin oral suspension 62.5 mg po tid c̄ food

   Stock strength available: cephalexin oral suspension 125 mg/5 mL
   What volume of medication is needed per dose?

   What is the equivalent in the household measurement system?

4. Prescribed: docusate sodium syrup 100 mg at bedtime prn dry, hard stools

   Stock strength: docusate sodium syrup—each teaspoon (5 mL) contains 20 mg docusate
   What volume of medication is needed per dose?

5. Prescribed: ranitidine syrup 150 mg bid q12h

   Stock available: ranitidine syrup 15 mg/mL
   What volume of medication is needed per dose?

6. Prescribed: fluoxetine oral solution 10 mg po bid

   Stock available: fluoxetine 20 mg/5 mL oral solution
   What volume of medication is needed per dose?

   What is the equivalent volume in the household measurement system?

   What types of medication administration devices could be used to administer this dose?

   _____

7. Prescribed: Lanoxin pediatric 75 mcg bid if P ↑ 60

   Stock available: digoxin 0.05 mg/mL solution
   What volume of medication is needed per dose?

   This medication increases the strength of heart contractions. Would it be appropriate to measure the dose with household utensils? Why or why not?
   _____

8. Prescribed: amoxicillin oral suspension 375 mg tid q8h

   Stock strength available: amoxicillin 125 mg/5 mL oral suspension
   What volume of medication is needed per dose?

   What is the equivalent in household measurements?

9. Prescribed: cefaclor oral suspension 250 mg tid c̄ food

   What volume of cefaclor oral suspension 125 mg/5 mL should be given per dose?

   What volume of cefaclor oral suspension 250 mg/5 mL should be given per dose?

   What volume of cefaclor oral suspension 375 mg/5 mL should be given per dose?

10. Prescribed: amoxicillin oral suspension 0.75 g *daily* in three divided doses

    Stock strength available: amoxicillin 250 mg/5 mL oral suspension
    What volume of medication is needed per dose?

Chapter 9 Calculation of Oral Liquid Doses   173

11. Prescribed: cephalexin oral suspension 0.375 g tid

    What volume of cephalexin oral suspension 125 mg/5 mL would be given per dose?

    What volume of cephalexin oral suspension 250 mg/5 mL would be given per dose?

12. Prescribed: acetaminophen 19 mg q4h prn fever and aching

    Stock strength available: acetaminophen liquid 160 mg/5 mL
    What volume of medication is needed per dose? (round to nearest tenth)
    Show the appropriate dose on the following dropper:

    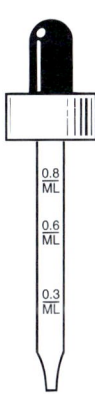

13. Prescribed: penicillin VK oral suspension 62.5 mg qid c̄ food

    Stock available: penicillin VK 125 mg/5 mL oral suspension
    What volume of medication is needed per dose?

! TECH ALERT

If the answer to a dose calculation does not agree with an anticipated answer based on the amount of medication prescribed and the dose of medication on hand, ALWAYS recalculate and ask for assistance as necessary. A dose that seems too large or too small should always be questioned.

RECONSTITUTION OF POWDERS INTO ORAL LIQUID MEDICATIONS

Medications that are unstable in liquid form for extended periods of time are manufactured in a powdered or **lyophilized** form that needs to be reconstituted before administration. **Reconstitution** is the process of dissolving the powdered medication, the **solute**, with the appropriate liquid **diluent**, the **solvent**. Follow the reconstitution instructions on medication labels *exactly* to prepare the correct strength. Before use, the dry medication must be completely dissolved or suspended into liquid form.

The most important step in reconstituting a powder is to read the label or package insert carefully because it provides the directions for reconstitution. The label states the total quantity of the drug in the container, the volume and type of diluent to use for reconstitution, and the final strength of the medication after reconstitution. The label also includes information on stability and storage needs after reconstitution. These directions must be read carefully and followed exactly each time a medication is reconstituted.

> **TECH NOTE**
> Tap the bottle of medication to be reconstituted to loosen any medication that may be attached to the side of the container before adding any diluent.

Many oral liquid antibiotics are supplied in powdered form. Most are manufactured in bottles that are larger than the final medication volume to allow space for shaking before administration. Because the usual vehicle for reconstitution of oral medications is distilled water, **graduates** are used to measure the quantity of liquid to be added (Fig. 9.7). The diluent should be added in increments according to the label, shaking after each addition. In some pharmacies, a computerized dispenser for distilled water is available.

The label on every medication to be reconstituted provides the necessary information for the volume of diluent to be mixed with the powder to provide the desired dosage per unit of volume. When medications are supplied in dry powder or crystalline form, the space occupied by the powder is known as **powder volume**. The powder actually displaces or takes the place of some of the liquid needed to achieve the correct total volume. For example, a powdered medication for oral suspension may require only 78 mL of diluent to be added to produce a total of 100 mL of suspension (Fig. 9.8). The powder displaces, or takes the place of, the other 22 mL. The total liquid volume of the medication will be that of the amount of powder medication displacement plus the amount of added liquid.

The product manufacturers have already calculated the powder volume, or **displacement value,** for medications, and the appropriate amount of diluent to add is listed on every bottle of medication. With medications supplied as reconstitutable powders, the manufacturer's container usually provides the volume needed for a normal course of therapy. For example, most oral antibiotic suspensions will provide enough medication for the necessary 7 to 10 day supply required. Sometimes a drug normally intended for pediatric use will be prescribed for an adult, and more than one bottle of the selected liquid medication may be needed to fill an entire prescription for the desired length of time. This will be covered in Chapter 13.

Before reconstitution, these medications are labeled with an **expiration date** from the manufacturer. Once the pharmacy reconstitutes the medication, the expiration date is no longer valid since these medications begin to degrade. The pharmacy must then assign a **beyond use date** or BUD according to the directions on the manufacturer's label regarding stability. The BUD should be clearly visible on the prescription label.

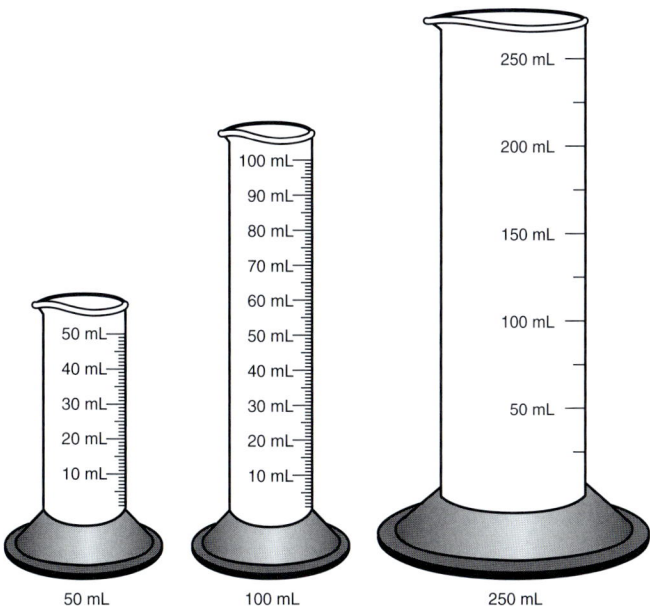

FIGURE 9.7 Examples of graduated cylinders.

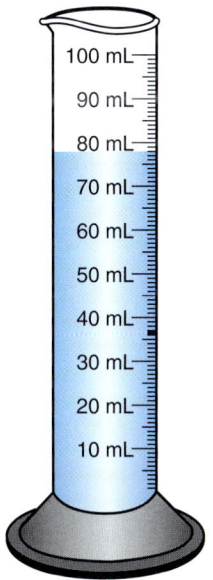

FIGURE 9.8 Graduated cylinder shows 78 mL of diluent.

EXAMPLE 9.5

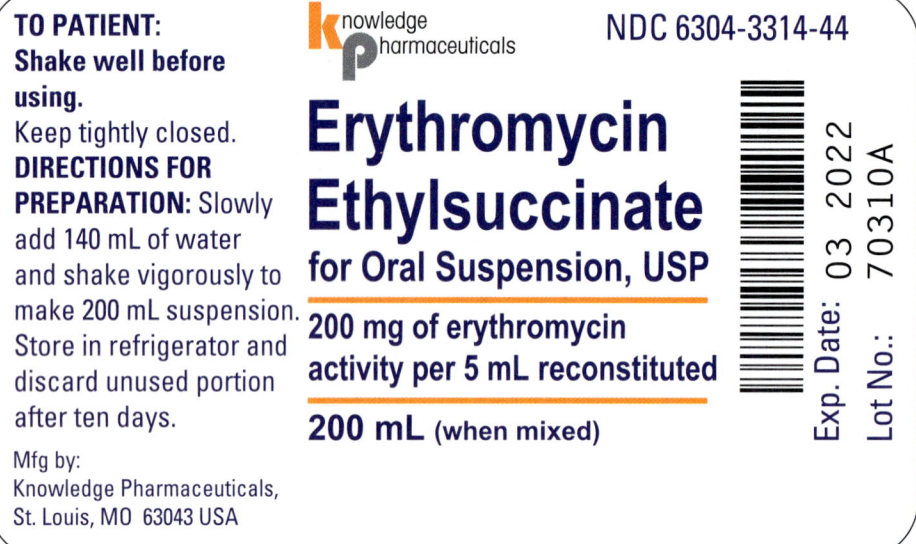

According to the "DIRECTIONS FOR PREPARATION," the bottle of erythromycin will contain a total volume of 200 mL after reconstitution with 140 mL of distilled water. It must then be kept refrigerated and any unused portion discarded after 10 days. The expiration date of 03 2022 must be replaced with a BUD of 10 days from the time of reconstitution. The strength will be 200 mg/5 mL.

The powder volume calculation is: 200 mL – 140 mL = 60 mL

Remember that the final volume of medication in the container will always be greater than the amount of diluent added due to the powder volume. Thus the total volume prepared should always be checked to ensure that there is an adequate amount for dispensing the prescription or order; if not, be sure the correct medication strength has been chosen and reconstituted as required to meet the order.

EXAMPLE 9.6

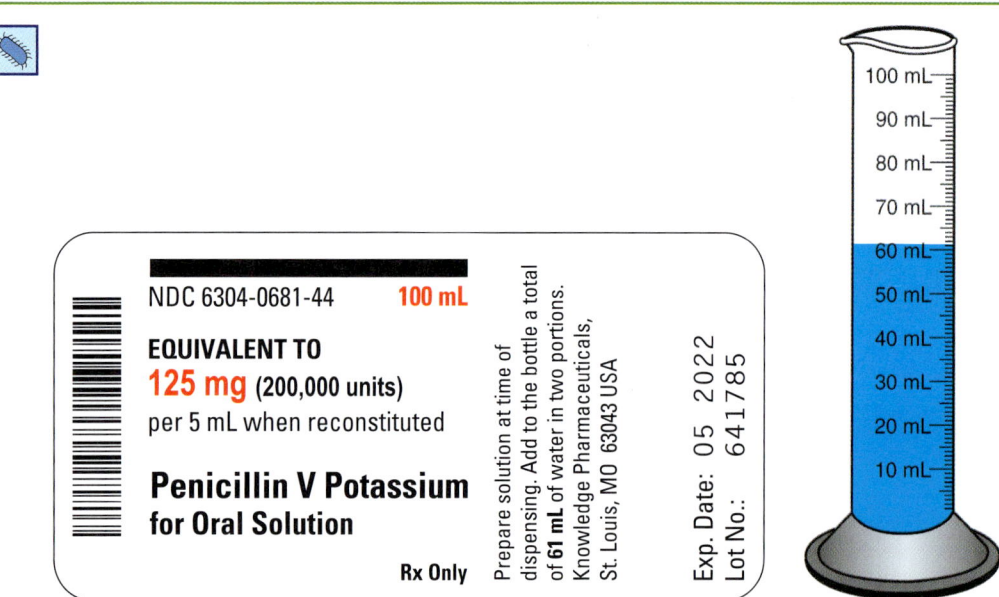

What is the total volume of medication after reconstitution? 100 mL

What diluent is indicated to be added to powder for reconstitution? Water

What volume of diluent is added to the powder? 61 mL

What is the powder volume? 100 mL − 61 mL = 39 mL

What special instructions are given for adding the diluent? Add water in two portions; shake well after each addition

What is the metric strength of the solution after reconstitution? 125 mg/5 mL

What is the medication strength in units? 200,000 units/5 mL

What volume of medication is necessary to provide 125 mg of medication? 5 mL

What volume of medication would be given for 62.5 mg?

$$\frac{125 \text{ mg}}{5 \text{ mL}} = \frac{62.5 \text{ mg}}{x} \quad 125x = 5 \cdot 62.5 \text{ mL} \quad 125x = 312.5 \text{ mL}$$

Divide both sides by 125: $x = 2.5$ mL

Practice Problems B

Answer the following questions. Show your calculations.

1. **FOR ORAL USE ONLY**
    Shake well before each use. Discard unused portion after 14 days.

    MIXING DIRECTIONS
    Tap bottle lightly to loosen powder. Add 24 mL of distilled water to the bottle. Shake well.

    NDC 6304-0002-44 35 mL when reconstituted

    FLUCONAZOLE for Oral Suspension, USP
    10 mg/mL
    *each teaspoonful (5 mL) contains 50 mg of fluconazole when reconstituted
    This package contains 350 mg of fluconazole in orange flavor

    knowledge pharmaceuticals

    Exp. Date: 03 2022
    Lot No.: 70310A

    What is the total volume of medication after reconstitution? _____

    What diluent is indicated to be added to powder for reconstitution? _____

    What volume of diluent is added to the powder? _____

    What is the powder volume?

    What special instructions are given for adding the diluent? _____

    _____

What is the metric strength of the suspension per milliliter after reconstitution? _____

What volume of medication is necessary to provide 50 mg of medication?

What volume of medication is necessary to provide 30 mg of medication?

2.

AMOXICILLIN
125 mg/5mL

Directions for mixing:
Tap bottle until all powder flows freely. Add approx. 2/3 of total water for re-constitution (total of 67 mL). Add remaining water and shake well Must be refrigerated. Discard after 10 days. .

Keep tightly closed.
Shake well before using.

125mg/5mL
NDC 6304-3314-44
AMOXICILLIN/ CLAVULANATE POTASSIUM
FOR ORAL SUSPENSION
When reconstituted, each 5 mL contains:
AMOXICILLIN, 125 MG,
as the trihydrate
CLAVULANIC ACID, 31.25 MG,
as clavulanate potassium
75 mL (when reconstituted)
kp Knowledge Pharmaceuticals

Mfg By:
Knowledge Pharmaceuticals
St. Louis, MO 63043

LOT 170508-A
EXP 05 2020

What two drugs are in this medication? _____

What is the total volume of medication after reconstitution? _____

What volume of diluent should be added? _____

On the graduate, show the volume of diluent to be added.

What is the powder volume?

On the label, what is the first direction necessary for reconstitution? _____

What special directions are necessary when adding the diluent? _____
_____

What volume of medication is necessary for a dose of 250 mg?

What is the volume of this dose in household measurements?

What instructions must be given to the patient when dispensing? _____
_____

3.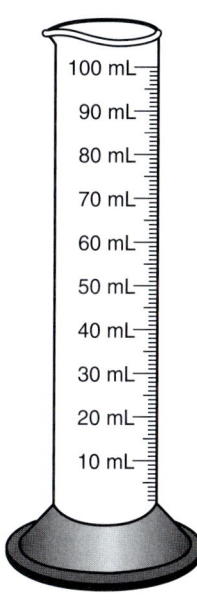

What is the total volume after reconstitution? _____

What diluent is used for reconstitution? _____

What diluent volume is added for reconstitution? _____

Show the amount of diluent on the graduate provided.

What is the powder volume?

What special directions are necessary for reconstitution? _____
_____

What is the medication strength after reconstitution? _____

What directions must be given to the patient? _____

How long can the medication be kept without loss of potency? _____

How many milliliters are necessary for a 375 mg dose?

4.

TO PATIENT:
Shake well before using.
Keep tightly closed.
DIRECTIONS FOR PREPARATION: Slowly add 140 mL of water and shake vigorously to make 200 mL suspension. Store in refrigerator and discard unused portion after ten days.

Mfg by:
Knowledge Pharmaceuticals,
St. Louis, MO 63043 USA

knowledge pharmaceuticals

NDC 6304-3314-44

Erythromycin Ethylsuccinate
for Oral Suspension, USP

200 mg of erythromycin activity per 5 mL reconstituted

200 mL (when mixed)

Exp. Date: 03 2022
Lot No.: 70310A

What is the diluent volume that should be added to the medication when reconstituting to the strength designated on the container? _____

What is the powder volume in the bottle?

What is the strength of the medication after reconstitution? _____

How long is the medication stable after reconstitution when stored in the refrigerator? _____

What information needs to be supplied to the patient when this medication is dispensed? _____

What volume of medication is necessary for a dose of 400 mg?

What is the dose in household measurements?

REVIEW

The same methods for calculation—R&P and DA—are used for oral solid and liquid dosing calculations. Liquid medications are dispensed using the measurements for liquids in the three systems—metric, household, and, rarely, apothecary. Conversions for the correct volume of medication depend on the measurement system to be used for administration. The household system is often used for home delivery of oral medications when a more accurate utensil for administration is not provided. The metric system is used in inpatient settings.

Reconstitution is necessary when a medication is unstable in a liquid form. Most oral antibiotic liquid medications come in powders that require reconstitution with a diluent. Distilled water or purified water USP are the usual diluents used. Always follow the reconstitution directions printed on the medication label exactly to attain the correct strength.

Liquid oral medications may be administered from a medicine cup, dosespoon, oral syringe, medicine dropper, or medication pacifier depending on the volume of medication and the age and ability of the patient. Always provide an appropriate dosage delivery device for oral medications. As with all medications, the proper calculation and appropriate containers for administration are important for patient safety, which should always be the utmost concern.

Posttest

Using the following labels, interpret the orders and calculate the ordered medication doses. Show your calculations. Round to the nearest tenth after completing all calculations. Always make sure the answer is a measurable volume.

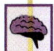
1. Prescribed: Dilantin-125 Suspension 100 mg q8h

   Stock strength available: phenytoin 125 mg/5 mL oral suspension

   What volume of medication is needed per dose?

2. Prescribed: phenobarbital elixir gr $\overline{ss}$ q4h for epilepsy

   Stock strength available: phenobarbital elixir 20 mg/5 mL

   Interpret the order: _____

   _____

   What volume of medication is needed per dose?

3. Prescribed: penicillin V potassium oral solution 0.25 g po qid

   Stock strength available: penicillin V potassium 125 mg/5 mL

   What volume of medication is needed per dose?

   What is the equivalent in household measurements?

   Indicate the amount of medication in the medication cup.

   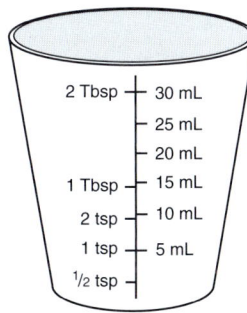

4. Prescribed: Keflex (cephalexin) oral suspension 32 mg q6h

   Stock strength available: 125 mg/5 mL

   What volume of medication is needed per dose?

Posttest, cont.

5. Prescribed: amoxicillin oral suspension 125 mg q8h

Stock strength available: amoxicillin 250 mg/5 mL

What volume of medication is needed per dose?

What is the equivalent in household measurements?

6. Prescribed: Zantac syrup 75 mg bid 30 min ac

Stock strength available: ranitidine 15 mg/mL

Interpret the order: _____

_____

What volume of medication is needed per dose?

What is the equivalent in household measurements?

Indicate the volume of medication on each of the utensils to be used for administration.

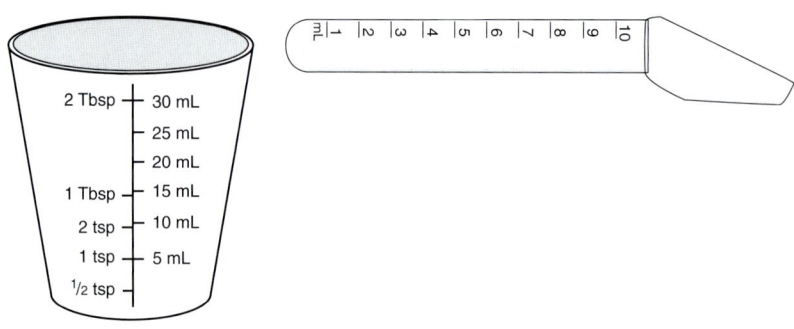

7. Ordered medication: Colace syrup 80 mg po at bedtime

Stock strength: docusate sodium syrup—each teaspoon (5 mL) contains 20 mg docusate

What volume of medication is needed per dose?

Posttest, cont.

8. Prescribed: Duricef Suspension 750 mg po stat then 0.5 g q12h

   Stock strengths available: cefadroxil 250 mg/5 mL and cefadroxil 500 mg/5 mL

   Interpret the order: _____

   _____

   Which strength should be used? _____

   What volume of medication should be given for the stat dose in the metric system?

   What volume of medication should be given for the stat dose in the household system?

   What volume of medication should be given q12h in the metric system?

   What volume of medication should be given q12h in household measurements?

   How would the answers differ if the other strength had to be used? _____

   _____

9. A physician orders Mycostatin Oral Suspension 300,000 units to be administered bid. Each bid dose is then divided evenly for each side of the mouth. The available medication is nystatin oral suspension 100,000 units/mL.

   What total volume of medication should be administered with each dose?

   The dose is to be divided between each side of the mouth; what volume of medication should be placed in each side? _____

Continued

Posttest, cont.

10.

[Label: NDC 6304-0002-19, 75 mL (when mixed), LORACARBEF FOR ORAL SUSPENSION, 200 mg per 5 mL. Directions for mixing - Add 45 mL of water in two portions to the dry mixture in the bottle. Shake well after each addition. Contains Loracarbef equivalent to 3 g of activity. Each 5 mL (Approx. one teaspoonful) will then contain: Loracarbef equivalent to 200 mg of activity. Store at room temperature. May be kept for 14 days without significant loss of potency. Knowledge Pharmaceuticals, St. Louis, MO 63043 USA. Exp. Date: 09 2019. Lot No.: 700509A. 150 mL CEFACLOR FOR ORAL SUSPENSION 200 mg per 5 mL SHAKE WELL BEFORE USE]

What is the total volume after reconstitution? _____

What is used as the diluent for reconstitution? _____

What volume of diluent is added? _____

Show the volume of diluent on the graduate.

What is the powder volume?

What is the medication concentration after reconstitution? _____

What volume of medication is needed for a 400 mg dose in milliliters?

What volume of medication is needed for a 400 mg dose in household measurements?

What are the storage requirements before reconstitution? _____
_____

What are the storage requirements after reconstitution? _____
_____

How long is the medication potent after reconstitution? _____
_____

CHAPTER 10

Calculation of Parenteral Doses

OBJECTIVES

1. Discuss parenteral medications and how they are administered.
2. Measure parenteral medications with the appropriate syringe.
3. Describe ampules and vials, and discuss their uses.
4. Discuss the rules for calculating parenteral medication doses, interpret orders and calculate the volume of parenteral medication necessary to administer doses using either ratio and proportion or dimensional analysis.
5. Describe the following related to reconstitution:
   - Interpret labels of reconstitutable medications to determine correct type and volume of diluent needed, expiration dates, storage conditions before and after reconstitution, and instructions for assigning beyond use dates.
   - Understand the importance of labeling multidose reconstituted medications with date, time, strength, and initials of person performing the reconstitution.
   - Determine the appropriate dilution concentration when more than one dosage strength is possible, and then determine amount of diluent necessary to achieve this concentration.

KEY WORDS

Act-O-Vial System Two-section vial divided by a seal holding a premeasured amount of active ingredient in the lower section and a premeasured diluent in the upper section; mixing occurs when the two sections of the vial are combined either through puncturing the seal or moving the seal through pressure; similar to Mix-O-Vial

Ampule Sealed glass container that holds a single dose of medication, usually for injection

Infusion Slow administration of fluids, other than blood, into a vein

Intradermal Into or within the dermis of the skin (ID)

Intramuscular Into or within the muscle (IM)

Intravenous Into or within a vein (IV)

Large volume parenteral IV bags that are larger than 250 mL; up to 3 L

Parenteral Administration outside the gastrointestinal tract; mostly considered to be by injection or infusion

Piggyback A small volume IV (50 to 250 mL) with added medication administered through an established IV line that is kept patent (open) by a continuous IV solution or by flushing

Subcutaneous Beneath the skin; medications injected into the subcutaneous tissue (Subcut)

Therapeutic range A dosage or blood concentration range that normally produces desired results; too much may be toxic, and too little may not achieve the desired effect and/or not be therapeutic

Vial Glass or plastic container with metal-enclosed rubber seal for injectable medications; may contain single or multiple doses

Pretest

If you are comfortable with the subject matter, perform the following calculations to test your knowledge. If not, work your way through the chapter and return to them for extra practice. Interpret each medication order that follows. Show your calculations. Round answers to nearest tenth.

1. A physician orders Zofran 2 mg IM 30 minutes before chemotherapy treatment. The available medication is Zofran (ondansetron) 2 mg/mL (20 mL multidose vial).

   Interpret the order:
   _____

   How many milliliters should be administered to the patient?

2. The physician orders vitamin B_{12} 500 mcg IM qwk.

   The available medication is cyanocobalamin injection 1,000 mcg/mL

   Interpret the order:
   _____

   How many milliliters should be administered to the patient as a weekly dose?

3. A physician orders meperidine 40 mg IM stat for pain.

   The available strength is meperidine injection 50 mg/mL (1-mL vial)

   Interpret the order: _____

   How many milliliters should be administered?

4. A physician orders 25 mg of meperidine and 25 mg of promethazine IM q4–6h prn for a postsurgical patient with pain and nausea. The drug strengths available are meperidine 50 mg/mL and promethazine 25 mg/mL.

   Interpret the order:
   _____
   _____

   How many milliliters of meperidine are needed per dose?

   How many milliliters of promethazine are needed per dose?

   What is the total amount of medication in milliliters if this is administered in one syringe?

Pretest, cont.

5. A physician ordered streptomycin 750 mg IM.

   After reconstitution, the strength of the medication is streptomycin 400 mg/mL.

   Interpret the order:

   _____

   How many milliliters should be administered for this dose?

6. Ordered medication: codeine phosphate gr s̄s̄ subcut q4h prn

   Stock available: codeine phosphate injection 30 mg (½ gr)/mL (1-mL ampule)

   Interpret the order:

   _____

   How many milliliters should be administered per dose?

7. A physician orders penicillin G 250,000 units IM q4h × 5 d for a child.

DILUENT	FINAL CONCENTRATION
9.6 mL	100,000 units/mL
4.6 mL	200,000 units/mL
1.6 mL	500,000 units/mL

   What is the appropriate concentration to prepare, from a multidose vial with the above choices, to keep the dose volume under 1 mL? _____

   What volume of diluent is needed to meet the requirement for this dose?

   _____

   After reconstitution, what volume of medication is needed per dose?

8. A physician orders ampicillin 500 mg IM q6h.

   The available medication is a 1-g vial with the following information on the label:

   Ampicillin Concentration: 250 mg/mL

   Amount of Diluent: 3.4 mL

   What is the total amount (weight) of medication in the vial?

   _____

   What is the total volume after reconstitution? _____

   What is the powder volume? _____

   What volume of medication is needed for the dose ordered?

INTRODUCTION

Parenteral medications technically include anything administered outside the gastrointestinal tract but are usually considered to be those given by injection or infusion. They are most commonly administered directly within the bloodstream (**intravenously**), within the muscle (**intramuscularly**), under the skin (**subcutaneously**), or within the skin (**intradermally**). With the exception of slow-release injectable medications, which are *never* given intravenously, parenteral medications have a quicker onset of action than oral medications. Injectable medications may be given if a person is unable to swallow solid medications, if a quicker effect is needed, if the person is combative, or if the particular medication would be degraded by stomach acid.

> **! TECH ALERT**
>
> All medications administered by injection must be in a sterile liquid form. Once these medications have been injected, the medication cannot be retrieved, so special care is needed to ensure that the medication and its dose are correct before administration.

Most parenteral medications are available in **ampules** or **vials** (Fig. 10.1) and are most often prepared as a liquid either in an aqueous (water) or occasionally in an oil base by the drug manufacturer. Some medications, especially those used for cardiac emergencies, are supplied as prefilled syringes from the manufacturer. Medications that are not stable in the liquid form come in powders and crystals that must be reconstituted before administration. These medications are not stable in liquid form for an extended period of time, so stability must be considered at the time of reconstitution and administration.

As with oral liquid medications, strengths of parenteral medications are identified as weight of medication in a specific volume of liquid. The weight is usually provided in the metric system—milligrams, grams, and micrograms—and the volume in milliliters. The apothecary system's units of grains per milliliter may also be used, although this is not as

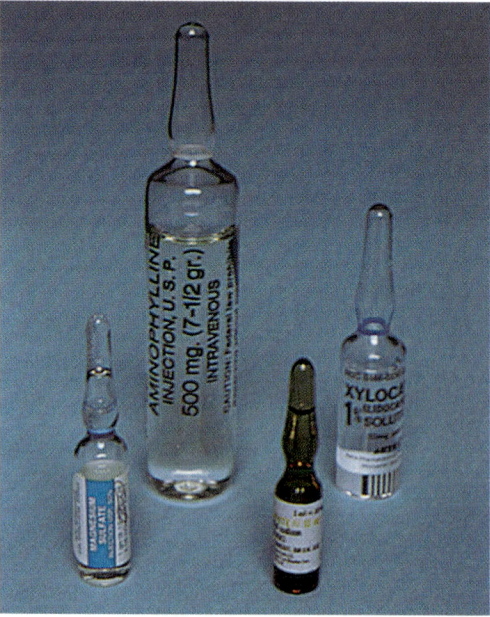 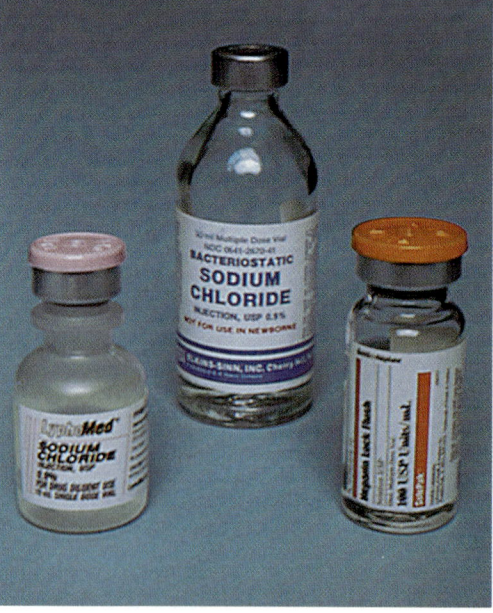

FIGURE 10.1 Typical ampule and vial containers. (Potter P, Perry A: *Fundamentals of Nursing*, ed 9, St. Louis, Mosby, 2017.)

common today as it was previously. International units and mEq are found with injectable medications as well. Some parenteral medications are expressed in percentage or ratio strengths, but these are usually also expressed on the manufacturer's label in weight per volume strengths.

> **TECH NOTE**
>
> The label will express weight per volume, such as mcg/mL, mg/mL, g/mL, units/mL, mEq/mL, and occasionally gr/mL.

Syringes

Because all parenteral medications must be prepared using sterile technique, sterile needles and syringes must be used. Pharmacy staff commonly use syringes ranging from 1 to 60 mL in size when preparing parenteral medication. Tuberculin (TB) syringes have a 1-mL capacity and are calibrated in 0.01-mL increments (Fig. 10.2). Three-milliliter syringes are calibrated in 0.1-mL increments (Fig. 10.3). Five-milliliter and ten-milliliter syringes are calibrated in 0.2-mL increments (Fig. 10.4). Twenty-milliliter syringes are calibrated in 1-mL increments. Sixty-milliliter syringes are calibrated in 2-mL increments.

> **TECH NOTE**
>
> The calibrations between markings on a syringe are usually found as four spaces, as in increments of 0.1 mL on the 3-mL syringe or 0.2 mL on the 5-mL syringe. Always be sure to understand the markings before using the syringe for preparing medications to ensure that the correct amount of medication is being prepared.

Once the parenteral dose has been calculated, the correct syringe must be chosen based on the amount of medication to be administered or added to other intravenous fluids. If the volume of a medication dose is less than 1 mL, it should be measured with a 1-mL TB syringe except in the case of insulin U-100, which is measured in specially calibrated insulin syringes (covered in detail in Chapter 11). Doses less than 1 mL that require rounding are generally rounded to the hundredth place because that is measurable on a TB syringe. A 3-mL syringe is the usual choice for measuring volumes between 1 mL and 3 mL, which would be rounded to the tenths position if necessary. A 5-mL syringe is used for doses between 3 and 5 mL, and a 10-mL syringe is used for doses between 5 and 10 mL. These doses should also be rounded to the tenths position if necessary. A 20-mL syringe is generally used when measuring medication to be added to a larger bag of IV fluid or for an IV push.

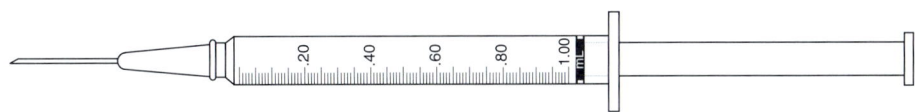

FIGURE 10.2 Typical tuberculin syringe measured in 0.01 mL. (Fulcher EM, Soto CD, Fulcher RM: *Pharmacology: Principles and Applications*, ed 3, St. Louis, Saunders, 2012.)

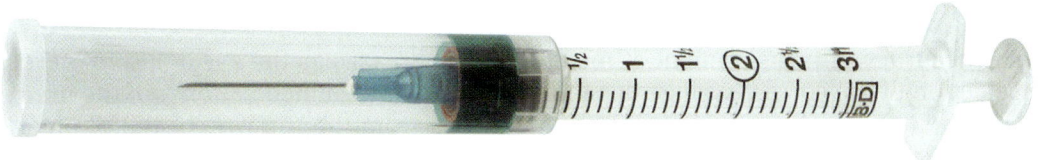

FIGURE 10.3 BD Safety-LOK 3-mL syringe. (Courtesy and copyright Becton, Dickinson and Company.)

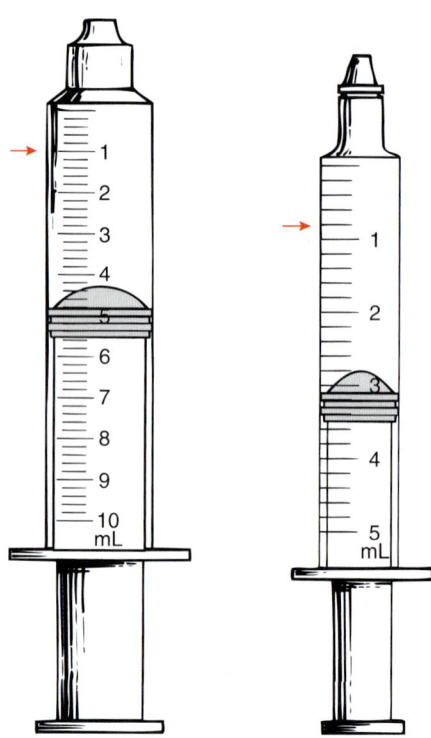

FIGURE 10.4 Measurement of liquids in larger syringes in 0.2-mL increments. (Brown M, Mulholland JM: *Drug Calculations: Process and Problems for Clinical Practice*, ed 8, St. Louis, Mosby, 2008.)

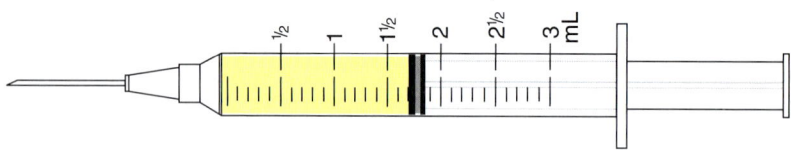

FIGURE 10.5 Syringe containing a volume of 1.7 mL. (Fulcher EM, Soto CD, Fulcher RM: *Pharmacology: Principles and Applications*, ed 3, St. Louis, Saunders, 2012.)

Parenteral medications may be prepared for direct administration to a patient or for addition to a **piggyback** (50-mL to 250-mL) or **large-volume** (over 250 mL) IV bag. Some medications *must be further diluted* to be safely administered to a patient.

> **TECH NOTE**
> Large syringes are seldom used for medication administration (other than an IV push) but are frequently used in the preparation of intravenous fluids.

The accuracy of measurement of medications decreases as the syringe size increases. The selection of the correct syringe depends on the volume of medication and the precision needed. The liquid volume in a syringe is measured from the top ring of the plunger, not the raised portion in the middle. In Fig. 10.4, the 10-mL syringe is pulled back to the 4.8-mL mark and the 5-mL syringe to the 3.1-mL position (halfway between the 3.0 mL and 3.2-mL marks). Fig. 10.5 indicates 1.7 mL, and Fig. 10.6 indicates 2.3 mL.

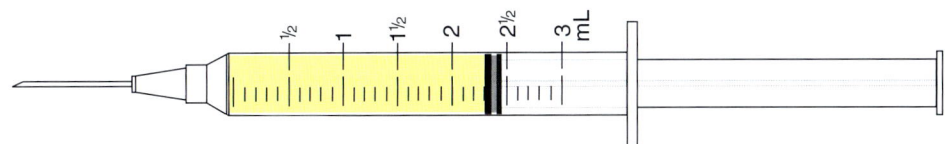

FIGURE 10.6 Syringe containing a volume of 2.3 mL. (Fulcher EM, Soto CD, Fulcher RM: *Pharmacology: Principles and Applications*, ed 3, St. Louis, Saunders, 2012.)

Practice Problems A

Record the amount in the syringes for numbers 1 through 4 and mark the correct amount on the syringes in numbers 6 through 10. Remember to write your answers with decimals, since mL is a metric measurement, even though some of the syringes are labeled with fractions!

1. The amount in the syringe is _____.

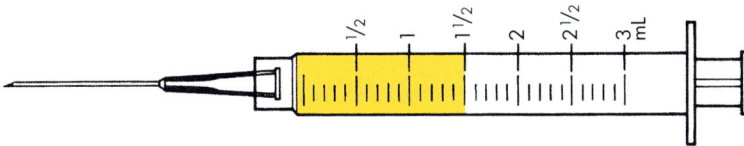

2. The amount in the syringe is _____.

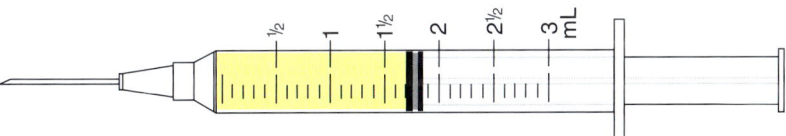

3. The amount in the syringe is _____.

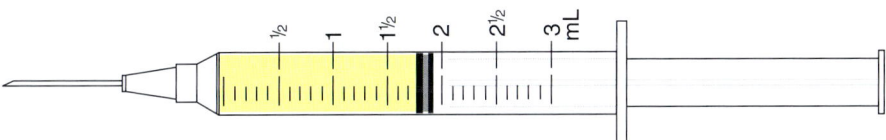

4. The amount in the syringe is _____.

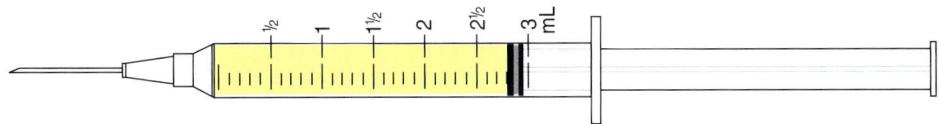

5. Indicate 9.4 mL.

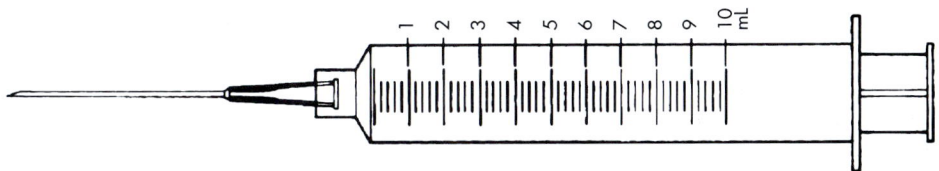

6. Indicate 0.64 mL.

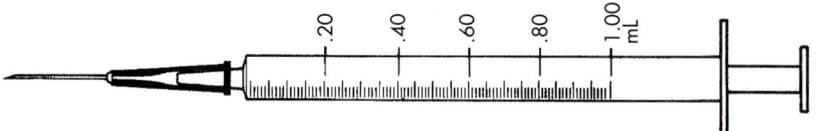

7. Indicate 6.8 mL.

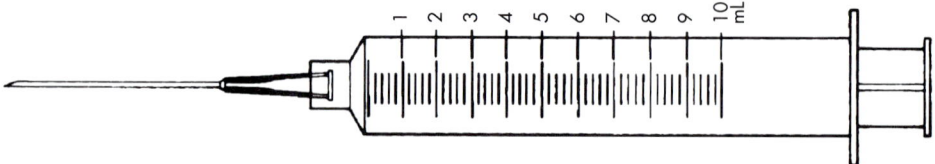

8. Indicate 1.8 mL.

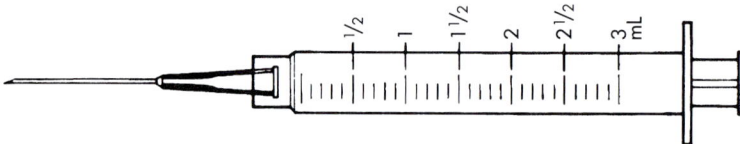

9. Indicate 3.4 mL.

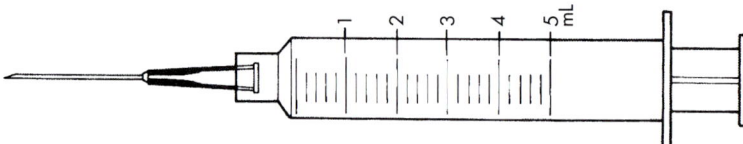

10. Indicate 8.6 mL.

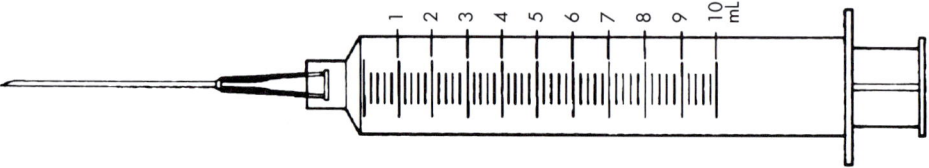

Ampules and Vials

Injectable medications are provided in vials or ampules (see Fig. 10.1). Some are also supplied in prefilled syringes. Ampules are sealed glass containers, which may only be used once because there is no way to ensure sterility after they have been opened. The use of a filter needle is required when withdrawing medication from ampules in case any glass shards entered the product when it was opened. Vials have a rubber top and are available in single-dose or multidose vials. Multidose vials contain preservatives, whereas single-dose vials do not. Single-dose vials and ampules are slightly overfilled, but the concentration is as written on the label. Powders for reconstitution may come in either multidose or single-dose vials or even in **Act-O-Vials** (Fig. 10.7). Most sterile liquids used for reconstitution are also supplied in vials.

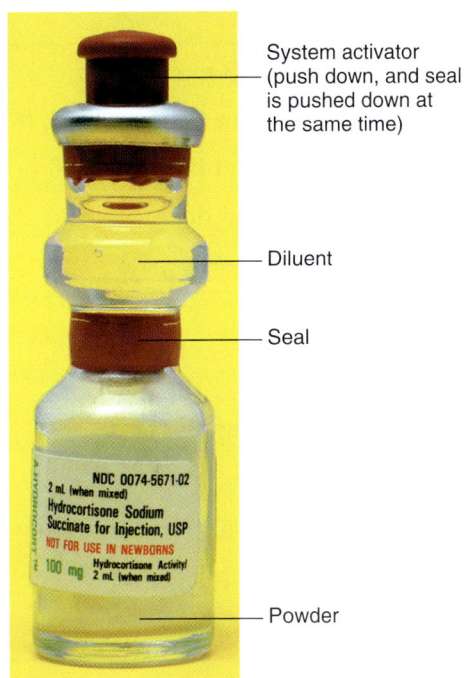

FIGURE 10.7 An Act-O-Vial.

Amounts of Medicine

When calculating parenteral doses, it is important to know the appropriate volumes for the various routes of administration. The intradermal injection limit is 0.1 mL. Medications given subcutaneously are usually less than 1 mL but may go as high as 2 mL in some instances. Small-volume IM injections are less than 3 mL, and IM injections into larger muscles can be up to 5 mL. If your calculations do not yield an answer within these parameters, there is most likely an error in your calculations or the prescribed amount.

CALCULATING PARENTERAL MEDICATION DOSES

The rules for calculating parenteral doses are the same as those for oral liquid medications. The same formulas are used, and the calculations are the same; however, the dose volume is generally not as large. If more than one dosage strength is available with parenteral medications, the strength that requires the smallest volume of medication to be administered is the dosage strength that should be used for that drug order, unless the medication is available in a strength that will provide an easily measurable amount to the exact readings for the markings on the syringe.

TECH NOTE

Many medications for IV use may not be given directly from the vial but require even further dilution in intravenous fluid before administration.

EXAMPLE 10.1

Prescribed: Tagamet (cimetidine HCl) 75 mg IM q6h

Stock available: cimetidine HCl injection 300 mg/2 mL (8 mL multidose vial)

Interpret the order: Tagamet 75 mg intramuscularly every 6 hours

Volume of medication to be given for a single dose:

Ratio and proportion (R & P) $\dfrac{300 \text{ mg}}{2 \text{ mL}} = \dfrac{75 \text{ mg}}{x}$ $300x = 150 \text{ mL}$ $x = 0.5 \text{ mL}$

OR

Dimensional analysis (DA) $\text{mL} = \dfrac{2 \text{ mL}}{300 \text{ mg}} \cdot \dfrac{75 \text{ mg}}{1}$
$= 0.5 \text{ mL}$

This is an IM dose, and it is within the allowable volume range.

What is the appropriate size syringe for administering this dose? 1-mL TB syringe

EXAMPLE 10.2

Prescribed: aminophylline 125 mg IV q6h

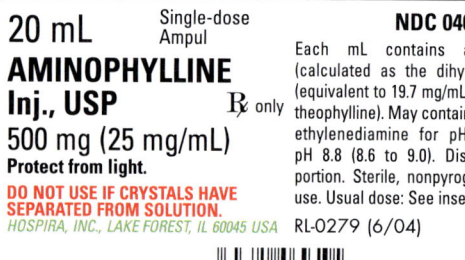

© Pfizer. Used with permission.

Interpret the order: aminophylline 125 mg intravenously every 6 hours

When interpreting this label, the strength of the medication can be read as 500 mg/20 mL or 25 mg/mL. These are equivalent fractions. The entire 20 mL ampule contains 500 mg, but only part of this is needed for each dose. Either strength designation may be used to calculate the dose, but the smaller numbers keep the calculations more simple. After reviewing the following examples, rework them replacing 500 mg/20 mL with 25 mg/mL to see that you reach the same answer.

What volume of medication needs to be given for a single dose?

R & P $\dfrac{500 \text{ mg}}{20 \text{ mL}} = \dfrac{125 \text{ mg}}{x}$ $500x = 2{,}500 \text{ mL}$ $x = 5 \text{ mL}$

OR

DA $\text{mL} = \dfrac{20 \text{ mL}}{500 \text{ mg}} \cdot \dfrac{125 \text{ mg}}{1} = 5 \text{ mL}$

Chapter 10 Calculation of Parenteral Doses

! **TECH ALERT**

If the answer to a dose calculation does not agree with an anticipated answer based on the amount of medication prescribed, the dose of medication on hand, or the intended route of administration, ALWAYS recalculate. Ask for assistance if necessary!

Some parenteral doses require rounding to a measurable quantity. Usually if an injectable dose is less than 1 mL, it should be rounded to the nearest hundredth. Once rounded, the dose should generally be within a 10% margin. Some medications require rounding to be within a much lower percentage of variation. This is due to the narrow *therapeutic range* between effectiveness and toxicity levels.

! **TECH ALERT**

Usually, if an injectable dose is less than 1 mL, it should be rounded to the nearest hundredth. If you have questions regarding acceptable rounding techniques, ask a pharmacist for assistance.

Practice Problems B

Use the method of calculation with which you are most comfortable, R&P or DA, to complete these problems. Remember that DA is best for multistep conversions to keep track of units. Round to the nearest tenth unless the dose is less than 1 mL, and then round to the nearest hundredth.

1. Prescribed: morphine sulfate 15 mg IM q4h prn pain

    Stock available: morphine sulfate 25 mg/mL (1-mL preservative-free vial)

    Interpret the order: _____

    _____

    What volume of medication is needed for one dose?

2. Prescribed: prochlorperazine 10 mg IM q6h prn N&V

    Stock available: prochlorperazine injection 5 mg/mL (2-mL vial)

    Interpret the order: _____

    _____

    What volume of medication is needed for one dose?

3. Prescribed: Nebcin (tobramycin) 60 mg IM q8h (This is an example of a medication with a narrow therapeutic range that requires monitoring of medication levels.)

   Stock available: tobramycin sulfate injection 80 mg/2 mL (2-mL vial)

   Interpret the order:

   _____

   What volume of medication is needed for one dose?

   Indicate the correct amount of medication on the appropriate syringe.

   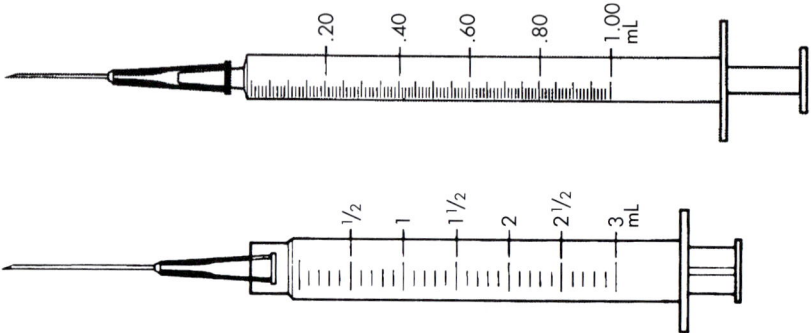

4. Prescribed: vitamin B_{12} 1 mg IM qwk × 4 wk

   Stock available: cyanocobalamin injection 1,000 mcg/mL (10-mL multidose vial)

   Interpret the order:

   _____

   What volume of medication is needed for one dose?

5. Prescribed: meperidine 75 mg IM q4–6h prn pain

   The following strengths are available:

   A. Meperidine injection 25 mg/mL (1-mL vial)

   B. Meperidine injection 50 mg/mL (1-mL vial)

   C. Meperidine injection 100 mg/mL (1-mL vial)

Interpret the order: _____

_____

Which strength should be used for this order? Hint: This is an IM injection. _____

Why did you choose this vial? _____

_____

What volume of medication is needed per dose?

Indicate the correct amount of medication on the appropriate syringe.

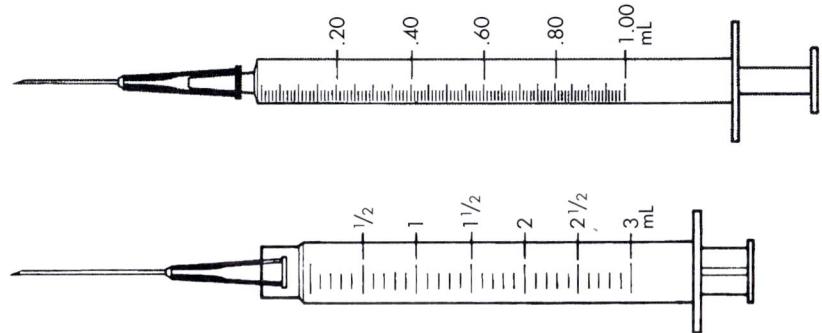

6. Prescribed: Cogentin 1.5 mg IM daily

Stock available: benztropine injection 2 mg/2 mL (2-mL single-dose vial)

Interpret the order: _____

_____

What volume of medication is needed for one dose?

Indicate the correct amount of medication on the appropriate syringe.

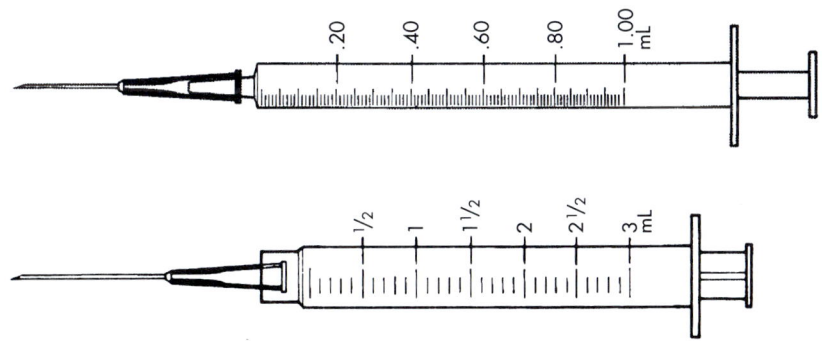

7. Dose ordered: vitamin K 2 mg IM stat

Stock available: vitamin K1 (phytonadione) injectable emulsion 10 mg/mL (1 mL single-dose ampule)

Interpret the order: _____

_____

What volume of medication is needed for the dose?

Indicate the correct amount of medication on the appropriate syringe.

8. Prescribed: amikacin 250 mg IM q8h

Stock strength: amikacin sulfate injection 500 mg/2 mL (2-mL vial)

Interpret the order: _____

_____

What volume of medication is needed for one dose?

9. Prescribed: hydroxyzine 75 mg and meperidine 50 mg IM stat

Stock strengths available:

Hydroxyzine HCl injection 50 mg/mL (10-mL multidose vial for IM use only)

Meperidine injection 100 mg/mL (1-mL ampule) CII

Interpret the order: _____

_____

What volume of hydroxyzine is needed for this dose?

What volume of meperidine is needed for this dose?

Indicate the volume of combined medication needed on the syringe.

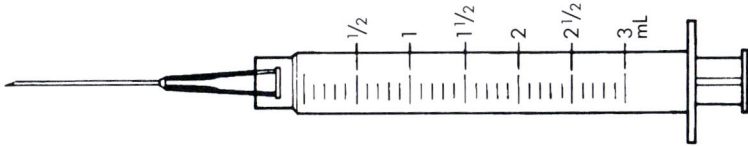

10. Prescribed: Cleocin 0.25 g IM stat then q8h

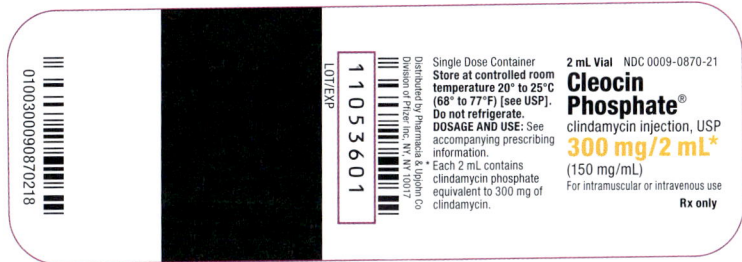

© Pfizer. Used with permission.

Interpret the order: _____

_____

What volume of medication is needed for one dose?

Indicate the correct amount of medication on the appropriate syringe.

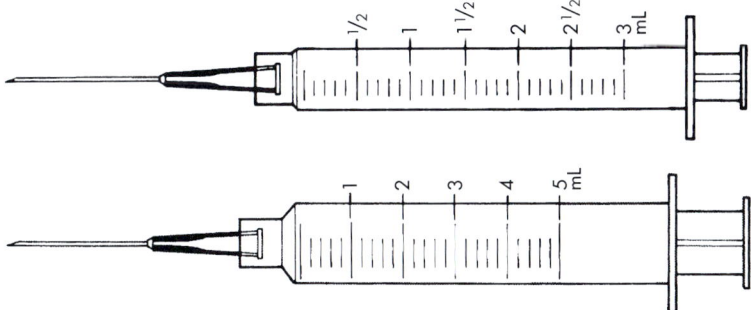

11. Prescribed: lincomycin 0.45 g IM stat

Stock available: lincomycin injection 300 mg/mL (2-mL vial)

Interpret the order: _____

_____

What volume of medication is needed for this dose?

12. **ENDO** Prescribed: Solu-Cortef 125 mg IM stat

Interpret the order: _____

_____

What volume of medication is needed for this dose?

13. Prescribed: Depo-Provera 0.3 g IM qmo

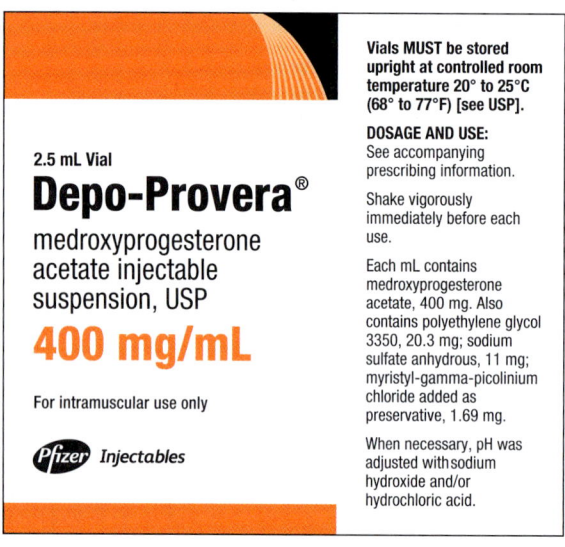

© Pfizer. Used with permission.

Interpret the order: _____

_____

What volume of medication is needed for one dose?

14. **PAIN** Prescribed: codeine gr ¾ IM q4h prn severe pain

   Stock strength: codeine phosphate injection 30 mg/mL (1-mL ampule) CII
   Interpret the order: _____

   _____

   What volume of medication is needed for one dose?

   What weight of medication in mg is needed for one dose?

RECONSTITUTION

Parenteral medications that are unstable in liquid form for extended periods of time are manufactured in a powdered form for reconstitution before use. The manufacturer's label states the total quantity of the drug in the container, the volume and type of diluent to use to attain the desired strength, the final strength of the medication after reconstitution, and the stability and storage requirements before and after reconstitution. To reconstitute a medication, follow the instructions on the medication label *exactly*. Before using, the dry medication must be completely dissolved in the diluent.

TECH NOTE
The directions on the label should be read carefully first and followed exactly to prevent errors in the reconstitution process.

Some injectable powders are manufactured with the diluent and powder in two separate chambers, such as hydrocortisone sodium succinate in Fig. 10.7. This particular system is called the Act-O-Vial system. In this case, when the plunger is dislodged by a push, the diluent drops from the upper chamber into the lower chamber, which contains the medication.

With injectable medications, the manufacturer may recommend the use of either sterile water for injection or sterile normal saline. Some drugs may require bacteriostatic water for IM injections or even require specific diluents, such as those with a small amount of anesthetic to prevent discomfort with IM administration. When a special diluent is necessary, this diluent may be packaged separately and supplied with the medication, as with some immunizations. If the solution for reconstitution is not indicated, consult a drug reference. Remember that the final volume of medication in the container will always be greater than the amount of diluent added because of powder volume.

Once the appropriate diluent has been identified, the amount of diluent for the desired dose must be verified. Vials of some multidose parenteral drugs may be diluted with different volumes of diluent to attain different concentrations for different routes of administration, as shown on the Pfizerpen label in Fig. 10.8. The directions on the label should be followed exactly to ensure that the correct type and amount of diluent are used. Read the possible concentrations or strengths after reconstitution, because the desired volume must match the intended route of administration.

! TECH ALERT
Never assume the directions are the same as previously found on the same medication—READ the label directions every time medication is reconstituted.

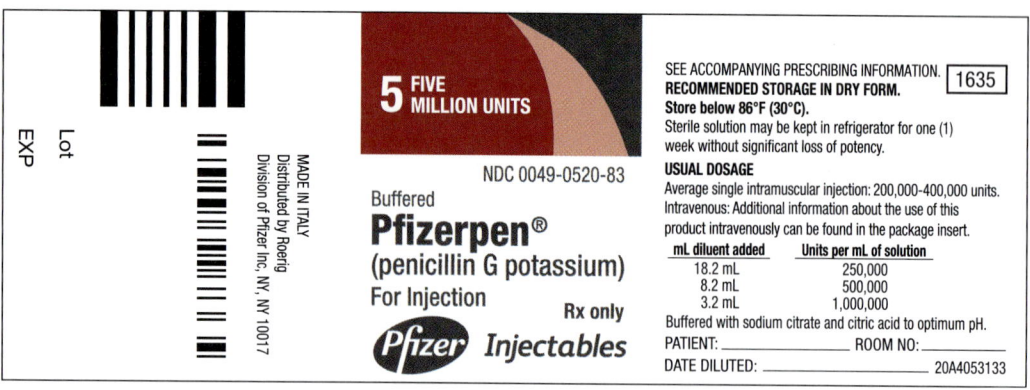

FIGURE 10.8 Label showing the volume of diluent necessary for reconstituting to a particular strength when multiple doses are a possibility. (© Pfizer. Used with permission.)

TECH NOTE

The less diluent added to a specific container of medication, the more concentrated the medication. When reconstituting medications with multiple strengths possible, choose the strength closest to the physician's order that will provide a dose appropriate for the intended route of administration and with the least chance for error.

Decide on the amount of diluent to add and prepare this for use. In Fig. 10.9, the label reads to add 2.7 mL of Sterile Water for Injection, USP. After injecting diluent, the mixing process for an injectable medication is accomplished by inverting the container slowly, unless otherwise indicated by the manufacturer. Shaking the container may decrease the effectiveness of some medication and may cause the liquid to foam. Foaming will make it difficult to withdraw the correct amount of medication.

Note the length of time that the medication is stable and the directions for storage both before and after reconstitution. In Fig. 10.9, the directions for storage read: Discard solution after 3 days at room temperature or 7 days under refrigeration. After the powder has been mixed, the person who reconstituted it should write the following on the label if it is to be used again:

- Their initials
- The date and time prepared
- The beyond-use date and time (For Fig. 10.9, indicate BUD based on whether it is stored at room temperature or in the refrigerator and include this on label)
- The strength to which it was reconstituted. (e.g., 500 mg/3 mL)

TECH NOTE

Patient safety is of utmost importance and should be safeguarded throughout each step of handling medications.

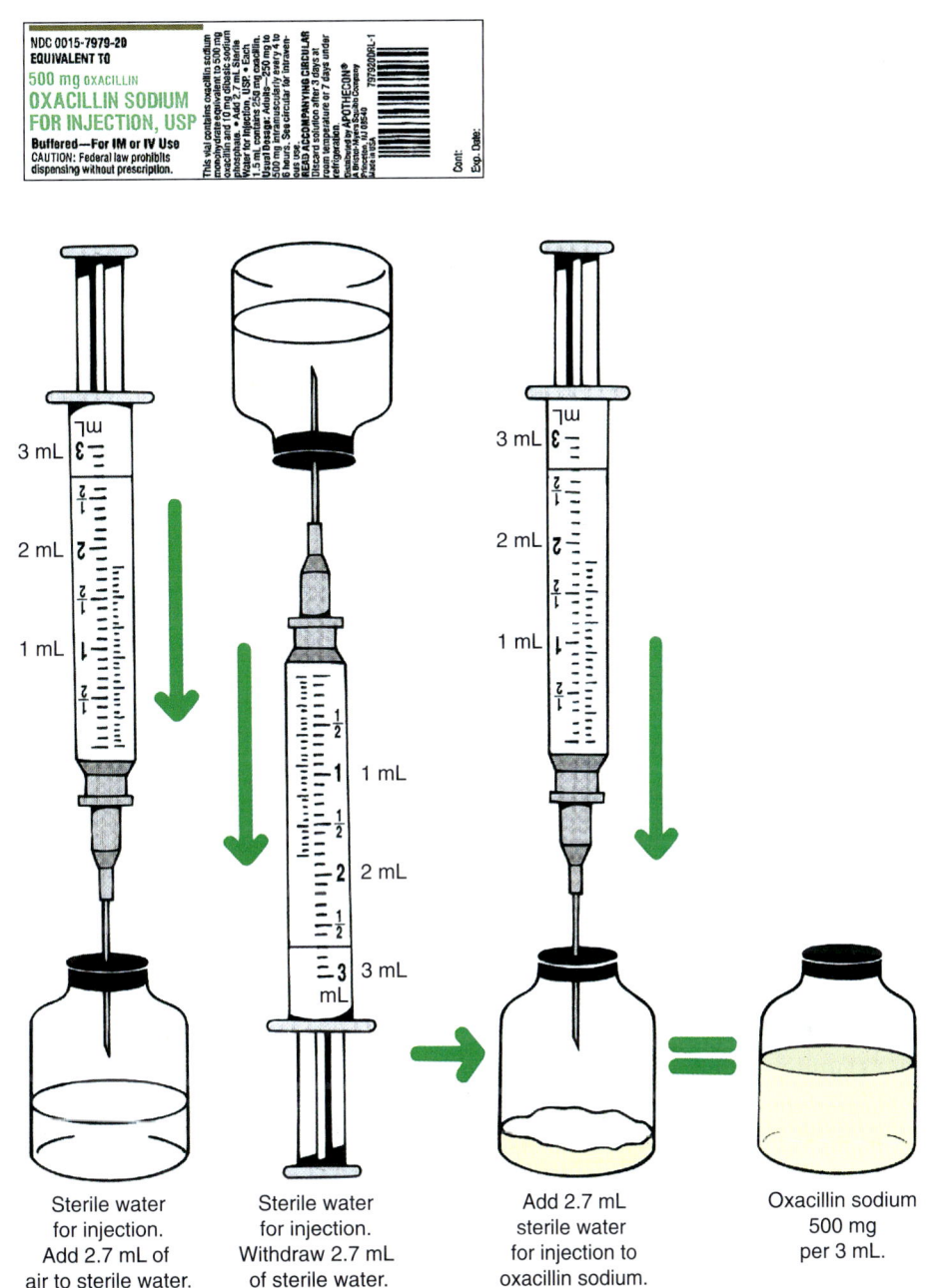

FIGURE 10.9 Diluting oxacillin sodium in sterile water for injection. (Brown M, Mulholland JM: *Drug Calculations: Process and Problems for Clinical Practice*, ed 8, St. Louis, Mosby, 2008.)

EXAMPLE 10.3

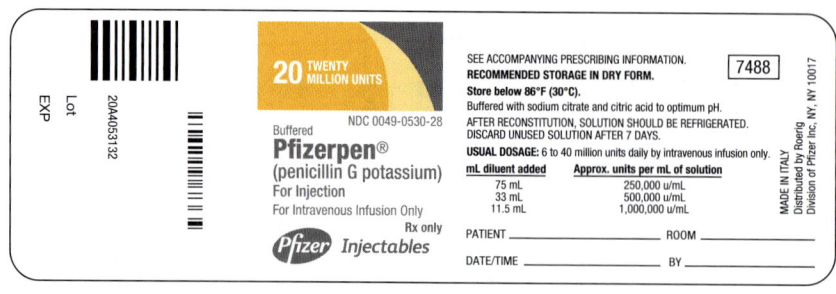

© Pfizer. Used with permission.

What is the total dosage found in the container? *20 million units or 20,000,000 units*

If 75 mL of diluent is added to the container, what is the strength per mL? *250,000 units/mL*

If 11.5 mL of diluent is added, what is the strength per mL? *1,000,000 units/mL*

What is the route of administration for this medication? *IV infusion only*

What diluent is needed for reconstitution? *Consult accompanying prescribing information*

How long is the medication stable in the refrigerator after reconstitution? *7 days*

If the medication is reconstituted to 250,000 units/mL, how many milliliters are needed for a dose of 375,000 units?

$$\frac{250,000 \text{ units}}{1 \text{ mL}} = \frac{375,000 \text{ units}}{x} \quad 250,000x = 375,000 \text{ mL} \quad x = 1.5 \text{ mL}$$

If reconstituted to 1,000,000 units/mL, how many milliliters would be needed for a dose of 2,500,000 units?

$$\frac{1,000,000 \text{ units}}{1 \text{ mL}} = \frac{2,500,000 \text{ units}}{x} \quad x = 2.5 \text{ mL}$$

! **TECH ALERT**

Be aware that medications for intramuscular (IM) and intravenous (IV) use are not interchangeable! The label on the medication will state its exact use. Some medications will indicate that IM or IV use is acceptable but will usually show a difference in the amount of diluent to be added.

Practice Problems C

Answer the following questions and make necessary calculations as indicated.

1.

Pfizerpen® (penicillin G potassium) For Injection
5 Million Units
NDC 0049-0520-83

mL diluent added	Units per mL of solution
18.2 mL	250,000
8.2 mL	500,000
3.2 mL	1,000,000

© Pfizer. Used with permission.

What is the total dosage of medication in this vial? _____

If 18.2 mL of diluent is added, what is the strength per milliliter? _____

If 8.2 mL of diluent is added, what is the strength per milliliter? _____

If 3.2 mL of diluent is added, what is the strength per milliliter? _____

What routes of administration can be used with this medication? _____

_____

After dilution, how long can the medication be stored in the refrigerator without a loss of potency? _____

What is the volume of the powder displacement?

If you reconstituted this medication on 9/20/20XX at 0130 with 8.2 mL of diluent, what information should you place on the label?

_____

_____

_____

_____

2.

Label information:
- NDC 0069-3150-84 Rx only
- Zithromax® (azithromycin for injection)
- 500 mg
- For I.V. infusion only
- STERILE equivalent to 500 mg of azithromycin
- No Latex No Preservative
- Store at or below 86°F (30°C).
- DOSAGE AND USE: See accompanying prescribing information.
- Constitute to 100 mg/mL* with 4.8 mL of Sterile Water For Injection.
- Must be further diluted before use. For appropriate diluents and storage recommendations, refer to prescribing information.
- *Each mL contains azithromycin dihydrate equivalent to 100 mg of azithromycin, 76.9 mg of citric acid, and sodium hydroxide for pH adjustment.
- MADE IN IRELAND
- DISTRIBUTED BY PFIZER LABS DIVISION OF PFIZER INC, NY, NY 10017
- Pfizer Injectables

© Pfizer. Used with permission.

What is the diluent to be used for reconstitution? _____

How much diluent should be added? _____

What is the strength after reconstitution? _____

What is the total volume of medication after reconstitution? _____

What is the route of administration for this medication? _____

What are the special administration instructions to follow after reconstitution?
_____

What volume of stock medication is needed to provide 0.5 g?

What volume of stock medication is needed to provide 300 mg?

REVIEW

Calculations with parenteral medications can be performed with ratio and proportion (R&P) or ratio and proportion (R&P) for single-step calculations and DA for multistep calculations. Parenteral medications are supplied in single-dose vials, multidose vials, ampules and prefilled syringes. Reconstitution is necessary when a medication is provided in powdered form due to instability in a liquid form. When medications are prepared for injectable routes, the required diluent may be sterile water for injection, bacteriostatic water for injection, 0.9% sodium chloride (normal saline) injectable, *or* a special solution provided with the medication by the manufacturer. After reconstitution, parenteral medications require special storage conditions and beyond use dates due to the instability of the liquid formulations. Some medications can be diluted to different strengths or concentrations as directed by the manufacturers, whereas others have only one dilution strength option. Always read medication labels before preparing parenteral products.

The necessary steps when reconstituting medications are as follows:

1. Read all of the directions on the medication label.
2. Tap the bottle to loosen the powder in the vial.
3. Use the diluent designated by the manufacturer in the amount appropriate for the strength of medication needed. If this information is not on the vial, use the package insert or drug reference to determine the appropriate diluent and amount.
4. After reconstitution of multidose vials, label the medication with the initials of the person who reconstituted it, the date and time of reconstitution, the strength of the medication, and the beyond use date and time.

Posttest

Using the following labels, interpret the orders and calculate the medication doses. Show all calculations. Round the final answer to the nearest tenth unless the dose is less than 1 mL, and then round to the nearest hundredth.

1. Medication order: butorphanol 1 mg IM stat for pain

    Stock available: butorphanol tartrate injection 2 mg/mL (1 mL vial)

    Interpret the order: _____

    _____

    What volume of medication is needed for the dose?

    Indicate the correct amount of medication on the appropriate syringe.

    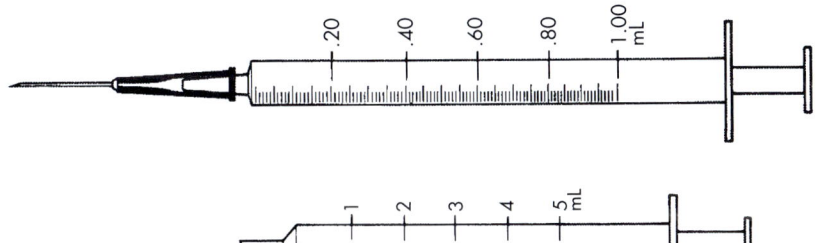

    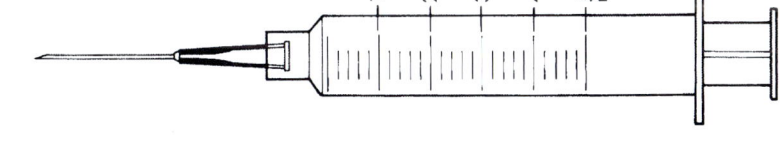

2. Medication order: gentamicin 0.06 g IM q8h

    Stock available: gentamicin injection 40 mg/mL

    Interpret the order: _____

    _____

    What volume of medication is needed per dose?

    Indicate the correct amount of medication on the appropriate syringe.

Continued

Posttest, cont.

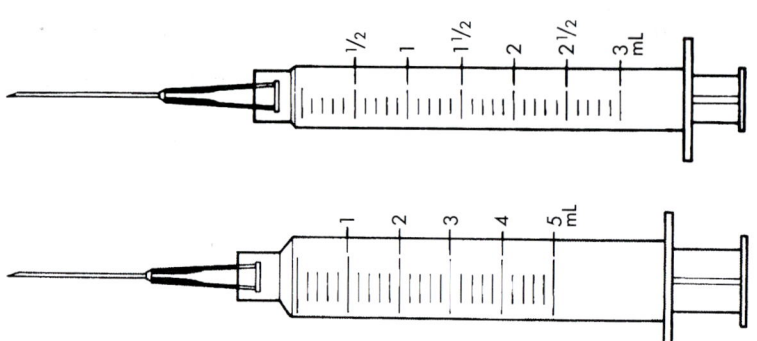

3. Medication order: Solu-Medrol 37.5 mg IM stat

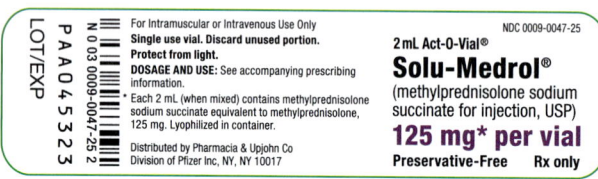

© Pfizer. Used with permission.

Interpret the order: _____

What volume of medication is needed per dose?

Indicate the correct amount of medication on the appropriate syringe.

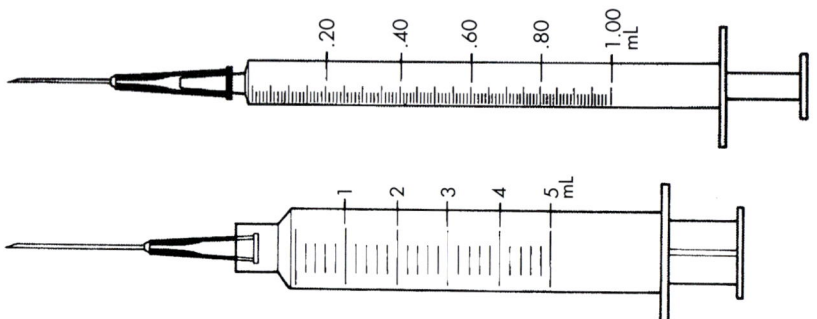

4. Medication order: diazepam 2 mg IM stat and then q6h prn for anxiety

Stock strength available: diazepam injection 5 mg/mL

Interpret the order: _____

_____

What volume of medication is needed per dose?

Posttest, cont.

5. Medication order: Dilaudid (hydromorphone) 500 mcg IM q4h prn severe pain

   Stock medication available: hydromorphone injection 2 mg/mL (1 mL vial)

   Interpret the order: _____

   _____

   What volume of medication is needed per dose?

   Indicate the correct amount of medication on the appropriate syringe.

   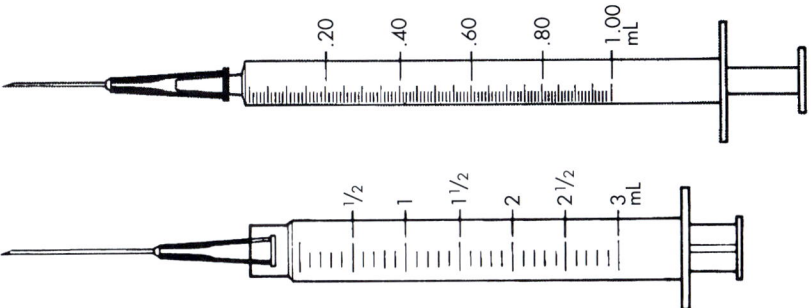

6. Medication order: digoxin 0.1 mg IM stat then daily

   Stock strength available: digoxin 500 mcg/2 mL injection

   Interpret the order: _____

   _____

   What is the stock strength in mg/mL? _____

   What volume of medication is needed per dose?

7. A physician orders Acthar Gel 50 units IM stat. The medication on hand is Acthar Gel-12 80 units/mL.

   Interpret the order: _____

   What measureable volume of medication should be given to the patient?

   What type of syringe should be used to administer this medication?

   _____

Continued

Posttest, cont.

8. Medication order: Garamycin 30 mg IM q8h
   Stock strength available: gentamycin 40 mg/mL injection (20 mL multidose vial)
   Interpret the order: _____
   What volume of medication is needed per dose?

9. Medication order: meperidine 50 mg IM q4h prn pain
   Stock strengths available: meperidine 75 mg/mL and meperidine 100 mg/mL
   Interpret the order: _____
   What volume of medication is needed per dose using meperidine 75 mg/mL?

   What volume of medication is needed per dose using meperidine 100 mg/mL?

   Which strength of meperidine would you choose to use? _____

10. A physician orders KCl 20 mEq in 1 L IV fluids for a patient with electrolyte imbalance.

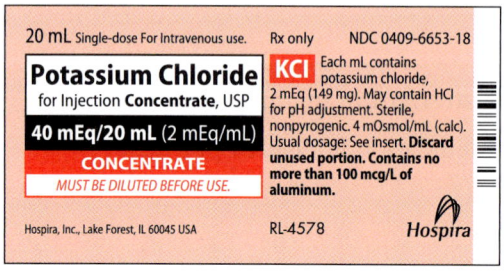

© Pfizer. Used with permission.

What is the mEq/mL strength of this vial? _____
What is the total *volume* of medication of the vial? _____
What is the total *amount (mEq)* of medication in the vial? _____
What volume of medication should be added to the liter of IV fluids for this order?

Indicate this amount on the following syringe.

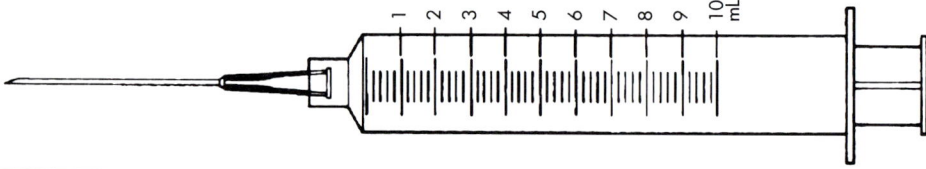

CHAPTER 11

Unit Calculations With Anticoagulants and Insulin

OBJECTIVES

1. Discuss calculating doses in units, and calculate insulin doses measured in units.
2. Calculate anticoagulant doses measured in units.

KEY WORDS

Anticoagulant Substance that stops or delays the clotting of blood

High-alert medications Medications that have a higher risk of causing significant harm to a patient if dosed or used incorrectly

International unit/Unit A *specific unit* of measurement used for biologicals; describes a standard amount of an *individual* drug that can produce a given biologic effect specific to that drug alone; a measurement of a medication's action as opposed to its weight; units of one substance are *not* equivalent to the same number of units of another substance

Patent Open and unobstructed as in IV lines or blood vessels

Pretest

If you are already comfortable with the subject matter, perform the following calculations to test your knowledge. If not, work your way through the chapter and return to them for extra practice. If syringes are included, indicate the volume of medication to be administered on the correct syringe, based on the route of administration, to provide the most accurate dose. Show your calculations. Round any dose less than 1 mL to the nearest hundredth and those over 1 mL to the nearest tenth.

1. A physician orders heparin sodium 1,500 units subcut stat.

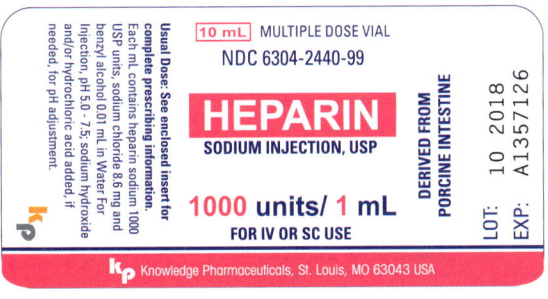

Interpret the medication order: _____

_____

What is the measurable volume of medication that should be given to the patient?

Continued

211

Copyright © 2019 by Elsevier, Inc. All rights reserved.

Pretest, cont.

What size syringe should be used to prepare this medication? _____

What is the total volume of medication in the vial? _____

What is the total number of units of heparin in the vial? _____

 2. A physician orders 2,500 units of heparin sodium subcutaneously. The medication strength available is 10,000 units/mL in a 1-mL vial. What volume of medication should the patient receive?

What volume of medication would be left in the vial after this dose has been prepared?

Indicate the desired volume on the syringe that would provide the most accurate dose.

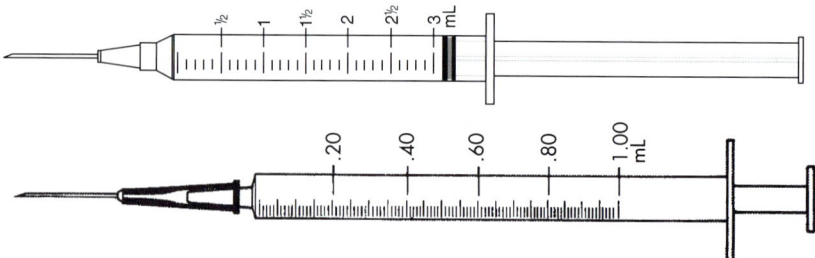

3. A physician orders Humulin R 50 units in IV fluid to make an insulin infusion.

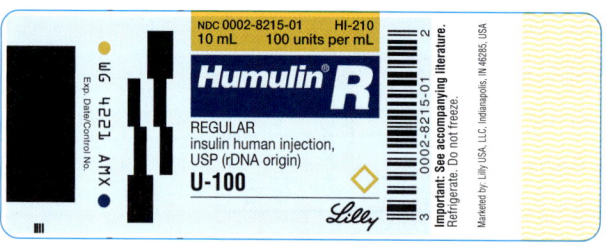

Eli Lilly and Company. All Rights Reserved. Used with Permission.

What volume of medication should be added to the fluid?

What volume of medication would be left in the vial?

Indicate the desired volume on the syringe that would provide the most accurate dose.

Pretest, cont.

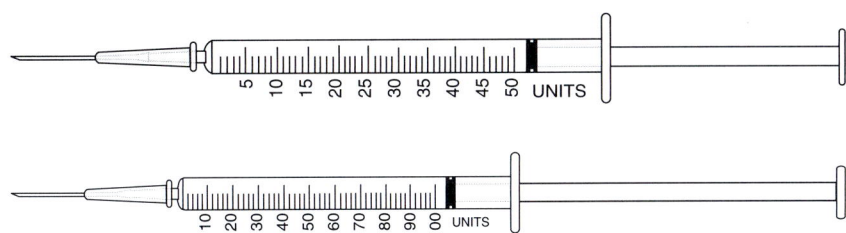

ENDO   **4.** A physician orders Humulin R 35 units subcutaneously stat. The available medication is shown on the previous label.

Indicate the desired volume on the syringe that would provide the most accurate dose.

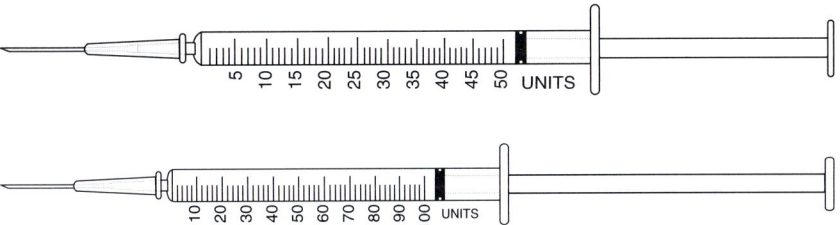

ENDO   **5.** A physician orders Lantus 55 units subcutaneously daily at bedtime.

Stock available: Lantus (insulin glargine) 100 units/mL

Can this medication be mixed with other insulin preparations? _____

Indicate the desired volume on the syringe that would provide the most accurate dose.

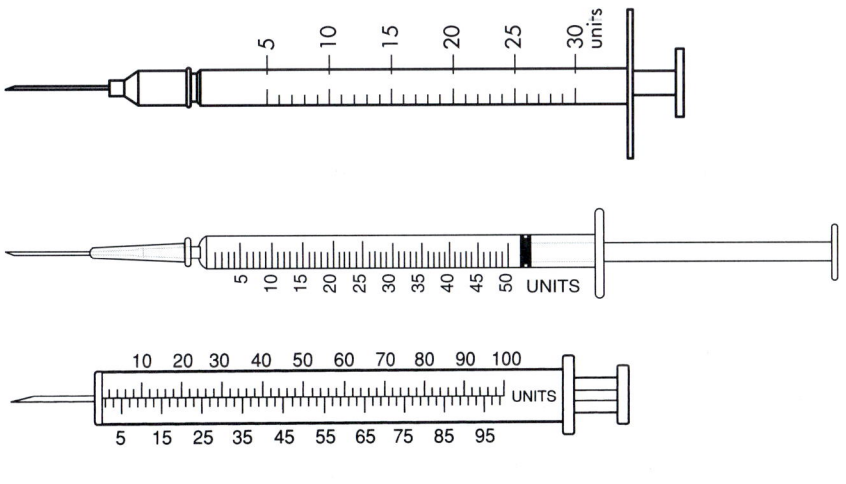

Continued

Pretest, cont.

6. A physician orders 17,000 units of heparin sodium subcutaneously as a stat dose. The available medications are shown on the following labels.

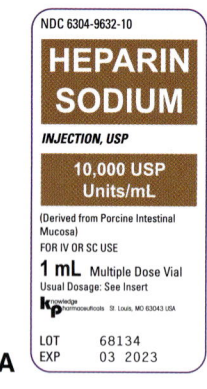
A

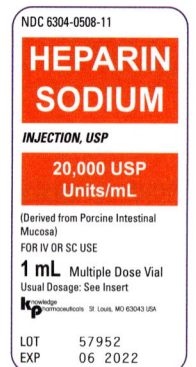
B

Which label strength of medication would provide the smallest volume dose?

_____

What volume of medication should the patient receive when using the selected vial?

Which syringe would be appropriate for administration of the medication?

_____

Indicate the amount of medication on the appropriate syringe.

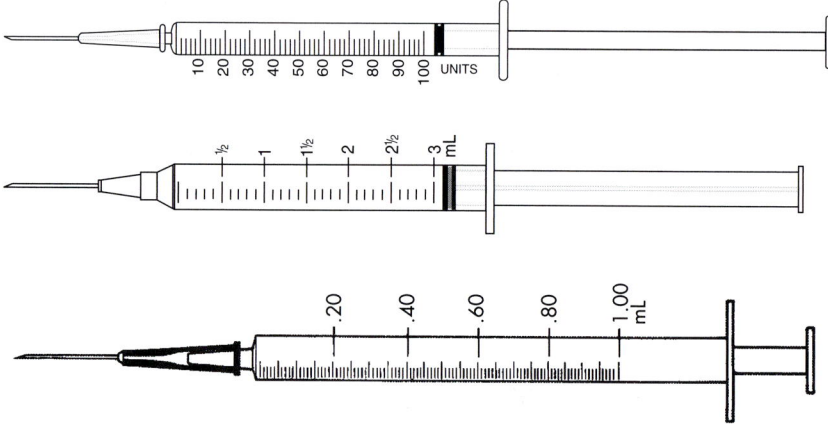

Chapter 11   Unit Calculations With Anticoagulants and Insulin   215

Pretest, cont.

 7. A physician orders heparin sodium 750 units subcutaneously as a stat dose.

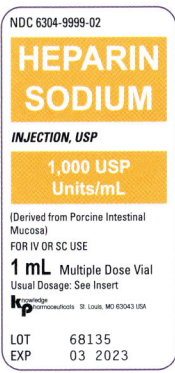

What volume of this medication should the patient receive? _____

Which syringe should be used for administration? _____

Indicate the amount of medication on the correct syringe.

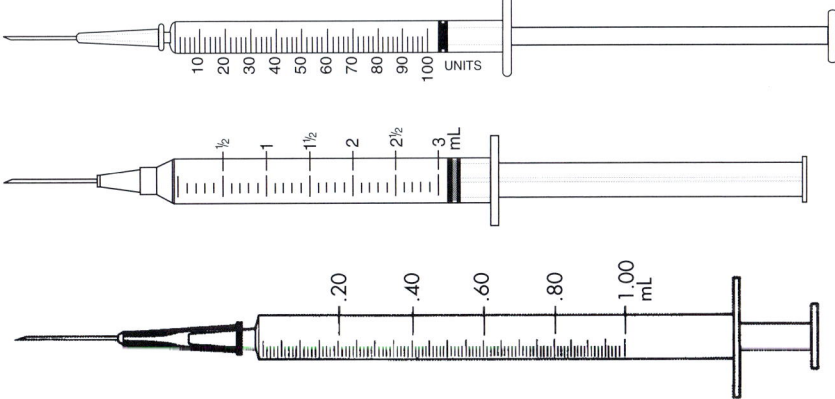

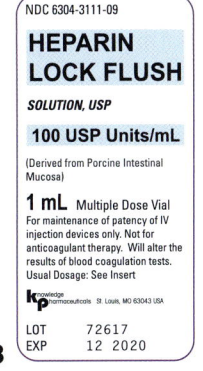 8. A physician orders heparin sodium flush 45 units to keep an intravenous site patent. The available strength flushes are shown on the following labels.

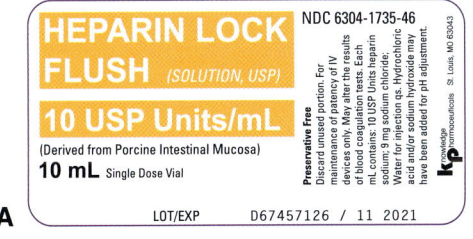

Continued

Pretest, cont.

Which strength of medication would provide the dose in the smallest volume?
_____

What volume of should be administered to the patient using this medication?

Indicate the desired volume on the syringe that would provide the most accurate dose.

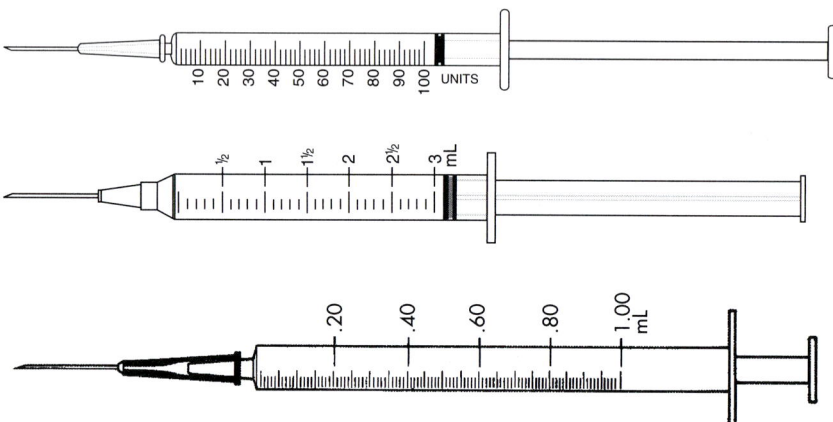

9. A physician provides a new prescription for Humulin R subcut 14 units tid ac.

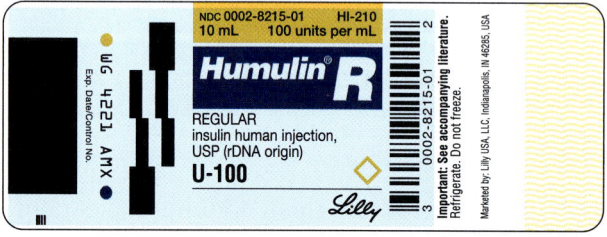

© Eli Lilly and Company. All Rights Reserved. Used with Permission.

Write the directions as they should appear on the prescription label:
_____

What syringe is most appropriate for this dose? _____

Pretest, cont.

10. A physician provides a new prescription for Humulin R 12 units and Humulin N 35 units subcutaneously qam.

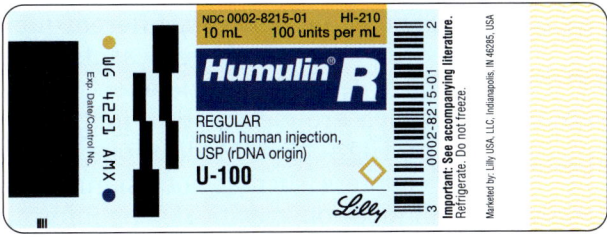

© Eli Lilly and Company. All Rights Reserved. Used with Permission.

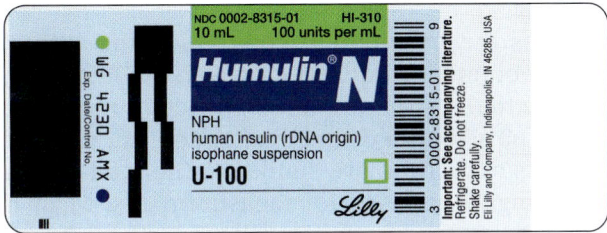

© Eli Lilly and Company. All Rights Reserved. Used with Permission.

What volume of regular insulin is needed per dose?

What volume of NPH insulin is needed per dose?

What total volume is needed if they are drawn in the same syringe? _____

What is the proper procedure for drawing them up in the same syringe?
_____
_____

Mark the amount of regular insulin needed on the first syringe, the amount of NPH insulin needed on the second, and the *total* amount of insulin needed on the final syringe.

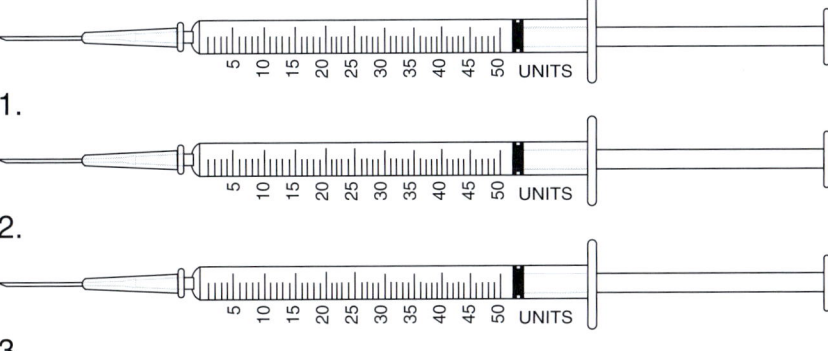

1.

2.

3.

INTRODUCTION

Medications such as insulin, heparin, and penicillin are measured in *international units*. Other, less used medications that have unit measurements include fat-soluble vitamin E, some forms of vitamins A and D, and the topical antibiotic bacitracin. With parenteral medications, the labels display the specific number of *units* per milliliter. The unit amounts are not interchangeable between different medications; rather, each medication unit is *specific* to the drug ordered and represents a standard amount of that particular medication that produces a desired biologic effect.

Insulin and heparin, both of which are measured in units, are considered *high-alert medications* on the ISMP List of High-Alert Medications. Although other high-alert medications are covered in other chapters, such as potassium chloride injection, which is measured in mEq, this chapter will focus on specific dosing information concerning these two commonly used medications.

Calculating Doses in Units

A unit measurement gives the information concerning the strength of medication in a given drug form, such as volume for liquids. A conversion factor is not necessary because a unit is the factor specific to the strength of the particular medicine. The medication label provides information on the strength of the medication, such as insulin U-100 (100 units/mL) or heparin 5,000 units/mL. These are similar to the medication strengths found with the metric system when mg/mL is used for measurements. Most important for you as a pharmacy technician is the need to be aware of the volume of the medication and strength for the dose as listed on medication labels. As with medication calculations in previous chapters, reading a drug label accurately is of utmost importance and is the basis for correct preparation and administration of medication to patients.

Calculating Insulin Doses in Units

Insulin is used to control type 1 diabetes mellitus and some stages of type 2 diabetes mellitus. It is prescribed and measured in units. Most insulin preparations are only available in U-100 strength, meaning that each milliliter of insulin contains 100 units of medication. While there is an ever-growing number of concentrated insulin products available (such as U-200 and U-300 products), most of these are available in pre-filled insulin syringes to help avoid dosing errors. Even insulin preparations that are combinations of regular insulin and intermediate-acting insulin and the newer long acting insulins are supplied as 100 units/mL. See Fig. 11.1 for labels of some different types of insulin preparations.

U-100 insulin syringes are used to administer U-100 insulin; *no other syringe is based in units for U-100 insulin.* (In an emergency, a tuberculin syringe can be used for U-100 insulins because it is also calibrated in hundredths of milliliters). U-500 syringes are now available *only* for use with U-500 insulin. The design of the syringe makes it easy to ensure that the exact dose of medication ordered is administered. Insulin syringes for U-100 insulin come in 30-unit, 50-unit, and 100-unit sizes (Fig. 11.2). Some of the 100-unit insulin syringes are marked in 2-unit increments, whereas others are marked in 1-unit increments with 2-unit increments of odd/even on each side of the syringe barrel. Note that the 30-unit and 50-unit insulin syringes are calibrated in 1-unit increments and are therefore easier to see for patients with vision problems, a common complication of long-term or uncontrolled diabetes mellitus. Insulin syringes *should not be used* for measuring *any* medication other than U-100 insulin.

Insulin preparations are labeled according to type. Each formulation has a specific onset, peak, and duration of action (see Table 11.1). An abbreviation of "**R**" for regular insulin, *a clear solution*, indicates that the medication is short-acting. An abbreviation of "**N**" for NPH insulin, *a cloudy suspension*, indicates that it is an intermediate-acting insulin

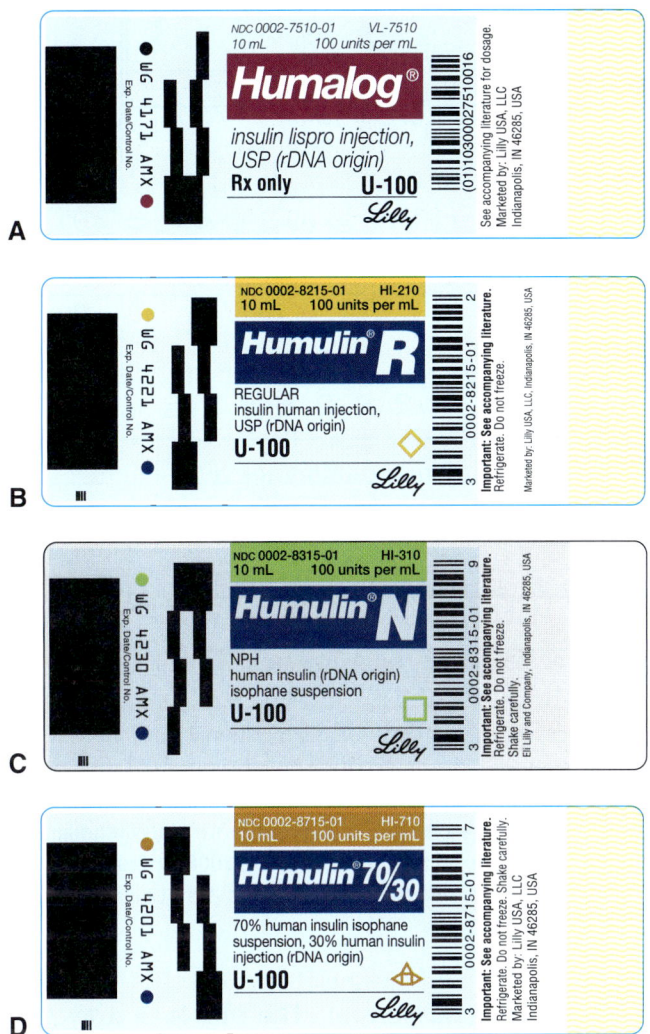

FIGURE 11.1 Labels for some different types of insulin used on a routine basis. **A,** Rapid-acting. **B,** Short-acting. **C,** Intermediate-acting. **D,** Intermediate- and rapid-acting mixture. Not depicted are long-acting insulins. (© Eli Lilly and Company. All Rights Reserved. Used with Permission.)

with a slower onset and longer duration of action. *Extreme care* must be taken to ensure that the correct insulin is chosen and delivered to the patient. For that reason, manufacturers have placed large letters on these two types of vials, emphasizing the exact type of insulin.

> **TECH ALERT**
>
> Always check the physician's insulin order with the insulin vial to be sure the correct type of insulin has been chosen. Do not confuse **R** and **N** on the labels.

All insulin formulations can be administered subcutaneously. *Only* regular insulin and some newer rapid-acting analogs are indicated for IV use. Regular insulin is typically used when insulin is prescribed intravenously. When mixing two types of insulin *in one syringe* for subcutaneous administration, one must be a clear short- or rapid-acting solution and

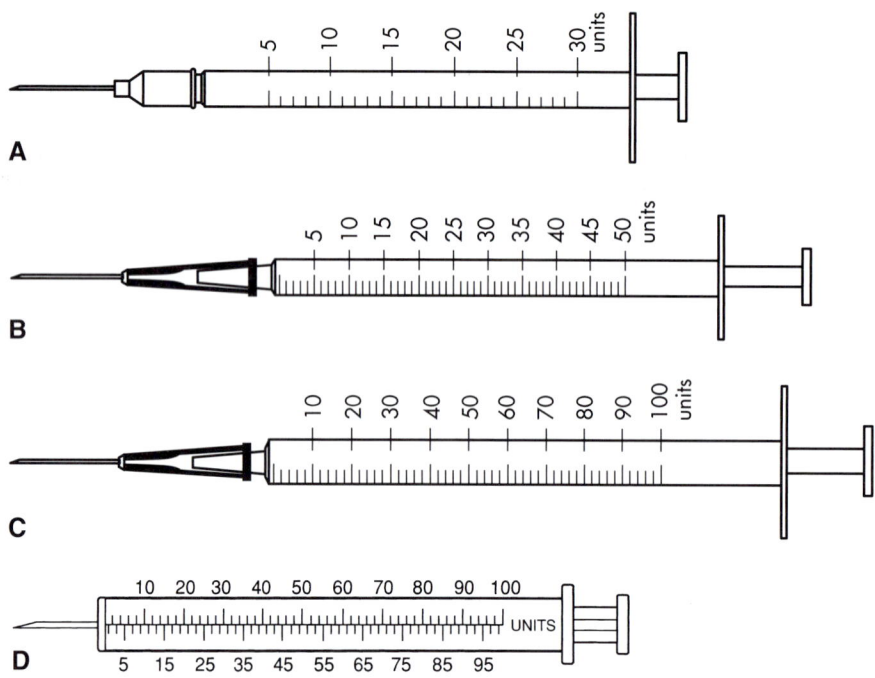

FIGURE 11.2 Insulin syringes for measuring 100 unit/mL strength insulin. The 30-unit insulin syringe **(A)** is recommended for measuring 30 units or less; the 50-unit syringe **(B)** should be used for measuring 31 to 50 units; and the 100-unit syringe **(C)** should be used for measuring 51 to 100 units of insulin. **D,** A 100-unit insulin syringe depicts single units on one syringe. (A–C, From Brown M, Mulholland JM: *Drug Calculations: Process and Problems for Clinical Practice*, ed 8, St. Louis, Mosby, 2008. D, From Kee JL, Marshall SM: *Clinical Calculations: With Applications to General and Specialty Areas*, ed 8, St. Louis, Saunders, 2017.)

the other a cloudy longer-acting suspension. The rule is to draw up clear insulin before cloudy insulin, so regular insulin must be drawn up in a syringe before NPH, which is a suspension. If different types of insulin need to be administered at the same time, the same source of the insulin, such as DNA or recombinant sources, must be used together. Different sources of insulin cannot be mixed in the same syringe. Lantus and Levemir, two long-acting insulins, can *never* be mixed with *any* other type of insulin.

> **! TECH ALERT**
> Be sure the person is aware that if the type of insulin changes from a previously ordered type, the newly ordered type of insulin cannot be combined with the old type in one syringe. Insulin from different sources or manufacturers may not be compatible. The old insulin should be discarded for patient safety.

All U-100 insulin contains 100 units/mL. Insulin syringes are designed for this strength. Usually the only thing that needs to be done is to choose the appropriate insulin and syringe for the dose ordered. A dose of 30 units or less should be measured in a 30-unit syringe, 31 to 50 units in a 50-unit syringe, and 51 to 100 units in a 100-unit syringe for the greatest accuracy.

> **! TECH ALERT**
> Only regular insulin and some rapid-acting analogs may be administered by the intravenous route!

TABLE 11.1 Approximate Action of Common Insulin Preparations

INSULIN TYPE	BRAND (GENERIC)	ONSET	PEAK	DURATION
RAPID-ACTING				
	Apidra (glulisine)	15 min	1 hr	2-4 hr
	Humalog (lispro)	15 min	1 hr	2-4 hr
	Novolog (aspart)	15 min	1 hr	2-4 hr
SHORT-ACTING REGULAR INSULINS				
	Humulin R	30 min	2-3 hr	3-6 hr
	Novolin R	30 min	2-3 hr	3-6 hr
INTERMEDIATE-ACTING NPH INSULINS				
	Humulin N	2-4 hr	4-12 hr	12-18 hr
	Novolin N	2-4 hr	4-12 hr	12-18 hr
LONG-ACTING				
	Lantus (glargine)	1-2 hr	Considered no peak	24 hr
	Levemir (detemir)	1-3 hr	Considered no peak	24 hr
ULTRA LONG-ACTING				
	Triseba (degludec)	1 hr	Considered no peak	up to 42 hours or more
COMBINATION				
NPH/R	Humulin 50/50	30 min	2-6 hr	16-24 hr
	Humulin 70/30	30-60 min	2-12 hr	18-24 hr
	Novolin 70/30	30-60 min	2-12 hr	18-24 hr
NPH/aspart	Novolog 70/30	15 min	1-7 hr	10-24 hr
NPH/lispro	Humalog 75/25	15 min	1-7 hr	10-18 hr

EXAMPLE 11.1

ENDO A physician orders 10 mL of Humulin N U-100, 12 units tid pc. What should the technician supply for the *administration* of this medication?

For maximum accuracy, the technician will provide 30-unit insulin syringes, because the dose is less than 30 units.

Other necessary calculations with insulin include determining the days' supply, both to input for insurance reimbursement and to know when to expect a refill request. This is covered in Chapter 13. When dealing with total parenteral nutrition or TPN, the number of units ordered may need to be converted to milliliters to calculate the volume of regular insulin that is added to the TPN. With U-100 insulin, this is a simple calculation. If any order is written to add regular insulin U-100 to an IV, remember the following:

$$\frac{100 \text{ units}}{1 \text{ mL}} = \frac{x \text{ units}}{x \text{ mL}}$$

After cross-multiplying, solving this equation for any amount of insulin involves dividing the number of units required by 100.

EXAMPLE 11.2

ENDO An order reads to add 80 units of regular insulin U-100 to a total parenteral nutrition IV bag. When calculating the total volume that has been added to the TPN, how many milliliters are equivalent to 80 units?

$$\frac{100 \text{ units}}{1 \text{ mL}} = \frac{80 \text{ units}}{x} \quad 80 \text{ mL} = 100x \quad x = 0.8 \text{ mL}$$

Likewise a 40-unit dose of U-100 is 0.4 mL, 95 units is 0.95 mL, 10 units is 0.1 mL, and so on.

> **! TECH ALERT**
>
> Although we will be working with U-100 insulin in this chapter, technicians should be aware of stronger concentrations of insulin, such as Humulin R U-500 (500 units/mL) and TOUJEO U-300 (300 units/mL), that are on the market. These formulations are more concentrated, allowing for more units to be delivered in a smaller volume than with U-100 insulin. This is important for diabetics requiring higher doses, to keep the volume small enough for subcutaneous injection. Specific attention is given to the U-500 insulin on the ISMP List of High-Alert Medications. It is five times more concentrated than U-100, and does come in a multidose vial, which has led to errors. U-500 insulin doses should be measured and administered using U-500 insulin syringes. Many pharmacies do not even store U-500 insulin near U-100 insulin to decrease the likelihood of errors.

> **! TECH ALERT**
>
> Only U-100 insulins should be measured in U-100 insulin syringes. Units are specific to the particular medication and strength.

Practice Problems A

Choose the correct label, and indicate the correct dose on the appropriate syringe. If two types of insulin are necessary to supply the order, indicate the volume of each, as well as the total volume to be administered, if they can be mixed, on a separate syringe and label each syringe.

Types of Insulin:

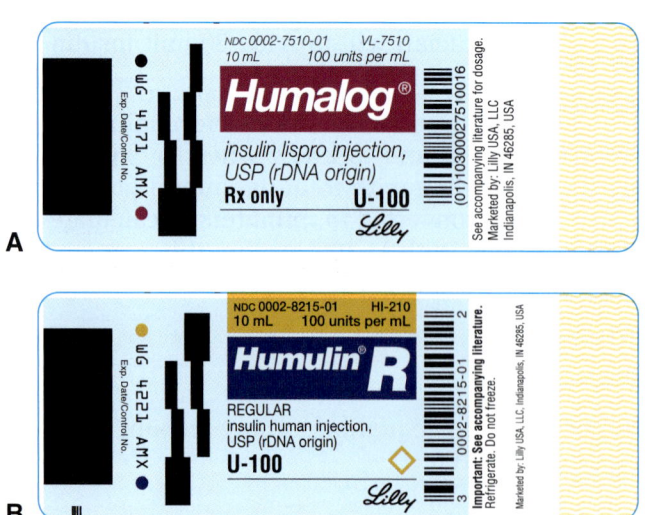

A. Humalog insulin lispro injection, USP (rDNA origin) U-100

B. Humulin R REGULAR insulin human injection, USP (rDNA origin) U-100

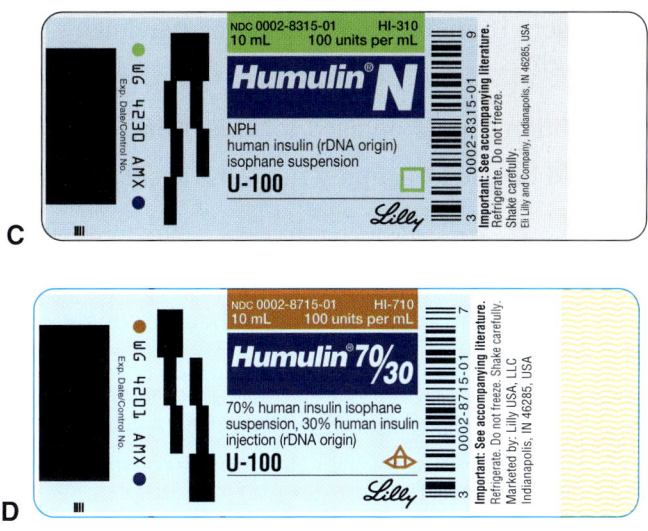

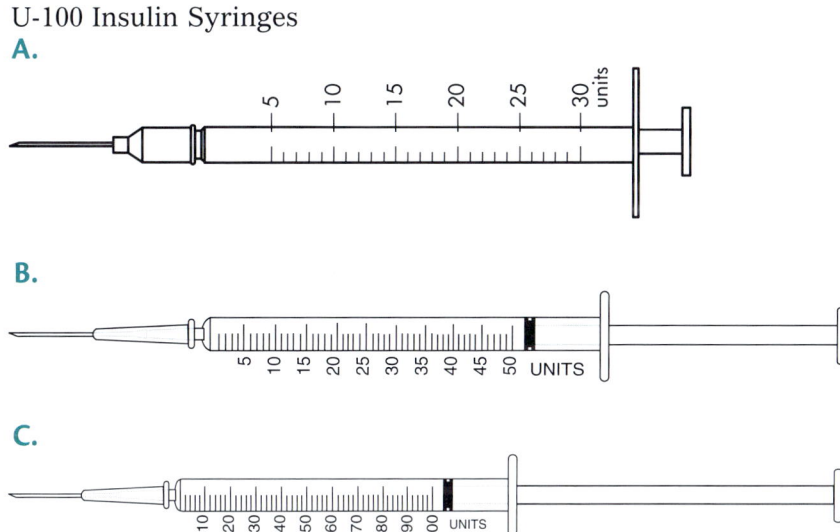

© Eli Lilly and Company. All Rights Reserved. Used with Permission.

1. A physician orders Humulin N insulin 45 units subcutaneously to be given qam.

   Which vial of insulin should be used for this order? _____

   Which syringe should be used to supply the most accurate dose of medication? _____

2. **ENDO** A physician orders Humulin R 30 units subcutaneously 30 min ac for a person with poor eyesight.

   Which vial of medication should be used for this order? _____

   Which syringe should be used to supply the most accurate dose of medication? _____

3. **ENDO** A physician orders Humulin N 55 units subcutaneously qam.

   Which vial of insulin should be used for this order? _____

   Which syringe should be used to supply the most accurate dose of medication? _____

4. **ENDO** A physician orders Humulin 70/30 42 units subcutaneously qam.

   Which vial of insulin should be used to fill this order? _____

   Which syringe should be used to supply the most accurate dose of medication? _____

5. **ENDO** A physician orders Humalog 66 units subcutaneously ac.

   Which vial of insulin should be used to complete this order? _____

   Which syringe should be used to supply the most accurate dose of medication? _____

6. **ENDO** A physician orders Humulin R 23 units subcutaneously qam for an elderly patient.

   Which vial of medication should be supplied to the patient? _____

   Which syringe should be used to supply the most accurate dose of medication? _____

7. **ENDO** A physician orders Humulin R 47 Units 30 min ac.

   Which vial of medication should be used to supply this medication? _____

   Which syringe should be used to supply the most accurate dose of medication? _____

Chapter 11 Unit Calculations With Anticoagulants and Insulin   225

8. **ENDO** A physician orders Humulin R 52 units to be added to a TPN.

   Which vial of medication should be used to supply this medication? _____
   How many mL of the total volume of the TPN are from regular insulin? _____

9. **ENDO** A physician orders Humulin 70/30 30 units and Humulin R 22 units qam.

   Which vials of medication should be used to supply this medication? _____ and _____
   Which syringe should be used to administer these medications together? _____

   70/30 means that in each dose of this insulin, 70% is NPH insulin and 30% is regular insulin.

   How many units of regular insulin would the patient receive per day?

   How many units of NPH insulin would the patient receive per day?

10. **ENDO** A physician orders Humulin N 21 units and Humulin R 36 units qam.

    Which vials of medication should be used to fill this order? _____
    Which syringe should be used to supply the most accurate dose of medication? _____
    How should this dose be drawn into the syringe? _____

11. **ENDO** A physician orders Humulin R 24 units and Humulin N 43 units qam.

    Which vials of medication should be used to fill this order? _____ and _____
    Which syringe(s) should be used to administer this medication? _____

12. **ENDO** A physician orders Humulin 70/30 40 units qam.

    Which vial of medication should be used to fill this order? _____
    Which syringe should be used to administer this medication? _____

    70/30 means that in each dose of this insulin, 70% is NPH insulin and 30% is regular insulin.

How many units of NPH insulin would be received per dose?

How many units of regular insulin would be received per dose?

Calculating Anticoagulant Doses in Units

Heparin is an injectable *anticoagulant* medication that is measured in units. Heparin may be used as a flush for an IV injection site to keep it *patent*, as an IV infusion additive, or as a deep subcutaneous injection into fatty tissue. The doses for heparin are highly individualized based on body weight and blood coagulation laboratory values. Because heparin prolongs bleeding time, the time that it takes for blood to clot, an accurate dose is of the utmost importance. A dose that is larger than necessary may cause hemorrhage, whereas a dose that is insufficient may not produce the necessary results to prevent clot formation and possible thrombi.

Heparin is available in 10 units/mL (pediatric heparin lock flush), 100 units/mL (heparin lock flush), 1,000 units/mL, 5,000 units/mL, 10,000 units/mL, and 20,000 units/mL strengths. Therefore it is *essential* to pay close attention to the strength of heparin chosen to provide the correct dose. Heparin doses should be measured using 1-mL tuberculin syringes for the greatest accuracy. The dose may be calculated using ratio and proportion (R&P) or dimensional analysis (DA), as with other dosage calculations.

> **! TECH ALERT**
>
> Heparin is never administered intramuscularly because of the danger of bleeding into the muscle tissue. It may be given subcutaneously and by IV infusion as a therapeutic dose or as a means of maintaining patency of an IV line.

Some low molecular weight heparins, such as dalteparin sodium (Fragmin), are also measured in units, although some, such as enoxaparin (Lovenox), are measured on a milligram basis. The low molecular weight heparins do not have the short half-life of heparin, but they are also primarily administered subcutaneously.

EXAMPLE 11.3

 A physician orders heparin sodium 2,500 units subcutaneously stat. The medication available is heparin sodium 5,000 units/mL. How much should be administered?

$$\text{R\&P} \quad \frac{5{,}000 \text{ units}}{1 \text{ mL}} = \frac{2{,}500 \text{ units}}{x}$$

$$5{,}000x = 2{,}500 \text{ mL}$$

$$x = 0.5 \text{ mL}$$

$$\text{DA} \quad \text{mL} = \frac{1 \text{ mL}}{5{,}000 \text{ units}} \times \frac{2{,}500 \text{ units}}{1} = 0.5 \text{ mL}$$

Because no conversion factors are needed with unit calculations, they are performed easily with R&P.

Practice Problems B

Calculate the following medication orders using the labels provided with each practice problem. Round your answers to hundredths for measurement on tuberculin syringes. Indicate the amount of medication on the syringe provided. Show your calculations.

1. A physician orders heparin sodium 5,000 units subcutaneously.

   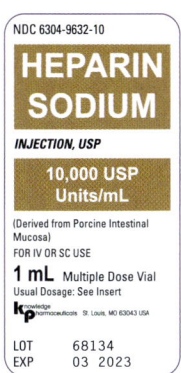

   What volume of medication should be given to the patient for this dose?

   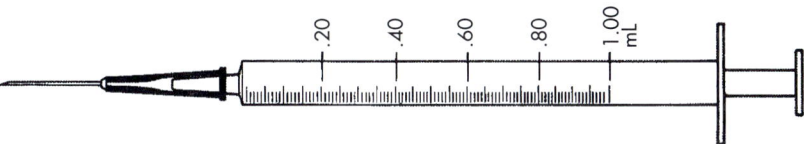

2. A physician orders heparin sodium 1,000 units subcutaneously.

   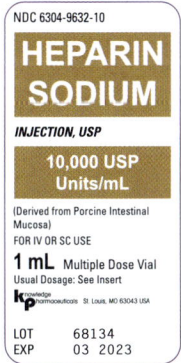

   What volume of medication should be administered for this dose?

   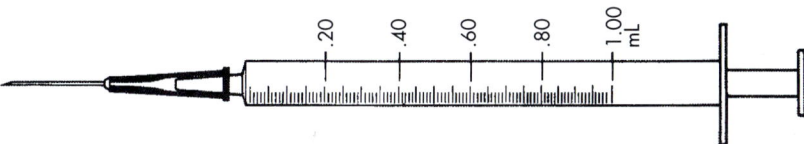

3. A physician orders dalteparin (Fragmin) 4,000 international units subcutaneously.

   Supplied: Fragmin 10,000 units/mL in a 9.5 mL vial

   What volume of medication should be given to this patient?

   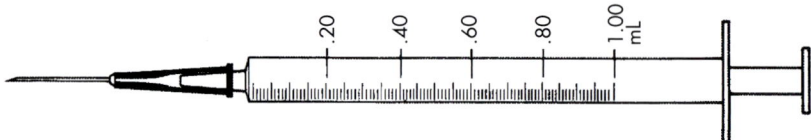

4. A physician orders heparin sodium 2,500 units subcutaneously stat.

   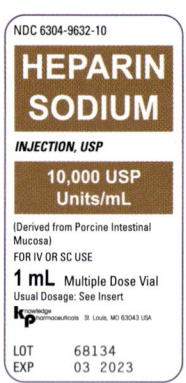

   What volume of medication should be administered to this patient? _____

   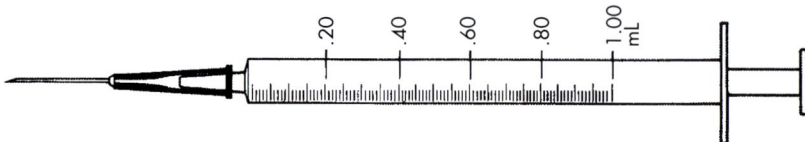

5. 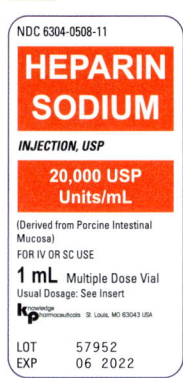 A physician orders heparin sodium 17,500 units subcutaneously stat.

What volume of medication should be administered to the patient? _____

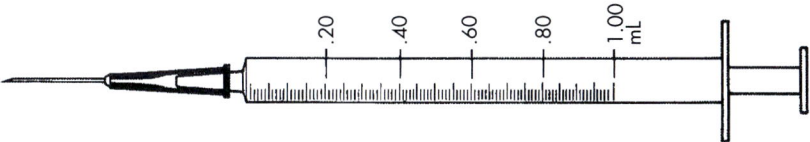

6. 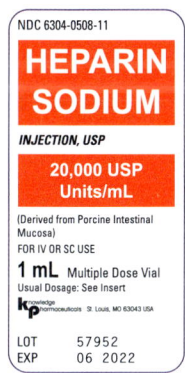 A physician orders heparin sodium 15,000 units subcutaneously.

What volume of medication should be administered? _____

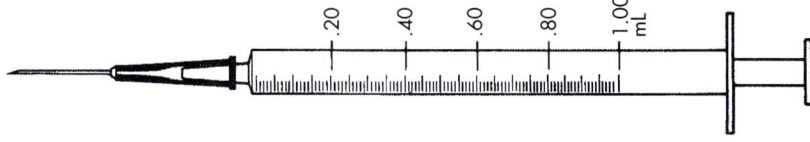

7. A physician orders Fragmin 2,500 international units subcutaneously stat.

   Supplied: Fragmin 10,000 units/mL in a 9.5 mL vial

   What volume of medication should be administered?

   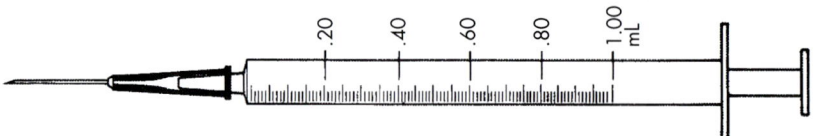

8. A physician orders heparin sodium 12,000 units subcutaneously.

   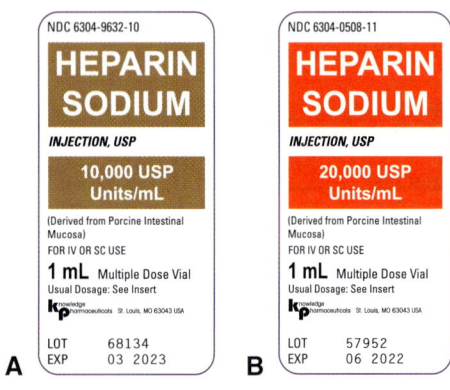

   Which strength vial of medication is more appropriate to be used to prepare this medication? _____

   What volume of medication should be administered? _____

   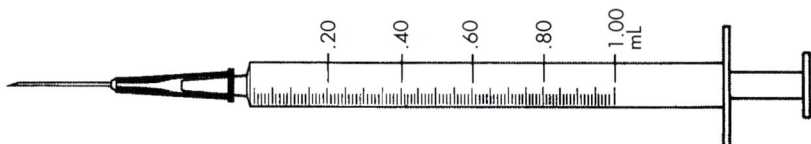

9. A physician orders heparin sodium 7,500 units stat.

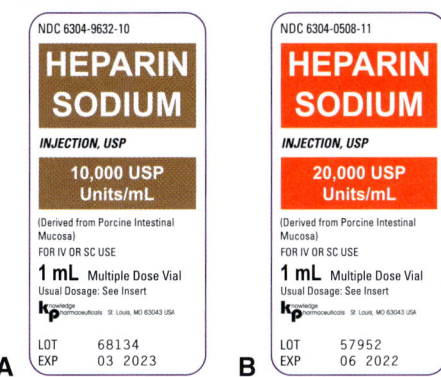

Which strength vial of medication can be used without rounding the dose? _____

What volume of the chosen medication should be given? _____

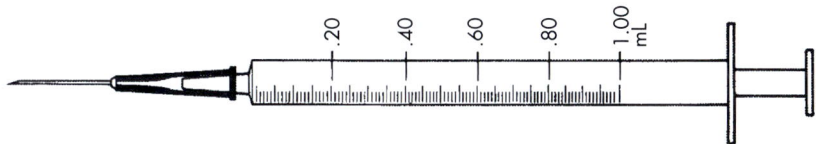

10. A physician orders heparin sodium flush 25 international units IV.

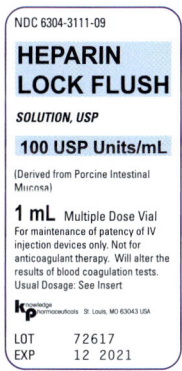

What volume of medication should be prepared for the flush? _____

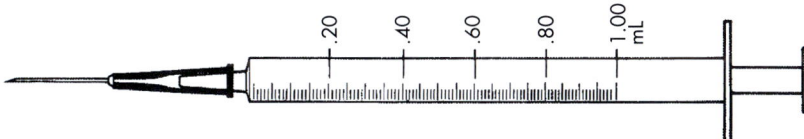

11. A physician orders heparin sodium 1,500 units subcutaneously daily.

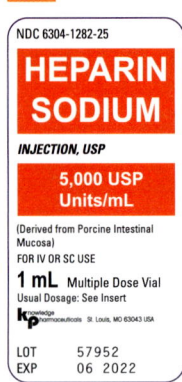

What volume of medication should be administered? _____

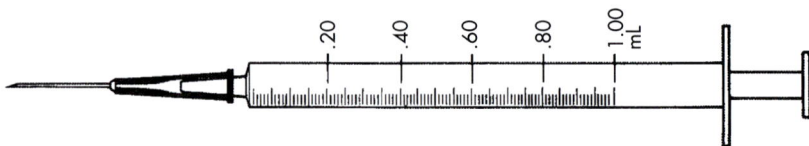

12. A physician orders heparin sodium 600 units subcutaneously stat.

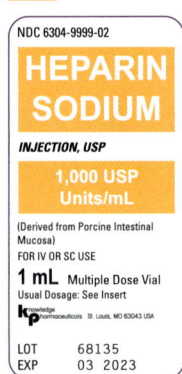

What volume of medication should be administered? _____

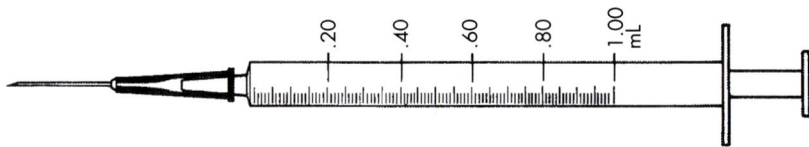

13. A physician orders Fragmin 6,000 international units stat.

    Supplied: Fragmin 10,000 units/mL in a 9.5 mL vial
    What volume of medication should be administered?

    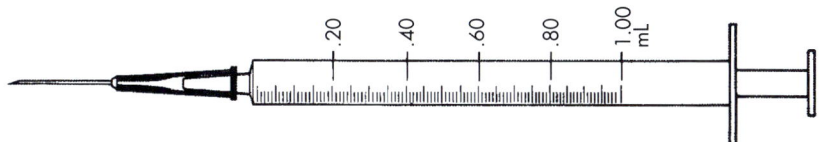

14. A physician orders Fragmin 1,200 international units subcutaneously stat.

    Supplied: Fragmin 10,000 units/mL in a 9.5 mL vial
    What volume of medication should be administered?

    What is the total volume of medication in the vial? _____

    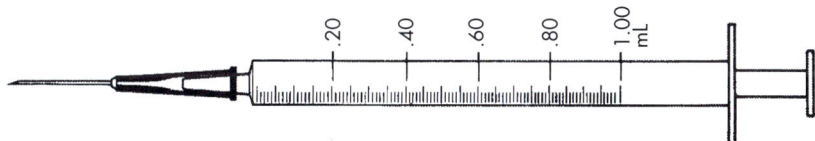

15. A physician orders heparin sodium 6,000 units stat.

    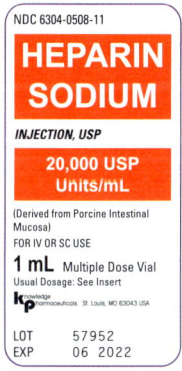

    What volume of medication should be administered? _____

234 SECTION III Calculations with Prescriptions and Medication Orders

REVIEW

Insulin, anticoagulants, and some antimicrobial agents are supplied in units per milliliter. Doses can be calculated using DA or R&P. Insulin products are supplied in a wide variety of preparations, mainly in U-100 strength. Heparin is supplied in a wide variety of strengths. You must read the label and physician's order carefully with either product, and prepare the medication that has been ordered for administration in the proper strength/dosage.

TECH NOTE
The important key in working with units is the careful interpretation of the label to ensure that the exact amount per milliliter is known before preparation of the dose to be given.

TECH ALERT
Parenteral medications in units per milliliter are specific for the medication being used and are not interchangeable between units per milliliter of other medications.

Posttest

Calculate the following doses. Show your calculations. If measuring devices are included, indicate the volume of medication on the appropriate measuring device(s). Round doses less than 1 mL to the hundredths place.

1. A physician orders heparin sodium 7,500 units subcutaneously stat.

   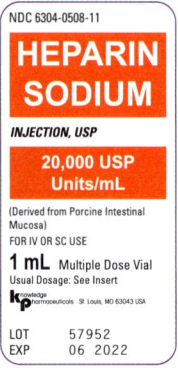

   What volume of medication should be administered? _____

Copyright © 2019 by Elsevier, Inc. All rights reserved.

Posttest, cont.

2. A physician orders Humalog 12 units ac.

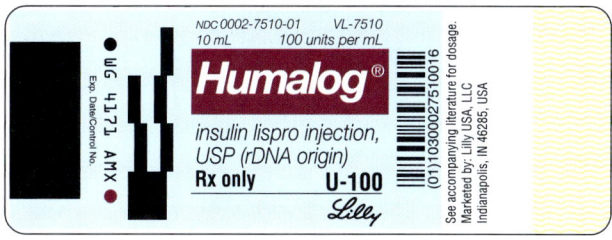

© Eli Lilly and Company. All Rights Reserved. Used with Permission.

Which of the following syringes would provide the most accurate dose? _____

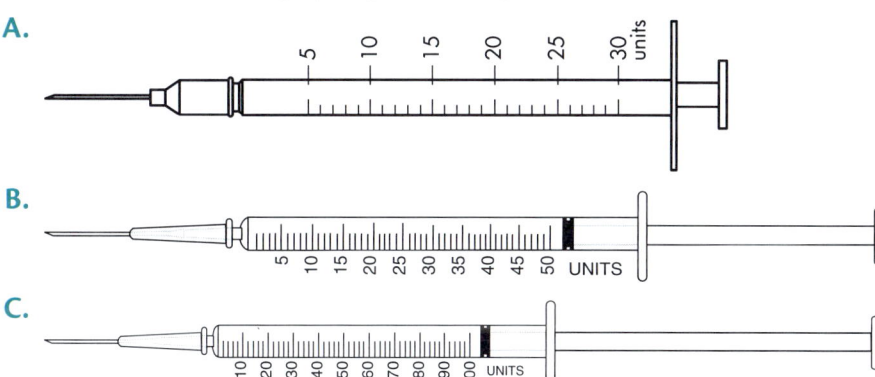

A.

B.

C.

3. A physician orders Fragmin 5,000 international units subcutaneously.

Supplied: Fragmin 10,000 units/mL in a 9.5-mL vial

What volume of medication should be given to this patient?

Which of the following syringes would provide the most accurate dose?

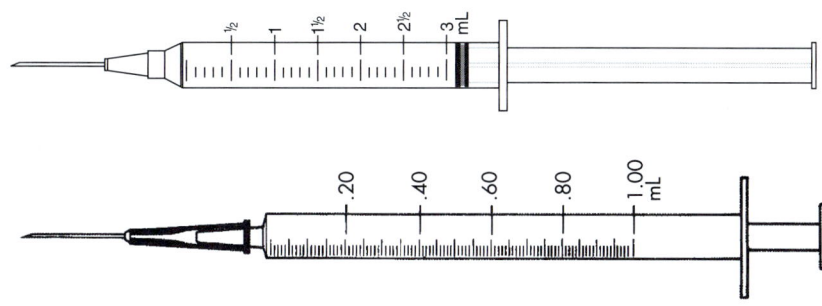

Continued

Posttest, cont.

4. A physician orders Humulin 70/30 40 units qam for an elderly patient.

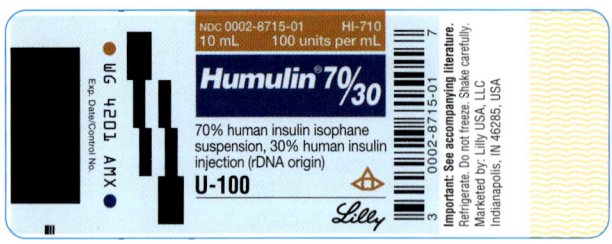

© Eli Lilly and Company. All Rights Reserved. Used with Permission.

Which of the following syringes would provide the most accurate dose? _____

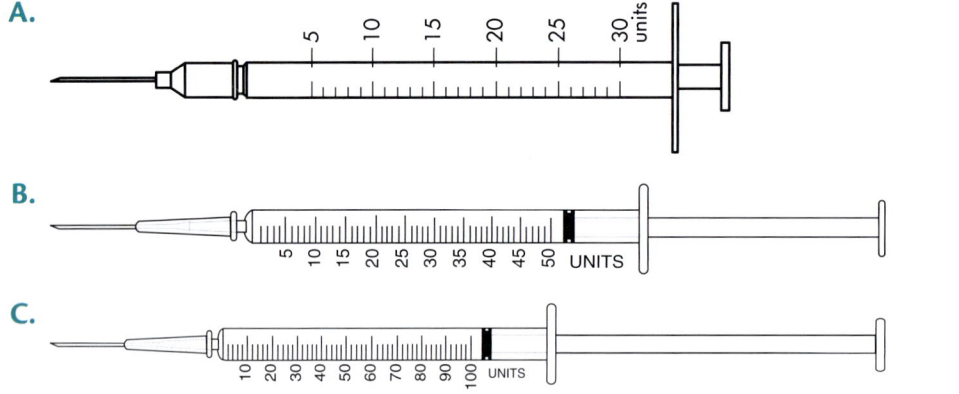

What is the composition of Humulin 70/30? _____
_____

How many units of NPH are supplied with this dose?

How many units of regular insulin are supplied with this dose?

Chapter 11 Unit Calculations With Anticoagulants and Insulin 237

Posttest, cont.

5. A physician orders heparin sodium 12,000 units subcutaneously stat.

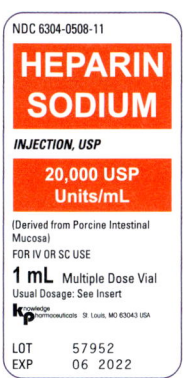

What volume of medication should be administered to the patient? _____

Which of the following syringes would provide the most accurate dose? _____

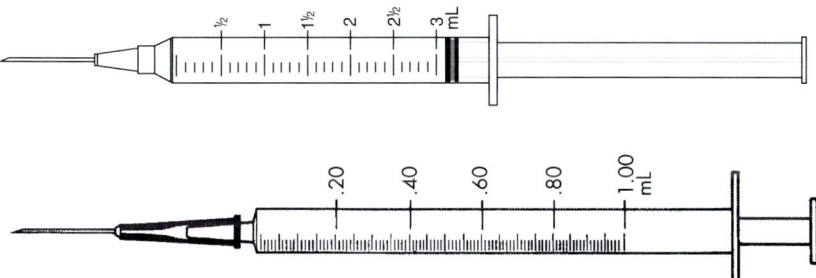

Continued

Posttest, cont.

6. A physician orders Humulin R 36 units and Humulin N 21 units qam to be mixed and administered as a single injection.

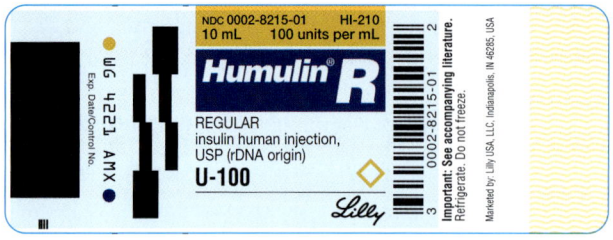

© Eli Lilly and Company. All Rights Reserved. Used with Permission.

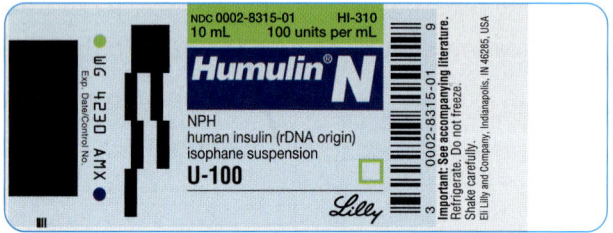

© Eli Lilly and Company. All Rights Reserved. Used with Permission.

Which syringe(s) should be used to administer this medication? _____

A.
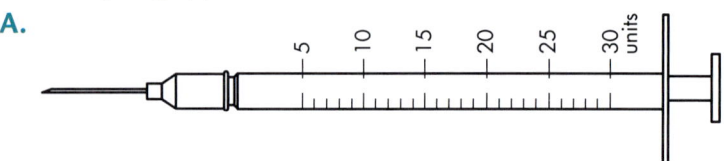

B.
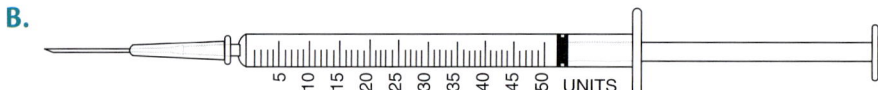

C.
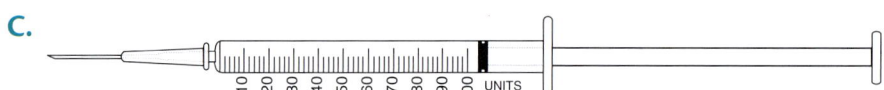

D.
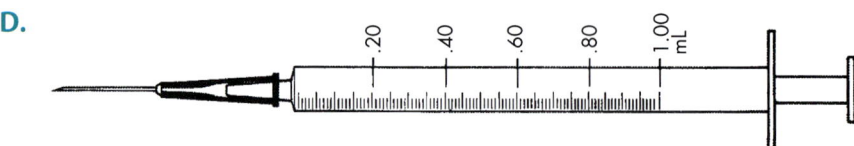

What is the rule for drawing up this dose in one syringe? _____

_____

Posttest, cont.

7. A physician orders Humulin 70/30 30 units and Humulin R 14 units qam 30 min ac to be mixed and administered as a single injection.

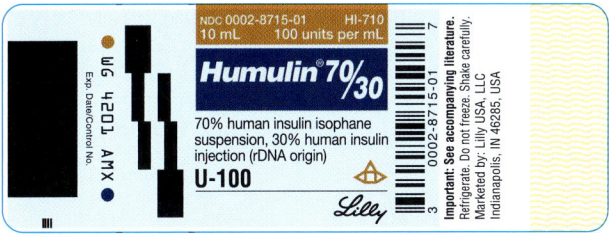

© Eli Lilly and Company. All Rights Reserved. Used with Permission.

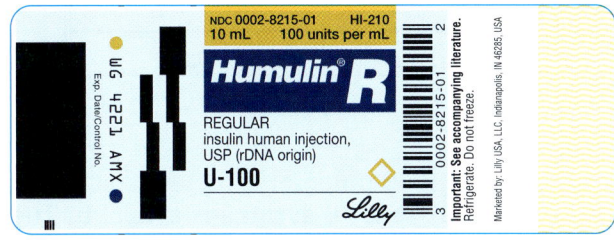

© Eli Lilly and Company. All Rights Reserved. Used with Permission.

What syringe should be used to administer the am dose? _____

How many units of regular insulin is the patient receiving in the morning?

How many units of NPH is the patient receiving in the morning?

Continued

Posttest, cont.

8. A patient is to receive Fragmin 2,500 international units subcutaneously daily. The label reads Fragmin 10,000 international units/mL.

   How many milliliters of medication should the patient receive daily?

   Indicate the desired volume on the syringe that would provide the most accurate dose.

   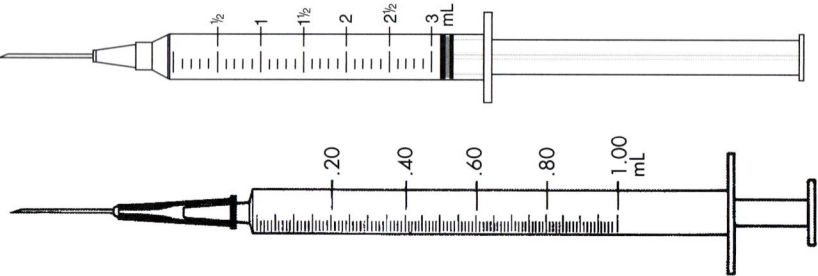

9. A physician orders Humulin R 30 units for a patient stat from a 10-mL vial of regular U-100 insulin. Only a 1-mL TB syringe is available. The physician approves its use in this instance.

   How many milliliters should be administered?

   Indicate the desired volume on the syringe.

   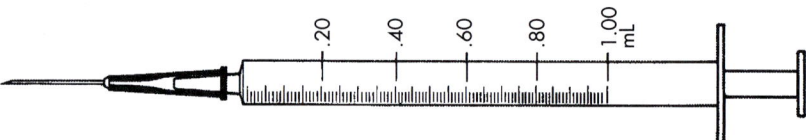

10. A physician orders regular insulin 70 units to be added to 500 mL of normal saline.

    How many mL of U-100 R should be added to the fluid?

REVIEW OF RULES

Calculations of Medications Measured in Units

- Liquid medications found in units are expressed as the number of units per milliliter.
- Medication labels in units/volume must be read carefully and interpreted for the strength of the medication.
- Use DA or R&P to calculate medications in units.

CHAPTER 12

Calculation of Medications by Age, Body Weight, and Body Surface Area

OBJECTIVES

1. Calculate doses of medications for children and adults using body weight.
2. Calculate doses of medications for children using Clark's rule.
3. Calculate doses of medication for special populations based on body surface area.
4. Calculate doses of medication for infants using Fried's rule.
5. Calculate doses of medication for children using Young's rule.

KEY WORDS

Adolescence From 11 through 21 years of age*
Body surface area (BSA) Measurement of total body area exposed to the environment; calculated from weight and height and expressed in square meters (m^2); used as a basis for calculating some medication doses
Childhood From 5 to 10 years of age*
Clark's rule Means of calculating a dose of medication for a child from an adult dose using weight in pounds
Early childhood From 1 through 4 years of age*
Fried's rule Means of calculating a dose of medication for an infant from an adult dose using age in months

Infant Prenatal to 1 year of age*
Neonate From birth to 1 month of age
Nomogram A graphic representation of two lines marked off to height and weight and arranged so that a straightedge, used to connect the known values on these two lines, intersects the corresponding BSA measurement on another line
Pharmacokinetics Movement of drugs through the body; absorption, distribution, metabolism, and excretion (ADME)
Young's rule Means of calculating a dose of medication for a child from an adult dose based on age in years

*According to the American Academy of Pediatrics (https://www.nichd.nih.gov/health/clinicalresearch/clinical-researchers/terminology/Pages/current.aspx)

Pretest

If you are already comfortable with the subject matter, complete the Pretest to test your knowledge. If not, work your way through the chapter and return to it for extra practice. Complete the following calculations for pediatric patients on the basis of age, body weight, or body surface area (BSA). Show your calculations. Round your answers to tenths if greater than 1 and hundredths if less than 1. Be sure your answer is a measurable dose.

Continued

Pretest, cont.

1. The adult dose of amoxicillin is 500 mg tid.

   What is the approximate dose for a child who is 2 years old?

2. The adult dose for Augmentin is 500 mg tid.

   What is the approximate dose for a 9-month-old infant?

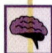
3. A child weighing 55 lb is to take phenobarbital. The physician orders 1 mg/kg tid.

   What is the dose to be given?

4. An 8-month-old infant is ordered Demerol following surgery. The normal adult dose is Demerol (meperidine) 50 mg.

   What is the approximate dose for the infant?

5. A child weighs 55 lb and has an order for acetaminophen. The adult dose is 325 mg.

   What is the approximate dose for the child?

6. A child has an order for digoxin based on 8 mcg per kilogram of body weight. The child weighs 35 lb. Stock strength: Lanoxin (digoxin) 50 mcg (0.05 mg)/mL

   How many mcg of Lanoxin should be administered to the child?

   What is the volume needed for one dose?

Chapter 12　Calculation of Medications by Age, Body Weight, and Body Surface Area　243

Pretest, cont.

　7. An 8-year-old child is to receive phenobarbital, and the adult dose is phenobarbital gr s̄s̄.

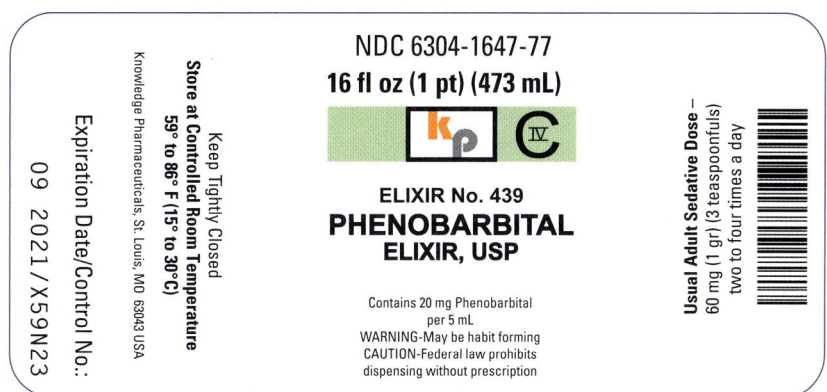

What is the child's dose in milligrams?

Using the label shown, what volume of medication would the child receive?

Show the correct dose of medication to be provided on the oral syringe.

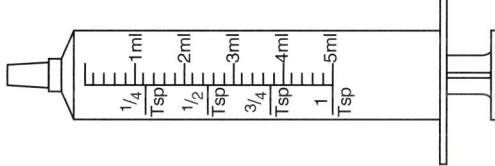

　8. A physician orders Zantac syrup for a 10-month-old child. The adult dose is 150 mg bid. Stock strength: Zantac (ranitidine) syrup 15 mg/mL

What is the approximate dose for the child in milligrams?

What volume of medication should be given to the child per dose?

Continued

Pretest, cont.

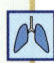

9. A child weighs 66 lb. The physician orders Benadryl (diphenhydramine) elixir. The adult dose is 50 mg q6–8h prn.

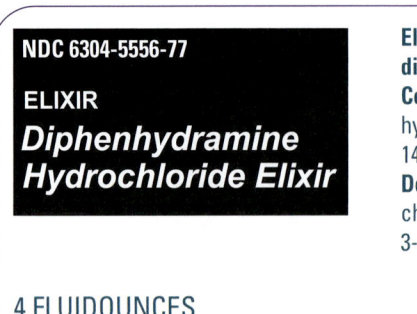

What is the approximate dose for the child in milligrams?

What is the measurable volume to be given per dose using the provided label?

Is this within the normal range for a child of this weight? _____

10. A 10-year-old child has bronchitis, and the physician orders Keflex suspension. The normal adult dose is 500 mg bid. Stock strength: Keflex (cephalexin) 125 mg/5 mL.

What is the approximate dose for the child in milligrams?

What volume of medication should be given per dose?

Pretest, cont.

11. A 5-year-old child is ordered Colace (docusate sodium) syrup for constipation. The adult dose is Colace 100 mg. Stock strength: docusate sodium 20 mg/5 mL

What is the approximate dose for the child in milligrams?

What is the volume of medication to be given?

What is the measurable dose volume in household measurements?

12. A child weighs 83 lb. The physician orders Biaxin oral suspension 10 mg/kg bid. Stock strength: Biaxin (clarithromycin) 125 mg/5 mL when reconstituted

What volume of medication should be given to the child per dose?

What is the measurable volume of medication in each of the following systems:
Metric: _____ Household: _____

Show the *measurable* volume of medication to be provided on the measuring devices.

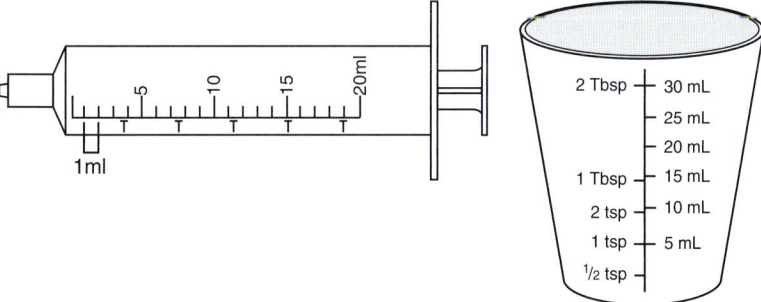

Continued

Pretest, cont.

13. A 10-year-old child weighs 56 lb and is 40″ tall. He has been diagnosed with epilepsy.

The physician orders Dilantin suspension for this child based on BSA. The normal adult dose is Dilantin 300 mg per day in three divided doses (100 mg per dose).

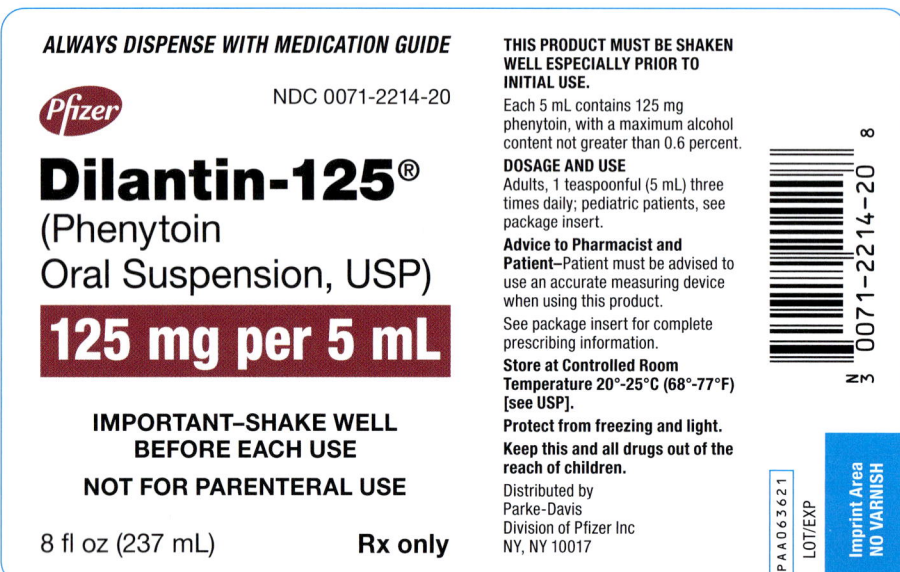

© Pfizer. Used with permission.

What is the child's BSA according to the nomogram on page 262? _____

What is the dose in milligrams to be given with each administration?

What is the volume of medication to be given for this dose?

Pretest, cont.

What is the approximate dose in milligrams using only the child's body weight and average adult dose?

What is the approximate dose in milligrams using only the child's age and average adult dose?

Considering that the BSA calculation is most accurate, are the last two very accurate methods of approximating doses? _____

14. A 75-pound child has otitis media. The physician orders Keflex tid.
    Stock strength: Keflex (cephalexin) 250 mg capsules
    What is the dose to be administered if the adult dose is 500 mg?

    How many capsules should be given to the child per dose?

Continued

Pretest, cont.

15. A 45-pound child is prescribed Lorabid (loracarbef) 15 mg/kg/*day* in divided doses bid.

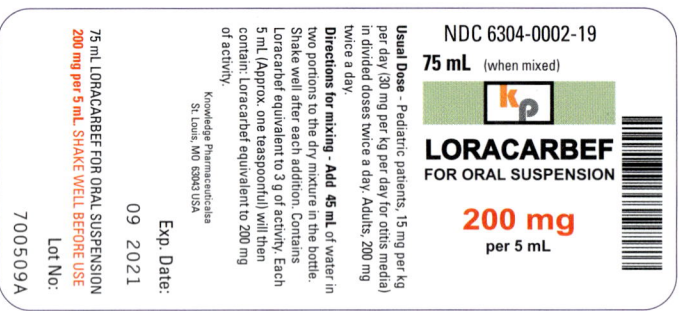

What is the strength per *dose* for the child using the label shown?

What is the measurable volume per dose of medication for administration?

What is the total dosage of loracarbef in milligrams per *day*?

Pretest, cont.

16. A physician orders nitrofurantoin suspension for a 59-pound child at 1.5 mg/kg/dose q6h × 7 days for a urinary tract infection.

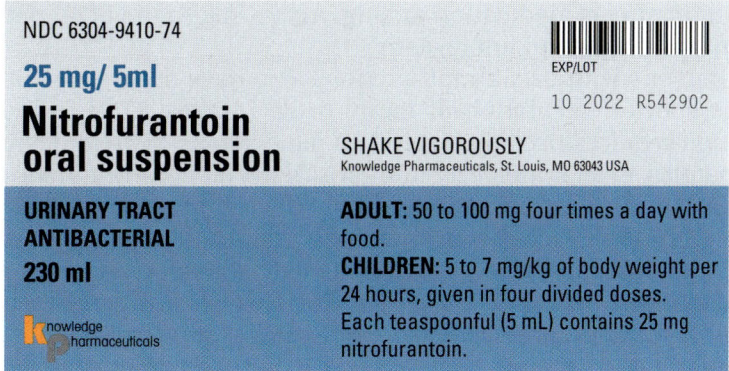

What is the strength of the dose for the child in mg? (*Round to a whole number.*)

What is the volume of medication that should be administered per dose?

Show the correct volume of medication to be provided on the measuring device.

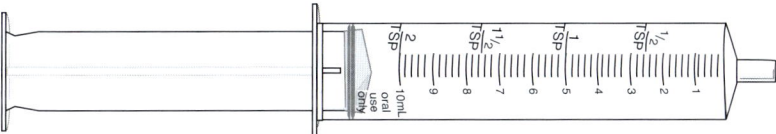

INTRODUCTION

Patients other than average adults may require special medication dosing. Children are not small adults but rather a distinct population of individuals that exhibits different **pharmacokinetics** (medication absorption, distribution, metabolism, and excretion rates) than adults. The growth and development of the child, or the focus of the field of pediatrics, significantly affects medication dosing. According to the FDA, pediatric stages include **newborn**; **infant**; **child**; and **adolescent**.

Geriatric persons and persons with organ malfunctions also have differences in pharmacokinetics requiring the special calculation of many drug dosages. Most individuals with renal or liver dysfunction require dose adjustments of medications. With toxic medications such as chemotherapeutics, even nonelderly adults with normal organ function may require the use of **body surface area (BSA)** based on height and weight for drug calculations. Emaciated patients, those who have excessively low body weight or muscle mass, and obese patients may also require dose adjustments for some medications. All of these groups are considered special populations because of the need for special dosage calculations. Since many dosing recommendations are standardized average adult doses, doses for special populations must be altered to meet the patient's needs according to age, body weight, BSA, and overall physical condition.

> **! TECH ALERT**
>
> If the manufacturer provides a recommended pediatric dose/dosage for a medication, the recommended dose/dosage should be used. Under these conditions, do not use any of the rules that provide estimates. If a physician's prescription does not agree with the manufacturer's indication, the pharmacist should contact the physician.

CALCULATING MEDICATION DOSES BY BODY WEIGHT

Pediatric doses of medications may be ordered according to body weight or body mass. The most common method of calculation uses grams, milligrams, or micrograms of drug per kilogram of body weight. The order therefore appears as g, mg, or mcg/kg. With this in mind, the child must be weighed with each visit to the hospital or physician's office to be sure the correct amount of medication is ordered. If weight is measured in pounds, it must be converted to kilograms. The conversion factor 2.2 lb = 1 kg is the basis for the conversion, which can be completed using ratio and proportion (R&P) or dimensional analysis (DA) (Example 12.1).

EXAMPLE 12.1

What is the weight of a 22-lb infant in kilograms?

R & P

$$\frac{1 \text{ kg}}{2.2 \text{ lb}} = \frac{x}{22 \text{ lb}} \quad 2.2x = 22 \text{ kg} \quad x = 10 \text{ kg}$$

DA

$$\text{kg} = \frac{1 \text{ kg}}{2.2 \text{ lb}} \times \frac{22 \text{ lb}}{1} = 10 \text{ kg}$$

> **TECH NOTE**
>
> Because the calculations in Example 12.1 are normally going to be included in multistep conversions to obtain the weight or volume of a dose, it is advisable to practice them using DA.

EXAMPLE 12.2

An infant weighs 18 lb 4 oz. What is the infant's weight in kilograms?

If a person is weighed in pounds and ounces, the ounces must be converted to pounds first.

Convert ounces to pounds using 16 oz = 1 lb.

$$lb = \frac{1\ lb}{16\ oz} \times \frac{4\ oz}{1} = \frac{1}{4}\ lb \quad so: 8\ lb + \frac{1}{4}\ lb = 18\frac{1}{4}\ lb$$

Fractions are *not* used in the metric system: $18\frac{1}{4}$ can be converted to 18.25 for the next step.

$$kg = \frac{1\ kg}{2.2\ lb} \times \frac{18.25\ lb}{1} = 8.3\ kg$$

> **! TECH ALERT**
> Conversions including a mixture of ounces and pounds need to be converted to pounds before using pounds in a DA or R&P equation because they involve addition.

Practice Problems A

Convert the following weights and round to the nearest hundredth of a kilogram. Show all of your calculations.

1. A child weighs 65 lb; what is the weight in kilograms? _____

2. An infant weighs 8 lb 12 oz; what is the weight in kilograms? _____

3. A child weighs 75 lb; what is the weight in kilograms? _____

4. A child weighs 112 lb; what is the weight in kilograms? _____

5. A child weighs 48 lb; what is the weight in kilograms? _____

Although body weight calculations can be performed with a series of R&P calculations, DA is the preferred method because one equation can be used to obtain the final answer. This is the best way to keep track of units throughout multistep problems.

TECH NOTE
ORDER FOR DIMENSIONAL ANALYSIS

1. Set up a DA equation so that the units needed in the numerator of the *final* answer are in the numerator of the first fraction of the DA equation—this unit will *never* be canceled.
2. Set up the next fraction in the equation so that the units of its numerator are the same as the units of the denominator of the first fraction (so these units will cancel when the fractions are multiplied).
3. If necessary, set up the next fraction in the equation so that the units of its numerator are the same as the units of the denominator of the second fraction (so these units cancel when the fractions are multiplied).
4. Repeat with additional terms as many times as needed to solve the problem.
5. Multiply the fractions, and cancel units.

EXAMPLE 12.3

A 53-lb child has been diagnosed with epilepsy. The physician orders Dilantin 30 mg Kapseals to be given at 2.5 mg/kg/*dose*. How many Kapseals should be given per dose?

As with any DA calculation, identify your intended answer and work from there. In this case the answer will be the number of Kapseals per dose.

$$\frac{\# \text{ Kapseals}}{\text{dose}} = \frac{1 \text{ Kapseal}}{30 \text{ mg}} \times \frac{2.5 \text{ mg}}{\text{kg/dose}} \times \frac{1 \text{ kg}}{2.2 \text{ lb}} \times \frac{53 \text{ lb}}{1} = 2.01 \text{ Kapseals/dose}$$

Therefore the child should be administered two Kapseals with each dose of medication because this is the measurable dose, given that capsules (Kapseals) cannot be divided.

EXAMPLE 12.4

A physician orders amoxicillin 20 mg/kg/*day* to be given q8h to a 42-lb child. The concentration of amoxicillin is 125 mg/5 mL.

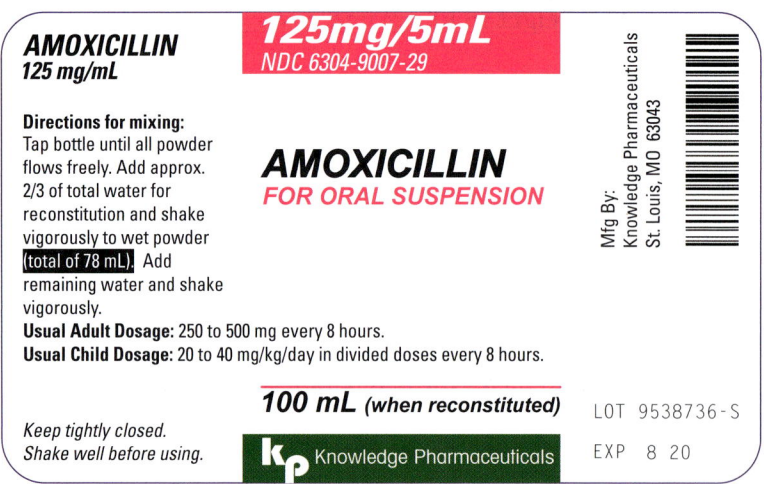

How many mg are needed *per dose*?

$$\frac{mg}{dose} = \frac{20\ mg}{kg/day} \times \frac{1\ day}{3\ doses} \times \frac{1\ kg}{2.2\ lb} \times \frac{42\ lbs}{1} = 127.27\ mg/dose$$

The more relevant question is what amount or volume of medication should be given per dose?

$$\frac{mL}{dose} = \frac{5\ mL}{125\ mg} \times \frac{20\ mg}{kg/day} \times \frac{1\ day}{3\ doses} \times \frac{1\ kg}{2.2\ lb} \times \frac{42\ lbs}{1} = 5.09\ mL/dose$$

The amoxicillin dose can be rounded to 5 mL rather than 5.1 mL for a measurable quantity. As a shorter method, because you already calculated the dose in mg, the volume can be determined as follows:

$$\frac{mL}{dose} = \frac{5\ mL}{125\ mg} \times \frac{127.27\ mg}{dose} = 5.1\ mL/dose$$

If the question had been what volume of medication would be given per dose in household measurements, the DA sequence would be as follows:

$$tsp = \frac{1\ tsp}{5\ mL} \times \frac{5\ mL}{125\ mg} \times \frac{20\ mg}{kg/day} \times \frac{1\ day}{3\ doses} \times \frac{1\ kg}{2.2\ lb} \times \frac{42\ lb}{1} = 1.02\ tsp$$

The measurable dose is 1 tsp.

EXAMPLE 12.5

A physician orders vancomycin 10 mg/kg IV (further diluted in 100 mL NS) to run over 60 minutes q6h. After reconstitution, the vancomycin strength is 500 mg/10 mL. The child weighs 50 pounds.

The way this order is written, the full 10 mg/kg is to be given four times a day, q6h, so use 10 mg/kg/*dose* in the DA calculation.

How many milliliters of reconstituted vancomycin for injection should be added to 100 mL of normal saline for injection to provide one dose?

$$\frac{mL}{dose} = \frac{10\ mL}{500\ mg} \times \frac{10\ mg}{kg/dose} \times \frac{1\ kg}{2.2\ \#} \times \frac{50\ \#}{1} = 2.27\ mL/dose$$

The measurable amount of 2.3 mL should be added to a 100-mL IV bag of normal saline.

TECH NOTE
Not all medications can be rounded to a whole number. Typically, the smaller the dose and the more potent the medication, the less rounding is recommended.

! TECH ALERT
Be sure to read orders carefully to distinguish whether medication is being ordered per dose or per day!

Practice Problems B

Use **body weight** calculations with DA to answer the following dosing questions.

1. A physician orders Veetids 10 mg/kg q8h for a child who weighs 55 lb. Note: *This dose is to be given every 8 hours for a total of three times per day.* The medication strength is 250 mg/5 mL.

   What volume of medication (mL) should be given per dose?

   How many milligrams will the child receive per dose?

   How many milligrams will the child receive in 1 day?

   Indicate the amount of medication to be administered per dose on each of the following measuring devices.

   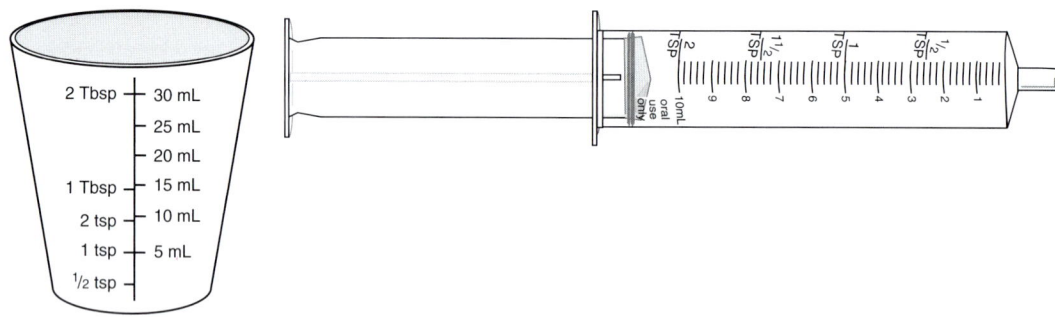

2. A physician orders Zithromax suspension 10 mg/kg daily for a 44-lb child with acute bronchitis. The medication available is 200 mg/5 mL.

   What is the dose in mg for the child?

   What is the volume of medication to be given to the child for this dose?

Indicate the amount of medication to be administered on each of the following measuring devices.

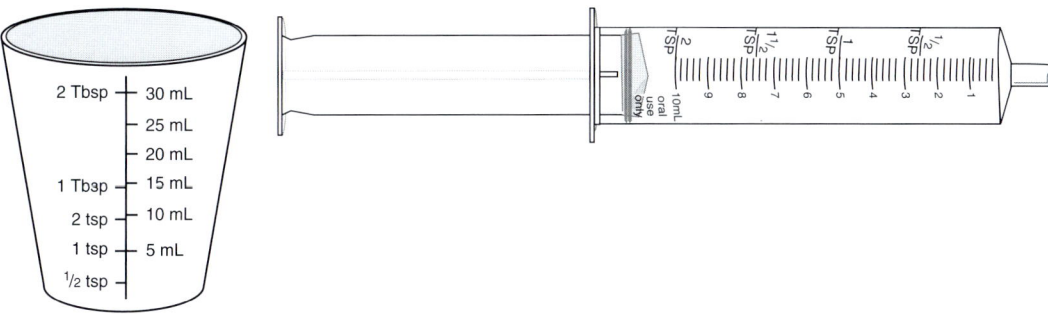

3. A physician orders Zyrtec syrup 0.1 mg/kg daily for a 55-lb child with allergies. The medication is available in 5 mg/5 mL.

What volume of medication in mL should be given to the child per dose?

What is this dose in the household measurement system?

Indicate the amount of medication to be administered on each of the following measuring devices.

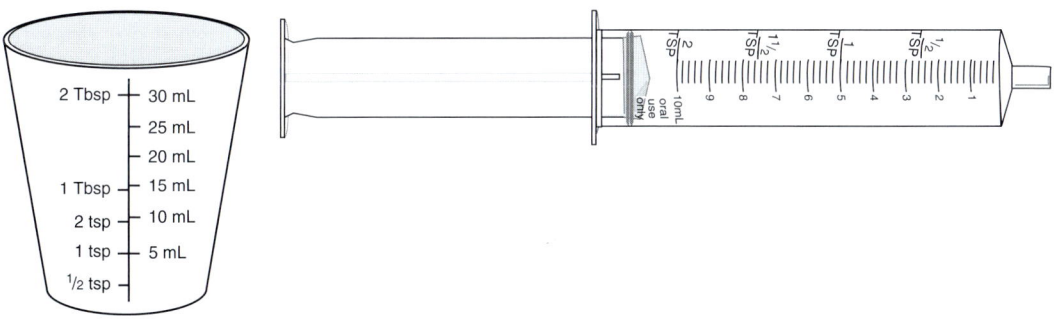

4. A physician orders Zarontin syrup 20 mg/kg/day in *divided* doses bid for a 54-lb child who has been diagnosed with seizures. Note: *The 20 mg/kg/day is the total daily dose.* The medication available is Zarontin syrup 250 mg/5 mL.

   How many milligrams should be given in a day?

   How many milligrams should be administered for a single dose?

   What is the volume (mL) of medication to be given to the child per dose?

5. A physician orders Lanoxin (digoxin) elixir 8 mcg/kg for a 55-lb child. The available medication is 50 mcg/mL.

   What is the dose in micrograms for the child?

   What volume of medication should be given for one dose?

6. A child has an order for Demerol (meperidine) syrup 1 mg/kg per dose for postoperative pain. The child weighs 88 lb. The medication available is meperidine 50 mg/5 mL.

   What volume of medication should be administered per dose to this child?

7. A physician wants a 53-lb child to have Tylenol (acetaminophen) elixir gr $\overline{ss}$/kg q8h prn high fever. The medication available is acetaminophen 325 mg/5 mL. *Hint: Use the conversion gr i = 65 mg.*

   What volume of medication should be given per dose?

8. A physician orders erythromycin 10 mg/kg q6h for an 88-lb child. The available medications are erythromycin suspension 400 mg/5 mL and erythromycin 200 mg chewable tablets.

   What strength of erythromycin should be given to the child q6h?

   What volume of the suspension would be given for one dose?

   How many chewable tablets would be administered for one dose?

9. A physician orders Tofranil (imipramine) 0.3 mg/kg hs for child with enuresis. The child weighs 72 lb. The available medication is 10 mg tabs.

   What dose strength of medication should be administered to the child each bedtime?

   How many tablets should be administered to the child for each dose?

10. A physician orders Ceclor (cefaclor) 50 mg/kg/day to be administered in divided doses qid to a 38-lb child. The available medications are 250 mg/5 mL and 125 mg/5 mL.

    What weight of medication should be administered to the child for a single dose?

    Which concentration should be chosen for this child and why?

    What volume of medication should be administered to the child per dose using the chosen concentration of the medication?

11. A physician orders ampicillin 100 mg/kg/day in four divided doses for an infant who weighs 12 lb. The available medication is 125 mg/5 mL.

What volume of medication should be given per dose?

What would be the measureable dose in household measurements?

What would be the measurable dose in household measurements if the concentration used was 250 mg/5 mL?

12. A physician orders aminophylline 2.5 mg/kg/dose q8h for a 40-lb child. The available medication is aminophylline oral liquid 90 mg/5 mL.

What is the strength of one dose (mg)?

What volume of medication should be administered per dose?

How many teaspoons of medication should be administered to the child per dose?

13. A physician orders acetaminophen elixir 6 mg/kg for a 45-lb child. The available elixir contains 160 mg/5 mL.

What volume of medication should be administered to the child?

What type of measuring device should be provided for the parent to administer this medication at home?

14. A 25-lb child has an order for Lasix (furosemide) 2 mg/kg IM stat. The available medication is Lasix 10 mg/mL.

    How many mg should be administered to the child?

    What volume of medication should be injected?

    What size syringe should be used to measure this dose? _____

15. A physician orders Demerol (meperidine) 1.25 mg/kg IM q6h prn for a 44-lb child. The available medication is meperidine 50 mg/mL.

    What is the strength needed per dose?

    What is the volume needed per dose?

Use of Clark's Rule for Pediatric Dosing

Clark's rule is a method for approximating pediatric doses based on the manufacturer's recommended average adult dose, by relating the child's body weight to an average adult's body weight. The assumption with the formula is that the average adult weighs about 150 lb. Because studies of body weight of adults have shown that the average adult now weighs more than 150 lb, Clark's rule is being phased out as a means for calculating pediatric doses. Technicians should still be aware of this method.

> **TECH ALERT**
> The pediatric dose recommended by a manufacturer should always be used!

Clark's rule:

$$\text{Child's dose} = \frac{\text{child's weight in pounds}}{150} \times \text{adult dose (AD)}$$

TECH NOTE
An answer obtained using Clark's rule is always an approximation; 150 pounds is an estimate of an average adult's weight.

! TECH ALERT
Clark's rule would never be used to determine the dose of medication with a narrow therapeutic range—that is, one where there is little difference between therapeutic and toxic levels!

EXAMPLE 12.6

 A physician orders Cefzil (cefprozil) for a 38-lb child with an upper respiratory infection. The adult dose for Cefzil is 500 mg q24h.

Because the physician did not order an amount per kilogram of body weight, calculating this medication by "mg/kg" body weight method is not possible.

How many milligrams should be given for one dose?

$$\text{Child's dose} = \frac{38}{150} \times 500 \text{ mg} = 126.7 \text{ mg}$$

If this prescription is filled with Cefzil 125 mg/5 mL, how many milliliters are needed per dose?

$$\text{mL} = \frac{5 \text{ mL}}{125 \text{ mg}} \times \frac{126.7 \text{ mg}}{\text{dose}} = 5.07 \text{ mL}$$

This dose should be rounded to 5 mL, which is a measurable amount. Remember this is already an approximation due to the use of Clark's rule.

Practice Problems C

Round all calculations to a measurable dose for the device to be used in the final step. Show your calculations.

1. A physician orders Benylin (dextromethorphan) syrup for a 30-lb child. The normal adult dose is 20 mg q6h. The medication on hand is Benylin syrup 15 mg/5 mL.

    How many milligrams should the child receive per dose?

    What is the volume of one dose of medication in the metric system?

What is the approximate volume of one dose in household measurements?

Mark the amount of medication in milliliters on one side of the oral syringe and teaspoons on the other side. Observe that they are very close but not exactly the same.

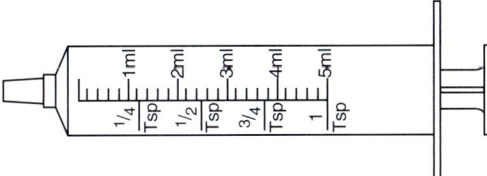

2. A 60-lb child is prescribed Biaxin (clarithromycin) suspension for sinusitis. The adult dose is 500 mg bid. The medication available is 125 mg/5 mL.

How many milligrams should the child receive per dose?

What is the volume of medication per dose?

3. A physician orders Benadryl (diphenhydramine) elixir q4h for a 60-lb child. The usual adult dose is 25 mg q4h. The available medication is diphenhydramine elixir 12.5 mg/5 mL.

How many milligrams should the child receive per dose?

What is the volume of medication per dose?

CALCULATING MEDICATION DOSES BY BODY SURFACE AREA (BSA)

Medications ordered based on an amount per square meter (m^2) provide the most accurate determination of therapeutic doses because they are based on both body weight and height. This form of calculation is often used for pediatric patients, elderly persons, and when dosing toxic medications such as chemotherapeutics. BSA refers to the total body area that is exposed to the environment and is expressed in square meters (m²). To calculate BSA in square meters, the weight and height of a person must be measured, either in the metric or household system, and applied to a **nomogram**, a chart on which height and weight are plotted to determine the BSA. The children's nomogram is seen in Fig. 12.1. A nomogram specific for adults is also available for use with adults who fall outside of what is considered normal weight for height or those who are being administered toxic medications (Fig. 12.2).

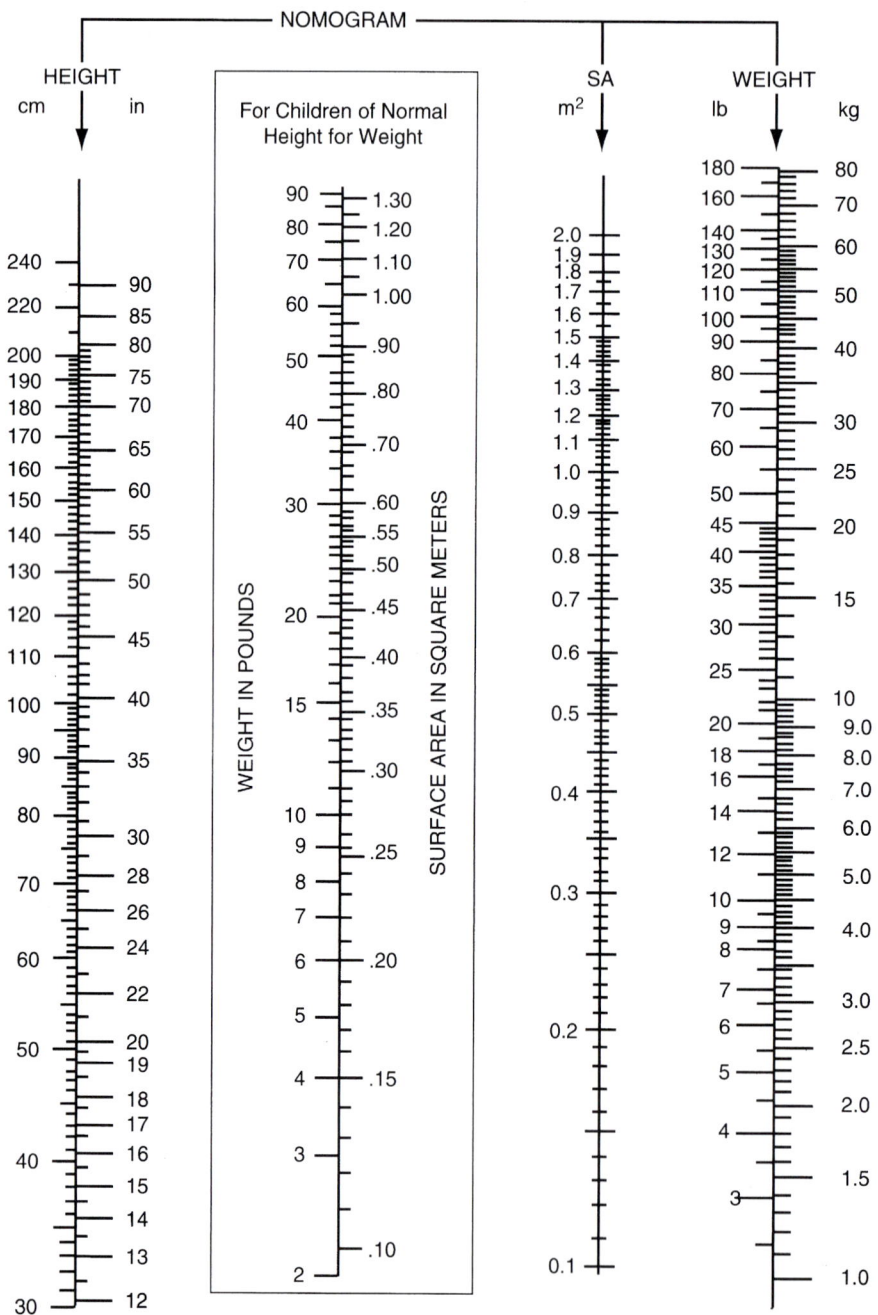

FIGURE 12.1 Nomogram for measuring body surface area for a child. (Modified from data by E Boyd and CD West. In Behrman RE, Vaughan VC: Nelson Textbook of Pediatrics, ed 14, Philadelphia, Saunders, 1992.)

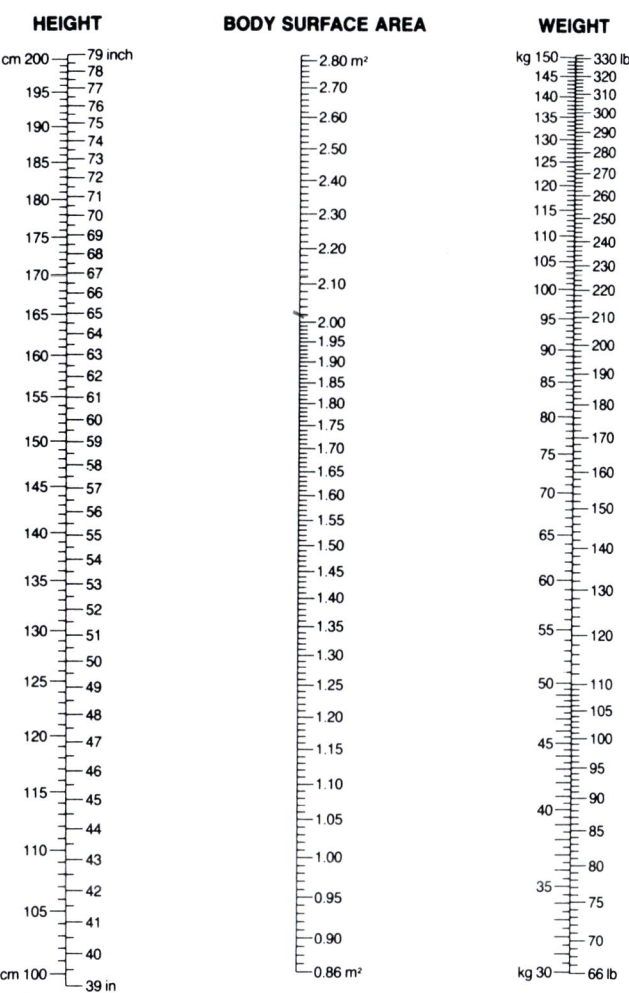

FIGURE 12.2 Nomogram for calculating body surface area for an adult. (Lentner C: Geigy Scientific Tables, ed 8, vol 1, Basel, Switzerland, Ciba-Geigy, 1981.)

To use a nomogram, locate the patient's height and weight, *in the same measurement system*, on the correct indication lines of the chart. Notice that the metric system is on the left side of the height measurement column and on the right side of the weight measurement column on the child's nomogram. On the adult chart, the metric system is on the left side of both the height and weight columns. After finding the height and weight for either the child or the adult, draw a straight line between the two points to find the measurement at the point of intersection on the surface area (SA) line. This is the estimated BSA. For the child who is of normal height and weight for age, the BSA may be calculated only by the child's weight. Notice that the child's nomogram has the added column within the center box that shows BSA indicated by weight in pounds for a child of normal height and weight. This box is not found on the adult nomogram.

Fig. 12.3 depicts the use of the nomogram. Notice that the person is 41″ tall and weighs 36 lb. The intersection of the straight line on the SA line is 0.68, so the estimated BSA for this patient is 0.68 m^2.

The pharmacy technician will rarely, if ever, have to use a nomogram, but once again, it is good to be familiar with the concept. They typically are used by a pharmacist or physician in a clinical hospital setting.

264 SECTION III Calculations with Prescriptions and Medication Orders

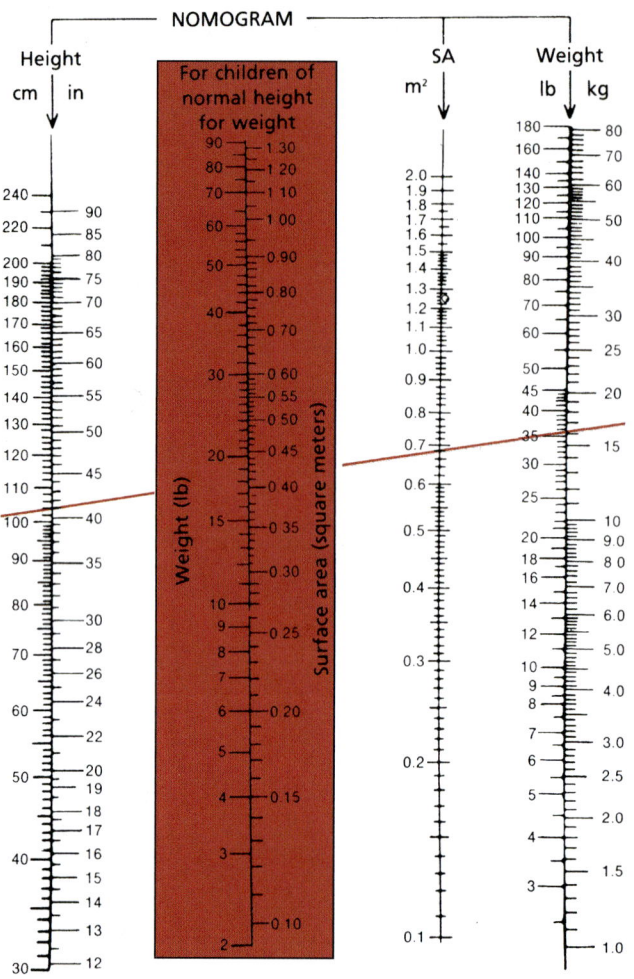

FIGURE 12.3 Reading an estimated body surface area at the point of line intersection on the surface area (SA) line. (Modified from data by E Boyd and CD West. In Behrman RE, Kliegman RM, Jenson HB: Nelson Textbook of Pediatrics, ed 16, Philadelphia, Saunders, 2000.)

Practice Problems D

Using the proper nomogram, calculate the following BSA as practice. Round to the nearest hundredth.

1. A child weighs 15 lb and is 24" tall.

2. A child is 48" tall and weighs 50 lb.

3. A child is 60 cm tall and weighs 5 kg.

Copyright © 2019 by Elsevier, Inc. All rights reserved.

4. A child is normal height for 40 lb.

5. A child weighs 20 kg and is 100 cm tall

The most accurate method of determining a dose using BSA is when the medication is ordered in micrograms, milligrams, or grams per square meter. For calculating doses in these instances, the BSA in square meters is multiplied by the dose ordered using DA.

EXAMPLE 12.7

 A physician orders the chemotherapeutic agent Cytoxan 50 mg/m²/dose IV for an adult who is 55" tall and weighs 160 lb. What dose should be given?

First, determine the BSA by plotting 55" and 160 lb on the nomogram. The BSA is 1.75 m².

If the vial of medication is 200 mg/10 mL, what is the volume of the dose?

$$mL = \frac{10 \text{ mL}}{200 \text{ mg}} \times \frac{50 \text{ mg}}{m^2/\text{dose}} \times \frac{1.75 \text{ m}^2}{1} = 4.375 \text{ mL/dose}$$

The measurable dose of this chemotherapeutic medication is 4.4 mL

If a medication for a child is not ordered in an amount per square meters, a formula similar to Clark's rule may be used to calculate the dose. The "normal" BSA of 1.7 m² for adults and the normal adult dose may be used to *estimate* the child's dose. After using the nomogram for a child, the following formula may be used for calculating the dose.

$$\text{Child's dose} = \frac{\text{child's BSA}}{1.7} \times \text{Adult dose}$$

EXAMPLE 12.8

A physician orders amoxicillin tid for a child who weighs 50 lb and is 45" tall. The normal adult dose is amoxicillin 500 mg tid.

What dose should be given to the child if the available medication is 250 mg/5 mL?

Determine the BSA of the child using the nomogram. The height and weight calculate to a BSA of 0.86 m².

Fill in the formula given earlier to obtain the desired strength of medication.

$$\text{Child's dose} = \frac{0.86}{1.7} \times 500 \text{ mg} = 252.94 \text{ mg}$$

Calculate the dose in milliliters.

$$mL = \frac{5 \text{ mL}}{250 \text{ mg}} \times \frac{252.94 \text{ mg}}{1} = 5.06 \text{ mL}$$

The measurable dose to be given is 5 mL.

Practice Problems E

Calculate the following based on BSA. Determine the BSA if required, and insert it into the proper formula. Use the same formula for BSA for adults who do not meet the standard height/weight sizes. Show your calculations. Round to the nearest hundredth for the dose in milligrams. Round to the nearest tenth for volume to be administered (measurable dose).

1. A child is 25″ long and weighs 15 lb. The physician orders Lanoxin (digoxin) elixir daily. The adult dose of Lanoxin is 0.25 mg/day. The available medication is Lanoxin pediatric elixir 0.05 mg/mL.

    What is the child's BSA? _____

    What is the daily dose of Lanoxin in milligrams for the child?

    What volume of medication would be administered per day? _____

2. A child has a BSA of 0.88 m². The physician orders Tegretol (carbamazepine) for epilepsy. The adult dose of the medication is 200 mg qid. The medication is available in Tegretol suspension 100 mg/5 mL.

    What is the single-dose strength for the child?

    What is the volume of medication per dose?

3. A physician orders prednisone for a child for an allergic reaction. The child weighs 41 kg and is 158 cm tall. The usual adult dose is 5 mg tid. The medication available is prednisone syrup 1 mg/1 mL.

    What is the child's BSA? _____

    What strength of medication should be administered to the child per dose?

    What volume of medication should be administered?

4. A 40-lb child is of normal height for weight. The physician orders Dilantin (phenytoin) suspension for the child for seizures. The available medication is Dilantin suspension 125 mg/5 mL. The normal adult dose is 100 mg tid.

   What is the child's BSA? _____

   What is the dose to be administered to the child?

   What is the volume of medication to be given to the child?

5. A physician orders erythromycin oral suspension for a child with acute bronchitis with a BSA of 1.08 m². The usual adult dose is erythromycin 250 mg qid. The medication is available as Ilosone oral suspension 250 mg/5 mL.

   What strength of medication should be given to the child in a single dose?

   What is the volume of medication to be given per dose?

6. A child who weighs 20 kg, is 114 cm tall, and has a BSA of 0.8 m² has an order for Demerol (meperidine) po q6h prn severe pain. The usual adult dose is 50 mg q6h. The medication is available as 50 mg/5 mL.

   What dose should be administered to the child q6h?

   What volume of medication should be given to the child per dose?

7. An adult is 64″ tall and weighs 120 lb. The physician has ordered Vancocin (vancomycin) 600 mg/m² IV q12h. The available medication is 1 g/10 mL after reconstitution. *Hint: Be sure to include the conversion factor between milligrams and grams in your DA setup.*

   What is the BSA? _____

   What volume of medication should be prepared for administration of the infusion?

8. An adult with a BSA of 1.78 m² has been diagnosed with a malignant neoplasm. The physician orders Oncovin (vincristine) 1.4 mg/m² IV. Oncovin is available as 1 mg/1 mL.

   What volume of medication should be given to this patient?

9. An adult with a BSA of 1.62 m² has severe herpes zoster. The physician has ordered Zovirax (acyclovir) 500 mg/m² q8h. Zovirax is available in 400-mg tablets.

   What dose of medication should be given to the patient q8h?

   How many whole tablets should be given to come closest to this dose?

10. A child has severe streptococcal pneumonia, and the physician orders Augmentin (amoxicillin/clavulanate) q8h. The child weighs 44 lb and is of normal height for weight with a BSA of 0.8 m². The usual adult dose is 500 mg q8h. The medication is available in Augmentin pediatric chewable tablets 250 mg and Augmentin suspension 250 mg/5 mL.

    What amount of medication should be administered to the child with each dose?

    How many chewable tablets should be given to the child?

    What volume of suspension should be given to the child per dose?

    Which form of medication would be the most accurate for the child? _____

Calculating Medication Doses for Pediatric Patients Based on Age

Pediatric doses have also been estimated by age using Fried's or Young's rules, which are based on the normal adult dose. These formulas will yield approximate answers and should not be used with medications that have a narrow therapeutic index. Age is no longer considered a valid criterion for determining pediatric dosing, but a technician should still be aware of the following formulas.

Fried's rule is used for infants up to 12 months:

$$\text{Infant's dose} = \frac{\text{age in months}}{150} \times \text{Adult dose}$$

EXAMPLE 12.9

 A physician orders amoxicillin for a 6-month-old infant. The usual adult dose is 500 mg. How many milligrams should the infant receive per dose?

$$\text{Infant's dose} = \frac{6}{150} \times 500 \text{ mg} = 20 \text{ mg}$$

If the medication available is amoxicillin 50 mg/mL, what dose would be given to the infant?

$$\text{mL} = \frac{1 \text{ mL}}{50 \text{ mg}} \times \frac{20 \text{ mg}}{1} = 0.4 \text{ mL}$$

Young's rule is used to calculate medications for children 1 year of age to 12 years of age.

$$\text{Child's dose} = \frac{\text{child's age in years}}{\text{child's age in years} + 12} \times \text{Adult dose}$$

EXAMPLE 12.10

A physician orders amoxicillin for a 5-year-old child. The adult dose is 500 mg per dose. What dose would be given to the child?

$$\text{Child's dose} = \frac{5}{5 + 12} \times 500 \text{ mg} = 147.06 \text{ mg}$$

If the medication is available as amoxicillin suspension 400 mg/5 mL, what dose would be given to the child?

$$\text{mL} = \frac{5 \text{ mL}}{400 \text{ mg}} \times \frac{147.06 \text{ mg}}{1} = 1.84 \text{ mL}$$

The measurable dose is 1.8 mL.

> **! TECH ALERT**
>
> If the manufacturer has a suggested amount for a pediatric dose, that dose should always be used. More and more physicians are using only medications that have suggested manufacturer's doses for children rather than using age or body weight as a basis for calculating prescriptions for special populations.

Practice Problems F

Calculate the following doses of medication. Show your calculations. Round to the nearest hundredth for weight calculations and the nearest tenth when providing volume calculations, unless otherwise noted.

1. A physician orders Milk of Magnesia for a 3-year-old child. The adult dose for Milk of Magnesia is 30 mL.

    What volume of Milk of Magnesia should be given to the child?

2. A physician wants a 6-month-old child to have phenobarbital. The usual adult dose is phenobarbital 30 mg. Medication is available in an elixir of 20 mg/5 mL.

   What dose of the medication should be given to the child?

   What volume of medication should be administered per dose?

3. A 6-month-old infant has an order for Demerol (meperidine) q4h. The usual adult dose is Demerol 50 mg q4h. The medication is available as meperidine 50 mg/5 mL.

   What dose should be given to the child?

   What volume of medication should be administered per dose?

4. A 6-year-old child has a severe case of hives. The physician wants the child to have prednisone for relief. The adult dose is 20 mg. The available medication is prednisone oral solution 5 mg/5 mL.

   What dose should be given to the child?

   What volume of medication should be administered to the child per dose?

REVIEW

Certain populations require special dosing considerations. In all cases, the manufacturer's suggested dosage should be the guideline for the amount of medication that is administered. Highly toxic medications also require special calculations for safe and accurate doses. In most cases today, BSA is the basis for calculating children's doses and chemotherapeutic medications. In the past, children's doses were estimated from adult doses based on weight or age using Clark's, Young's, or Fried's rules. These methods are not common now. With other medications, the physician may write adult or children's dosages to be given on the basis of the amount of medication per body weight, such as milligrams per kilogram.

! **TECH ALERT**

Remember that "normal" for an adult is not always "normal" but must be adjusted for certain characteristics of patients, such as body weight, organ function, and other parameters.

Posttest

Calculate the following problems using the correct formula for each situation provided. If measuring devices for administration are included, indicate the volume of medication on the appropriate measuring device(s). Show your calculations. If the volume of medication is less than 1 mL, the answer should be rounded to the hundredths position.

1. A 66-lb child is ordered Benadryl (diphenhydramine) elixir 0.4 mg per kilogram of body weight.

   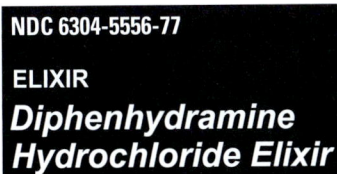

   NDC 6304-5556-77
   ELIXIR
   Diphenhydramine Hydrochloride Elixir

   Elixir K-P 5556 for prescription dispensing only.
   Contains-12.5 mg diphenhydramine hydrochloride in each 5 mL. Alcohol 14%.
   Dose-Adults: 2-4 teaspoonfuls; children over 20 lb: 1-2 teaspoonfuls; 3-4 times daily

   4 FLUIDOUNCES
   KNOWLEDGE PHARMACEUTICALS
   St. Louis, MO 63043 USA
   5556A406   10 2021 P67419N
   Exp date and lot

   What is the strength of medication to be given in mg?

   What dose should be given in mL using the diphenhydramine label?

   What is the measurable dose in household measurements?

Continued

Posttest, cont.

2. A child weighs 66 lb, and the physician orders prochlorperazine (Compazine) syrup 0.5 mg/kg/day *in three divided doses*. Prochlorperazine syrup is available in a 5 mg/5 mL strength.

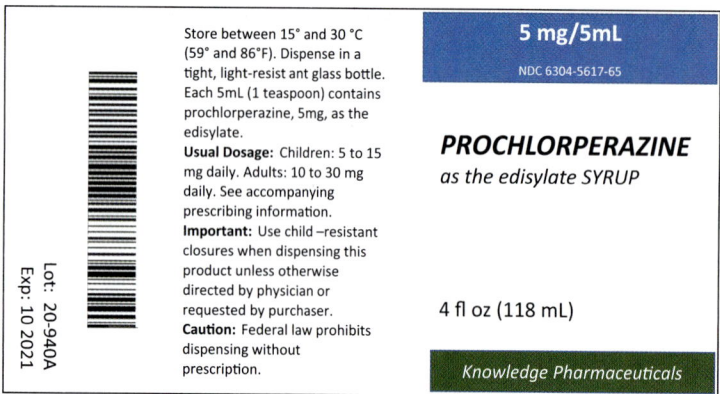

What volume of medication should be administered *per dose*? _____

3. A child weighs 55 lb and is normal height for weight. The physician orders amoxicillin for this child. The normal adult dose is amoxicillin 500 mg tid. The medication is available as amoxicillin 125 mg/5 mL and 250 mg/5 mL.

   What is his BSA? _____

   How many mg should be administered per dose?

   Which strength is the most appropriate for this dose? _____

   What volume of the chosen medication should be administered?

4. A child has a BSA of 0.54 m². The physician wants this child to have Claritin for hay fever. The normal adult dose is 10 mg. The available medication is 1 mg/1 mL.

   What volume of medication should be administered to the child?

Posttest, cont.

5. The recommended dose of meperidine for a child is 6 mg/kg/day for pain. The physician orders this to be given every 4 hours for a 66-lb child. The medication is available as 50 mg/5 mL.

   What is the total amount of medication that the child can receive in a day?

   How many mg should be given per dose?

   What volume of medication would provide one dose?

6. An emaciated 100 lb adult has a maintenance order for aminophylline 3 mg/kg/dose every 8 hours. The medication available is aminophylline oral liquid 105 mg/5 mL.

   What strength of medication should be given to this patient every 8 hours?

   What volume of medication should be administered for each dose?

7. An 8-year-old child has an order for Tofranil. The usual adult dose is Tofranil 50 mg. The medication is available in 10 mg tablets.

   What rule is needed for this calculation? _____

   What strength of medication should be administered to the child?

   How many tablets are needed for the dose? _____

Continued

Posttest, cont.

8. A 12-year-old child has an order for ibuprofen for elevated temperature. The usual adult dose is 400 mg q6h. Ibuprofen is available as 100 mg/5 mL.

   What rule is needed for this calculation? _____

   What strength of medication should be given per dose?

   What volume of medication should be administered for each dose?

   If the medication is available in 50 mg chewable tablets, how many tablets should be given per dose? _____

9. A 6-month-old infant is to be given acetaminophen q4h for a high fever related to cellulitis. The usual adult dose is 325 mg q4–6h. The medication available is acetaminophen 160 mg/5 mL.

   What rule is needed for this calculation? _____

   What strength of medication should be given to the infant?

   What volume of medication should be given to the infant?

10. A 64-lb child has a severe allergic reaction to a bee sting. The physician orders Decadron. The normal adult dose is Decadron 4 mg. The available medication is dexamethasone elixir 0.5 mg/5 mL.

    What rule is needed for this calculation? _____

    What strength of medication should be administered to the child?

    What volume of medication should be administered to the child?

Posttest, cont.

11. A physician orders dexamethasone IM for a child with a BSA of 0.84 m². The normal adult dose is Decadron 4 mg. The available injection is Decadron 10 mg/mL.

What volume of medication is needed?

Show the dosage on the syringe.

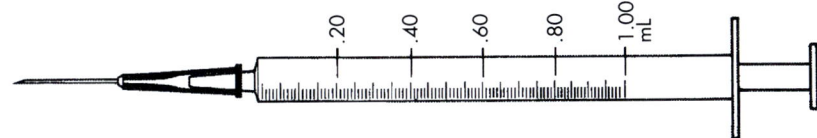

12. A 48-lb child has an order for dexamethasone 0.08 mg/kg every 12 hours. The medication is available as an oral liquid at 0.5 mg/5 mL and an injection at 4 mg/mL.

What strength of medication should be given to the child with each dose?

What volume of medication should be given to the child *orally*?

What volume of medication should be administered *parenterally*?

Continued

Posttest, cont.

13. A 7-year-old child weighing 78 lb is being treated for status epilepticus with diazepam 0.3 mg/kg. The medication is available in 5 mg and 10 mg tablets, 5 mg/5 mL oral solution, and 5 mg/mL injectable solution.

What strength of the medication should be administered to the child?

How many tablets would be given orally for this dose? _____

What volume of medication should be administered if the oral solution is used?

What volume of medication should be administered parenterally?

14. A male patient who is 5′ 11″ tall and weighing 185 lb is being treated with cisplatin IV for testicular cancer. The dosage for cisplatin is 20 mg/m^2 per day × 5 days of each cycle. The medication is available as a powder in 10-mg and 50-mg vials. The medication is reconstituted to a concentration of 1 mg/mL.

What is the patient's BSA? _____

What strength of medication should be administered per dose?

Which vial of medication should be reconstituted to provide the ordered dose? _____

What is the volume of reconstituted medication to be administered?

Show the amount of medication to be administered on the following syringe.

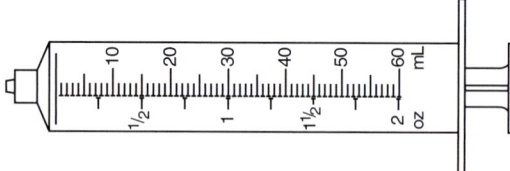

Chapter 12 Calculation of Medications by Age, Body Weight, and Body Surface Area

Posttest, cont.

 15. A patient with a BSA of 1.75 m² is being treated for Hodgkin's disease with doxorubicin 65 mg/m² every 21 days. The medication is available in 5, 10, 25, 75, and 100 mL vials in a 2 mg/mL strength.

How many milligrams of medication should this patient receive per dose?

What volume of medication would be used to provide the patient's dose?

Which vial of medication would be the best choice for use? _____

Continued

278   SECTION III   Calculations with Prescriptions and Medication Orders

Posttest, cont.

 16. A 56-lb child has an order for azithromycin oral suspension to prevent complications of influenza. The amount of medication to be given is 10 mg/kg/day for the first day and 5 mg/kg/day for the next 4 days. Use the label shown for the calculations of doses to be given.

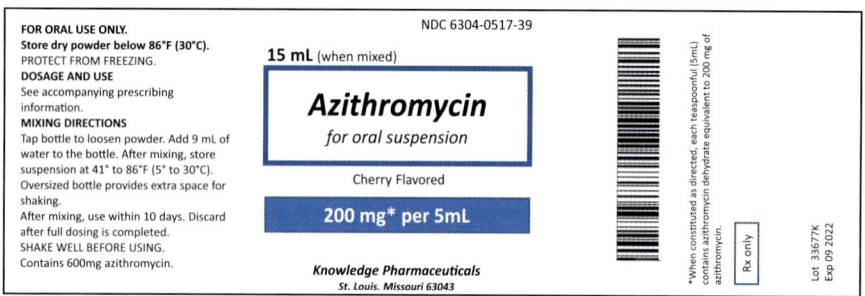

What strength of medication should be given to the child on the first day?

What is the measurable amount of suspension that should be given the first day?

Show this amount on the following oral syringe:

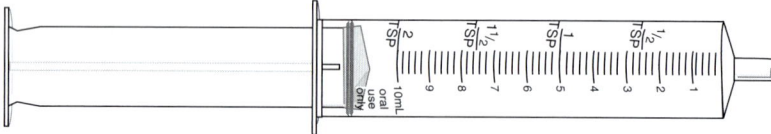

What strength of medication should be given to the child on subsequent days?

What volume of medication should be given to the child on subsequent days?

Show this amount on the following oral syringe:

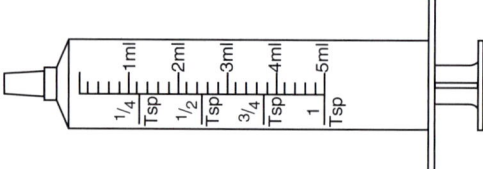

Copyright © 2019 by Elsevier, Inc. All rights reserved.

Chapter 12   Calculation of Medications by Age, Body Weight, and Body Surface Area   279

Posttest, cont.

17. A 4-month-old child is being treated with ampicillin for a strep infection. The normal adult dose is ampicillin 500 mg per dose. The medication is available as an oral suspension 125 mg/5 mL.

What rule is needed for this calculation? _____

What strength of medication should be administered to this child?

What volume of medication should be ordered for the child?

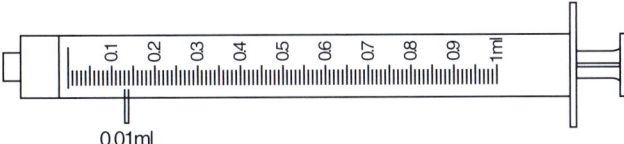

18. A 55-lb child has a prescription for penicillin V potassium to be given q8h. The normal adult dose is penicillin V potassium 500 mg q8h. Use the following label for calculations.

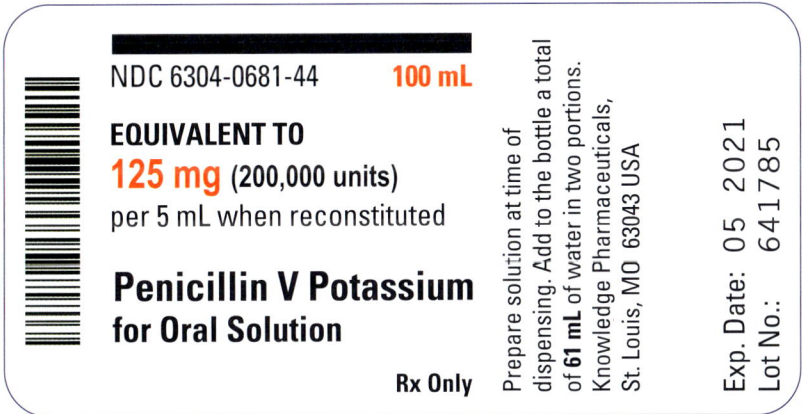

What rule is needed for this calculation? _____

What strength of medication should be administered per dose?

What is the volume of medication to be administered per dose?

Continued

Copyright © 2019 by Elsevier, Inc. All rights reserved.

Posttest, cont.

19. A child has a BSA of 0.9 m². A physician orders codeine 15 mg/m² q6h for a severe aching related to influenza not to exceed 60 mg per day. The medication strength available is 15 mg/5 mL.

What strength of medication should be administered per dose?

What volume of the oral liquid should be administered per dose?

Is the dosage within acceptable range if the child receives the medication every 6 hours? _____

CHAPTER 13

Interpreting Physicians' Orders for Dosages and Days' Supply

OBJECTIVES

1. Calculate the amount of medication needed when quantity is not indicated.
2. Calculate the number of doses of medication in a container.
3. Calculate the length of time a prescription will last.

KEY WORDS

Days' supply Number of days a prescription will last; important to input for insurance reimbursement

Inhaler A device used to deliver medicine by breathing it in through the mouth or nose

Nebulizer A device used to produce a fine spray of medication for inhalation

Pretest

If you are already comfortable with the subject matter, perform the following calculations to test your knowledge. If not, work your way through the chapter and return to them for extra practice. Calculate the doses or dosages for the prescriptions as appropriate. All doses will be administered on the first day as ordered, and a month means 30 days unless otherwise stated. Round answers to measurable doses depending on the utensil to be used or the available form of medication. Show your work.

1. A physician prescribes amoxicillin suspension 250 mg/5 mL 150 mL Sig: 1 teaspoonful three times a day until the entire amount has been taken. Include a dosespoon.

   How many days will the medication last?

2. A physician prescribes Lasix (furosemide) 20 mg po daily × 1 mo.

   How many furosemide 40 mg tablets are needed for a month's supply? _____

Continued

Pretest, cont.

3. Interpret the following prescription:
   _____

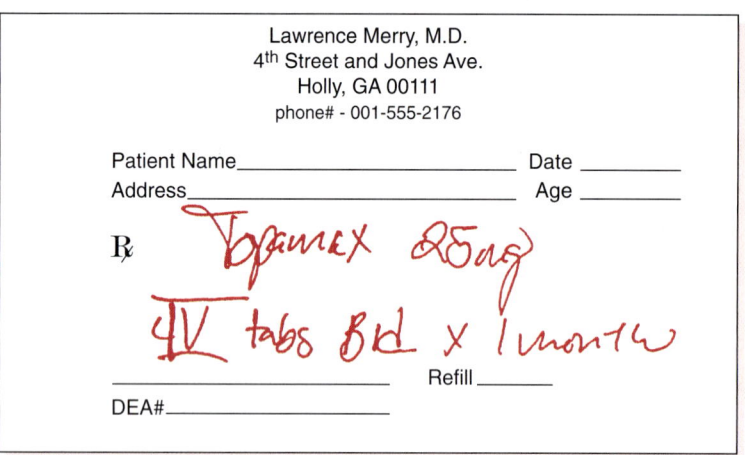

How many 25 mg tablets are needed to fill the prescription?

Write the directions as they should appear on the customer's bottle:
_____

4. A physician prescribes Vibramycin 100 mg po tab ii stat and repeat in 12 hours, then 100 mg qd for 1 week.

How many Vibramycin 100 mg tablets should be supplied to fill the prescription?

How many milligrams should the patient receive for the first dose?

Write the directions as they should appear on the customer's bottle:
_____

Pretest, cont.

5. A physician orders ampicillin 0.2 g/kg/d IV to be delivered in *divided doses* q6h. The patient weighs 110 lb.

    How many mg are needed *per dose*?

    How many grams of ampicillin would the patient receive daily?

    The physician wants each dose placed in 5% Dextrose and delivered in a total of 500 mL of fluid.

    How many total milliliters of fluids would the patient receive daily?

6. Stock strength: Toprol-XL 25 mg scored tablet *(unlike most extended-release tablets, Toprol XL can be split as long as the ½ tablet is not crushed or chewed)*

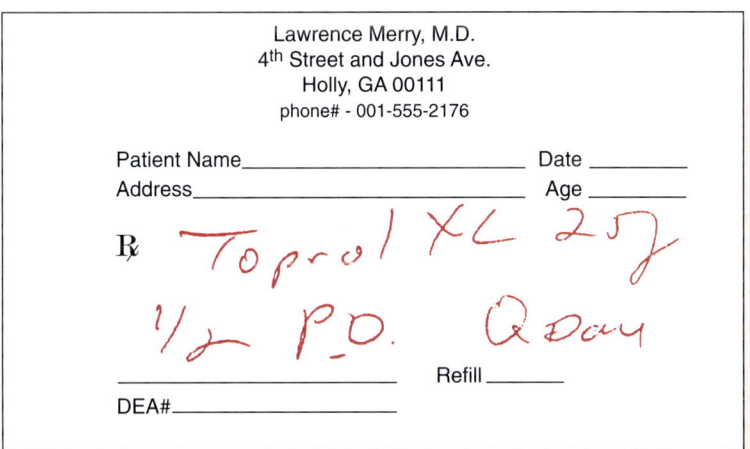

How many tablets are needed to fill the prescription for a month's supply?

What metric weight of drug would the patient receive with each dose?

Write the directions as they should appear on the customer's bottle:

_____

Continued

Pretest, cont.

7. A physician prescribes ibuprofen liquid 10 mg/kg to be administered po qid prn for pain for a child who weighs 66 lb. The available medication is 100 mg/5 mL. The volume of medication to be dispensed is 8 ounces.

   How many milliliters of medication are needed per dose?

   How many milliliters of medication would be needed for 1 day?

   How many doses of medication are available in this prescription?

   Indicate the prescription label directions using household utensils.
   _____

8. A physician prescribes amoxicillin 62.5 mg po tid for 10 days for a child weighing 44 lb. Amoxicillin 125 mg/5 mL is in stock in 100-mL and 150-mL containers.

   What quantity of the medication should the parents give per dose?

   Which container of amoxicillin should be provided for the prescription?

   How much medication would be discarded if the order was followed correctly?

   Write the directions as they should appear on the customer's bottle:
   _____

Chapter 13 Interpreting Physicians' Orders for Dosages and Days' Supply 285

Pretest, cont.

 9. A patient weighing 198 lb is to receive chloramphenicol 50 mg/kg/d in *divided doses* q4h to be administered in D5NS 500 mL for a *Salmonella typhi* infection. The available medication is chloramphenicol 1-g vials 100 mg/mL. *Hint: Only full vials are available for use.*

How many milliliters of chloramphenicol are in a full vial?

How many milliliters of chloramphenicol should be added to each bag of fluids *per dose*?

How many vials of chloramphenicol are needed for *1 day*?

Explain your answer.

_____

 10. A child has a streptococcal infection of the throat. The child weighs 66 lb. The prescription reads as follows: erythromycin 40 mg/kg/d in *divided doses* q6h for 10 days.

The medication is available as erythromycin 200 mg chewable tablets.

How many mg are needed *per dose*?

How many chewable tablets are needed to complete the 10 day order?

Write the directions as they would appear on the prescription label:

_____

Continued

Pretest, cont.

The parent states that the child will not chew the tablet but will take oral liquids. Erythromycin is also available as 400 mg/5 mL. After obtaining the physician's permission for the change, how many milliliters should be dispensed?

How many milliliters would be needed per dose? *(Round to the nearest tenth.)*

11. A patient presents the following prescription, has no drug insurance coverage, and wants a 1-month supply. The medication is available in 40 mg capsules.

Interpret the prescription:
_____

```
              Lawrence Merry, M.D.
              4th Street and Jones Ave.
                  Holly, GA 00111
                phone# - 001-555-2176

   Patient Name_____   Date _____
   Address_____   Age _____

         ℞      Strattera 40mg
                ĪĪ PO Qevening


   _____    Refill prn x 1 yr
   DEA#_____
```

How many capsules should be dispensed?

12. A physician prescribes atenolol 75 mg po qam and 25 mg po at bedtime. The available stock medication is atenolol 50 mg.

How many tablets are needed for a 30-day supply?

Write the directions as they should appear on the prescription label:
_____
_____

INTRODUCTION

The objective of this chapter is to bring together mathematical skills learned in previous chapters to accurately prepare medication for dispensing, given the information provided on a prescription. In some instances the medical professional omits the number of doses of medication necessary or the dose to be given from a total dosage. In many instances, because only one element is missing, pharmacy staff can make the necessary calculation from the prescription without contacting the physician. This chapter provides the knowledge base needed for making accurate decisions for doses and dosages.

Determining the Appropriate Quantity for Dispensing (Dosage)

As long as the physician provides a time frame for a prescription, the pharmacy staff is responsible for ensuring that the patient has sufficient medication to complete the desired medication cycle. Basically, the total dosage needed is the number of doses needed per day times the total number of days prescribed. This can be calculated with dimensional analysis (DA) or, in the case of solid medications, ratio and proportion (R&P).

EXAMPLE 13.1

 A physician orders amoxicillin 500 mg tid × 10 days. Available stock is 500 mg capsules.

This order reads as follows: dispense amoxicillin 500 mg capsules to be taken three times a day for 10 days. Amoxicillin is available in 500 mg capsules. Three capsules per day × 10 days = 30 capsules.

The pharmacy technician in a retail pharmacy would prepare 30 capsules for the pharmacist to check for dispensing. In an inpatient setting, such as a nursing home, the date of the order and the ending date would be noted, so the medication would be discontinued 10 days later.

This example essentially involves applying R&P or DA as follows:

$$\frac{3 \text{ caps}}{1 \text{ day}} = \frac{x \text{ caps}}{10 \text{ days}} \quad x = 30 \text{ caps} \quad \text{or} \quad \text{caps} = \frac{3 \text{ caps}}{1 \text{ day}} \cdot \frac{10 \text{ days}}{1} = 30 \text{ caps}$$

With prescriptions such as this, most pharmacists will expect a quick mental calculation of the answer because it is simple multiplication. Never forget to use common sense when looking at an answer. If a prescription is written for 4 capsules a day for 7 days, simple multiplication gives you the answer of 28 capsules. You are using the process of DA or R&P mentally.

EXAMPLE 13.2

A doctor prescribes cefdinir 125 mg bid for 10 days for a staph infection. The stock strength available is 125 mg/5 mL. How many mL are needed for the entire course of therapy? Using DA will help keep track of the units.

$$\text{total mL required} = \frac{5 \text{ mL}}{125 \text{ mg}} \cdot \frac{125 \text{ mg}}{1 \text{ dose}} \cdot \frac{2 \text{ doses}}{1 \text{ day}} \cdot \frac{10 \text{ days}}{1} = 100 \text{ mL}$$

EXAMPLE 13.3

 A physician prescribes phenobarbital gr i po q6h for epilepsy. Provide a month's supply.

Stock strength: phenobarbital 30 mg tablets

Interpret the prescription: phenobarbital one grain by mouth every 6 hours for epilepsy

How many tablets should be provided to fill the prescription?

$$\text{tablets} = \frac{1 \text{ tablet}}{30 \text{ mg}} \cdot \frac{60 \text{ mg}}{\text{gr i}} \cdot \frac{\text{gr i}}{\text{dose}} \cdot \frac{4 \text{ doses}}{\text{day}} \cdot \frac{30 \text{ days}}{1} = 240 \text{ tablets}$$

How many tablets are needed for a single dose?

$$\text{tablets} = \frac{1 \text{ tablet}}{30 \text{ mg}} \cdot \frac{60 \text{ mg}}{\text{gr i}} \cdot \frac{\text{gr i}}{\text{dose}} = 2 \text{ tablets}$$

What is the dose in milligrams? By definition, gr i = 60 mg with phenobarbital.

Write the directions as they would appear on the customer's bottle:

Take two tablets by mouth every 6 hours for epilepsy.

EXAMPLE 13.4

 On Friday a doctor orders Tagamet 300 mg IM q6h to be sent to the floor for the weekend.

Stock strength: cimetidine (Tagamet) 300 mg/2 mL injection in 8 mL multidose vials

Interpret the medication order:

Tagamet 300 mg intramuscularly every 6 hours

How many vials of medication should be sent to the floor for Friday noon through the weekend, with a sufficient amount to provide the medication on Monday 6 a.m.?

The medication will be administered every 6 hours or 1200, 1800, 0000, 0600

Friday: 2 doses 1200 and 1800

Saturday: 4 doses

Sunday: 4 doses

Monday: 2 doses 0000 and 0600

Total doses = 12

$$\text{vials} = \frac{1 \text{ vial}}{8 \text{ mL}} \cdot \frac{2 \text{ mL}}{300 \text{ mg}} \cdot \frac{300 \text{ mg}}{1 \text{ dose}} \cdot \frac{12 \text{ doses}}{1} = 3 \text{ vials}$$

EXAMPLE 13.5

 After adding 5.7 mL of sterile water for injection (SWI) to a vial of powdered oxacillin 1 g for injection, the resulting strength is oxacillin 250 mg/1.5 mL

How many vials are needed to prepare a 24-hour supply of an order for 750 mg IM q6h?

$$\# \text{ vials} = \frac{1 \text{ vial}}{1 \text{ g}} \cdot \frac{1 \text{ g}}{1{,}000 \text{ mg}} \cdot \frac{750 \text{ mg}}{\text{dose}} \cdot \frac{4 \text{ doses}}{\text{day}} = 3 \text{ vials}$$

Practice Problems A

Show your calculations. A month means 30 days unless otherwise stated.

1. A physician prescribes Voltaren (diclofenac) 50 mg po tid with meals or snack.

   Stock strength: diclofenac 50 mg tablets

   How many tablets are needed to fill this prescription for one month?

   Write the directions as they should appear on the customer's bottle:
   _____

2. A physician prescribes Keflex (cephalexin) oral suspension 62.5 mg po q6h × 10 days.

   Stock strength: cephalexin 125 mg/5 mL oral suspension/60 mL bottle (once reconstituted)

   How many milliliters are needed for the entire course of therapy?

   How many bottles would need to be dispensed for this prescription?

   How many milliliters should be remaining after 10 days?

   What volume of medication should be administered with each dose?

   What is the dose in household measurements?

   Write the directions as they should appear on the customer's bottle:
   _____

3. A physician prescribes nitrofurantoin 0.1 g po qid × 7 d for a urinary tract infection.

   Stock strength: nitrofurantoin 50 mg capsules

   How many capsules are needed to fill this prescription?

   Write the directions as they should appear on the customer's bottle:

4. Interpret the following prescription:

   _____
   _____

   ```
   Lawrence Merry, M.D.
   4th Street and Jones Ave.
   Holly, GA 00111
   phone# - 001-555-2176

   Patient Name_____ Date_____
   Address_____ Age_____

   ℞   Trileptal (150 mg/tab)
       iii po bid
       # 1 month supply
                                    Refill_____
   DEA#_____
   ```

   How many tablets are needed to fill the prescription?

5. What volume of medication is needed to fill the following prescription?

> Lawrence Merry, M.D.
> 4th Street and Jones Ave.
> Holly, GA 00111
> phone# - 001-555-2176
>
> Patient Name_____ Date _____
> Address_____ Age _____
>
> ℞ Keflex 250mg/5mL
>   7 days
>   5mL po qid
>
> _____ Refill _____
> DEA#_____

Write the directions as they should appear on the customer's bottle:

_____

6. During a severe influenza epidemic, a physician writes the following prescription as a prophylaxis against a secondary bacterial infection in an older adult with COPD.

Interpret the order:

_____

> Lawrence Merry, M.D.
> 4th Street and Jones Ave.
> Holly, GA 00111
> phone# - 001-555-2176
>
> Patient Name_____ Date _____
> Address_____ Age _____
>
> ℞ Amoxicillin 500 mg bid
>   × 10 days.
>
> _____ Refill _____
> DEA#_____

The only amoxicillin in stock is amoxicillin 250 mg/capsule. How many capsules should be dispensed to the patient to complete this order?

Write the directions as they should appear on the customer's bottle:

_____

7. A patient presents the following prescription:

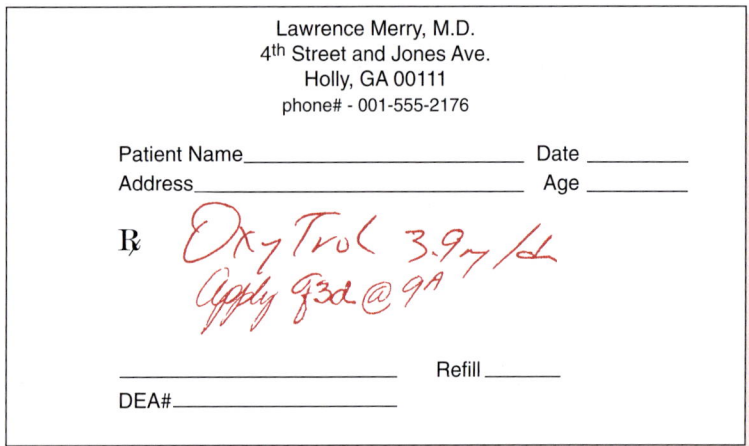

How many patches does the patient need for one month's supply?

Write the directions as they should appear on the customer's box:
_____

8. A physician orders Solu-Cortef 150 mg IM q8h for a patient with severe allergic dermatitis. How many vials should be sent to the floor for a 24-hour period?

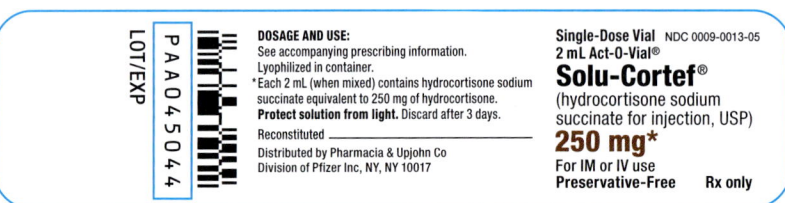

9. A physician prescribes cyanocobalamin 1.5 mg subcutaneously twice a week for 4 weeks. Stock supply: cyanocobalamin 1,000 mcg/mL injection/10 mL multidose vials

How many vials of cyanocobalamin are needed for this order?

How many milliliters are needed for one dose?

10. A physician prescribes cephalexin 500 mg po qid × 2 wk

    Stock strength: cephalexin 500 mg capsules
    How many capsules should be supplied for 2 weeks?

    Write the directions as they should appear on the customer's bottle:
    _____

11. How many tablets are needed for a 14-day supply of Paxil 20 mg tablets?

    ```
    Lawrence Merry, M.D.
    4th Street and Jones Ave.
    Holly, GA 00111
    phone# - 001-555-2176

    Patient Name_____  Date _____
    Address_____  Age _____

    ℞    Paxil 20 mg
         Ti po Qday

    _____  Refill _____
    DEA#_____
    ```

    Write the directions as they should appear on the customer's bottle:
    _____

12. A physician prescribes Lasix (furosemide) 80 mg po stat, then Lasix 40 mg po daily thereafter.

    Stock available: furosemide 40 mg tablets
    How many tablets are needed for the first month's supply?

    Write the directions as they should appear on the customer's bottle:
    _____

Determining the Number of Doses in a Container

If the size and frequency of the dose and the amount of medication in a container are known, the number of doses in the container can be calculated to ensure that the patient has a sufficient amount of medication for the expected time of administration. Basically, the number of doses in a container is the total amount of medication divided by the dose size.

EXAMPLE 13.6

  Prescription: furosemide 80 mg po daily for 1 month

How many doses are provided in a 100-count stock bottle of 40 mg tablets?

$$\text{doses} = \frac{1 \text{ dose}}{80 \text{ mg}} \cdot \frac{40 \text{ mg}}{\text{tablet}} \cdot \frac{100 \text{ tabs}}{1} = 50 \text{ doses}$$

Write the directions as they should appear on the customer's bottle:

Take 2 tablets by mouth daily.

How many tablets are needed to fill this order?

$$\frac{2 \text{ tabs}}{1 \text{ day}} = \frac{x}{30 \text{ days}} \quad x = 60 \text{ tabs for a 1-month supply}$$

EXAMPLE 13.7

A physician prescribes cephalexin suspension 125 mg q6h for 10 days.

Stock available: 60-mL bottles of celphalexin for oral suspension 125 mg/5 mL after reconstitution

How many doses are in one bottle?

$$\text{doses} = \frac{1 \text{ dose}}{125 \text{ mg}} \cdot \frac{125 \text{ mg}}{5 \text{ mL}} \cdot \frac{60 \text{ mL}}{1} = 12 \text{ doses}$$

Will one bottle be sufficient for the prescription?

No. Because 4 doses are needed per day for 10 days, 40 doses are needed.

How many 60 mL bottles of Keflex 125 mg/5 mL would be needed?

$$\text{bottles} = \frac{1 \text{ bottle}}{12 \text{ doses}} \cdot \frac{40 \text{ doses}}{1} = 3.3 \text{ bottles}$$

Dispense four bottles to cover the entire length of therapy.

Write the directions as they should appear on the customer's bottle:

Take 5 mL every 6 hours for 10 days.

Practice Problems B

Determine the number of doses in the container. Note that a month means 30 days unless otherwise stated. Show your work.

1. A physician orders erythromycin ethylsuccinate 200 mg po qid for a child with acute bronchitis.

    Stock supply: 60-mL bottles of erythromycin ethylsuccinate for oral suspension 400 mg/5 mL when reconstituted

    How many doses are in one 60-mL bottle?

    How many days would this container provide the necessary medication?

    How many containers would be needed for 10 days of therapy?

    Write the directions as they should appear on the customer's bottle:
    _____

2. A physician prescribes Halcion (triazolam) 0.25 mg at bedtime prn sleep.

    Stock supply: triazolam 0.125 mg tablets

    How many doses are in one 10-tablet stock bottle?

    Write the directions as they should appear on the customer's bottle:
    _____

3. A physician prescribes Rifadin (rifampin) 600 mg daily 1 hr before a meal for tuberculosis.

   Stock supply: rifampin 150 mg capsules

   How many full doses of medication are found in one 30-capsule stock bottle?

   How many containers are needed for a one month supply?

   Write the directions as they should appear on the customer's bottle:
   _____

4. One 10-mL multidose vial of Compazine (prochlorperazine) 5 mg/mL has been provided to the medical floor for a patient with postoperative emesis.

   How many 10 mg doses can be obtained from this vial?

5. Meperidine 50 mg has been given to four patients over the past 24 hours from the box of 25 ampules in the narcotic floor stock. Each 1-mL ampule contains 75 mg of meperidine.

   How many ampules should be left in the box if the floor stock supply has only been used for these injections?

   Explain your answer.
   _____
   _____

6. **PAIN** A physician prescribes ibuprofen 0.8 g tid pc for a patient with osteoarthritis.

    Stock supply: 100-tablet bottle of ibuprofen 400 mg tablets

    How many full doses are in one stock bottle?

    Write the directions as they should appear on the customer's bottle:
    _____

7. A physician orders lincomycin 0.6 g IM q12h. Stock available: 10-mL vial of lincomycin 300 mg/mL injection

    How many doses of medication are in this vial?

8. A patient is prescribed cephalexin 62.5 mg qid. Stock available: 60-mL bottles of cephalexin oral suspension 125 mg/5 mL

    How many doses of medication are in one 60-mL bottle?

Determining the Length of Time a Prescription Will Last

It is important to know how to calculate the length of time a prescription will last if taken appropriately, which is also called the **days' supply**. The pharmacist uses this information to monitor patients' compliance with their medications. Additionally, insurance claims for refills will only be approved after a specified period of time following the last dispensing. If an attempt is made to refill too soon, the claim will be rejected. The pharmacist or pharmacy technician needs to know if the medication has been taken properly and when the medication can be refilled through insurance.

> **! TECH ALERT**
>
> If the proper length of time between prescription refills is inappropriate, the pharmacist should be notified. The pharmacist should consult with the patient and contact the physician for further directions if necessary.

When entering new prescription information in the computer, care must be taken to input the correct days' supply. This can affect whether the insurance company reimburses or rejects the claim. One of the reasons claims are frequently rejected is for incorrect days' supply. This type of calculation can be solved with DA or R&P.

Determining days' supply for tablets and capsules is the simplest of these calculations. Oral and IV liquids, insulin, eye and ear drops, and inhaler calculations require more steps. Labels for **inhalers**, which are used to deliver medication through the mouth or nose, will state how many inhalations are present in each container. Some medications intended for inhalation need to be placed in a **nebulizer**, which is a device used to produce a fine spray of medication. These calculations will depend on whether the medication is supplied in single or multidose containers.

> **TECH NOTE**
> When calculating days' supply for insurance purposes, always round down to the closest whole number if you calculate a partial day. This will help avoid "Refill too soon" responses.

EXAMPLE 13.8

A physician orders 60 tablets of antibiotic to be administered qid. What is the days' supply?

$$R\&P \quad \frac{4 \text{ tablets}}{1 \text{ day}} = \frac{60 \text{ tablets}}{x \text{ days}}$$

$$4x = 60 \text{ days}$$

$$x = 15 \text{ days}$$

$$DA \quad days = \frac{1 \text{ day}}{4 \text{ tablets}} \cdot \frac{60 \text{ tablets}}{1} = 15 \text{ days}$$

This is basically dividing the total amount of medication by the number of doses to be administered per day.

> **TECH NOTE**
> Use 20 gtt = 1 mL for calculating days' supply of ophthalmic and otic medications for insurance purposes unless your pharmacy specifies something different.

EXAMPLE 13.9

```
                Lawrence Merry, M.D.
              4th Street and Jones Ave.
                   Holly, GA 00111
                phone# - 001-555-2176

Patient Name_____  Date _____
Address_____   Age _____

   ℞         Ocuflox Ophthalmic Solution
             5 mL
             Sig: i gtt each eye qid x 5 d

_____   Refill _____
DEA#_____
```

What is the days' supply? *Even though the medication is only ordered for 5 days, it is best to enter the actual days' supply in the computer for insurance purposes.*

$$days = \frac{1 \text{ day}}{4 \text{ doses}} \cdot \frac{1 \text{ dose}}{2 \text{ gtt}} \cdot \frac{20 \text{ gtt}}{1 \text{ mL}} \cdot \frac{5 \text{ mL}}{1} = 12.5 \text{ days}$$

Days' supply would be 12 full days.

Note the use of 2 gtt per dose because the prescription is written for *both* eyes.

TECH NOTE
Pay close attention to whether directions are for one or both eyes/ears when interpreting prescriptions for ophthalmic and otic medications.

EXAMPLE 13.10

 A physician prescribes Dilantin Suspension 100 mg tid.

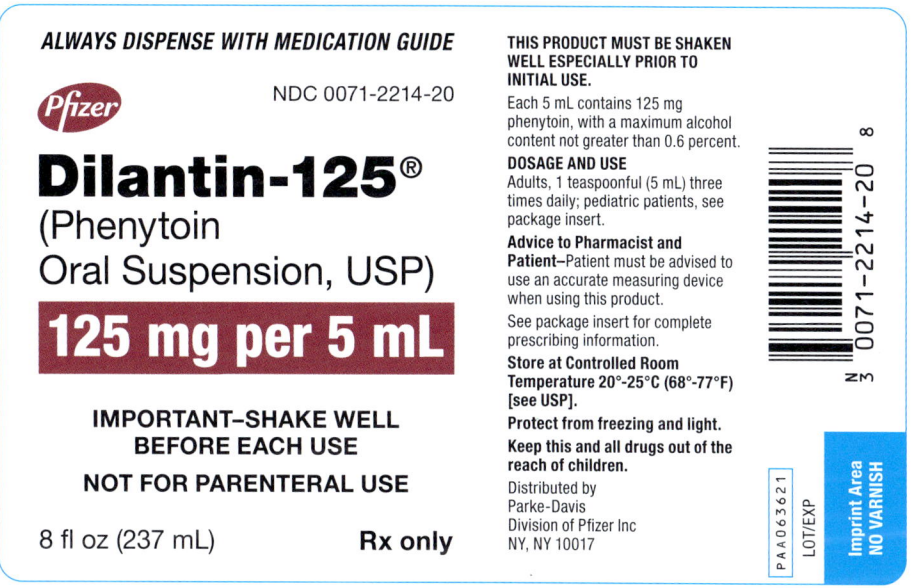

© Pfizer. Used with permission.

How many *full* days should this bottle of medication last?

$$\text{days} = \frac{1 \text{ day}}{3 \text{ doses}} \cdot \frac{1 \text{ dose}}{100 \text{ mg}} \cdot \frac{125 \text{ mg}}{5 \text{ mL}} \cdot \frac{237 \text{ mL}}{1} = 19.75 \text{ days} = 19 \text{ days}$$

Indicate the prescription label directions: Take 4 mL three times a day.

EXAMPLE 13.11

A physician prescribes Humulin R 50 units subcutaneously at breakfast and 40 units subcutaneously before the evening meal.

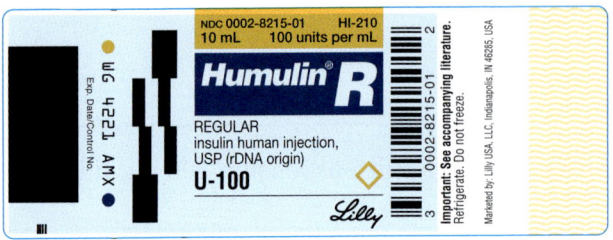

© Eli Lilly and Company. All Rights Reserved. Used with Permission.

How many *full* days should this vial last?

$$\text{days} = \frac{1 \text{ day}}{90 \text{ units}} \cdot \frac{100 \text{ units}}{1 \text{ mL}} \cdot \frac{10 \text{ mL}}{1} = 11.1 \text{ days}$$

Days' supply for one vial is 11.

How many 10-mL vials of Humulin R should be dispensed for a month's supply?

$$\text{\# vials} = \frac{1 \text{ vial}}{10 \text{ mL}} \cdot \frac{1 \text{ mL}}{100 \text{ units}} \cdot \frac{90 \text{ units}}{\text{day}} \cdot \frac{30 \text{ days}}{1} = 2.7 \text{ vials}$$

Three vials are needed for a 1 month supply.

> **TECH NOTE**
> Always round the days' supply of insulin **down** to the whole number of days and the needed amount of vials **up** to the next whole number.

EXAMPLE 13.12

 What is the days' supply for the following prescription? Proventil (albuterol) inhaler 2 puffs qid

Stock supply: albuterol inhaler 200 metered inhalations/17 g

A "puff" is the equivalent of an inhalation, and this inhaler contains 200 metered inhalations.

$$\text{days} = \frac{1 \text{ day}}{4 \text{ doses}} \cdot \frac{1 \text{ dose}}{2 \text{ inh}} \cdot \frac{200 \text{ inh}}{1} = 25 \text{ days}$$

EXAMPLE 13.13

 What is the days' supply for the following prescription?

acetaminophen with codeine elixir

Sig: 5 to 10 mL q4–6h prn pain

120 mL

When calculating days' supply for insurance purposes, it is best to base it on the maximum possible dose. In this case the patient *may* take a maximum of 10 mL six times a day, or 60 mL. Therefore the 120 mL bottle will provide a 2-day supply.

TECH NOTE

Never enter a days' supply that extends past the beyond use date of a medication. For this reason, if the days' supply for one vial of Lantus insulin was calculated to be 45 days, it would need to be reduced to 28 days.

Dealing with days' supply for topical medications is not an exact process. Generally, 1 g of cream is considered to be an amount that would cover four flat hands of area. This requires knowing how much of an area is to be covered, which could be an uncomfortable question. Most pharmacies will have general guidelines to follow for days' supply of creams, ointments, and lotions.

Practice Problems C

Complete the following, showing calculations. A month means 30 days unless otherwise stated.

1. Interpret the prescription for Zaroxolyn (metolazone) tablets. _____

   _____

   ```
   Lawrence Merry, M.D.
   4th Street and Jones Ave.
   Holly, GA 00111
   phone# - 001-555-2176

   Patient Name _____   Date _____
   Address _____   Age _____

   Rx   Zaroxolyn 2.5
        T po q3d

        #30
        _____     Refill _____
        DEA# _____
   ```

   What is the days' supply?

2. How long would the medication in the provided prescription last?

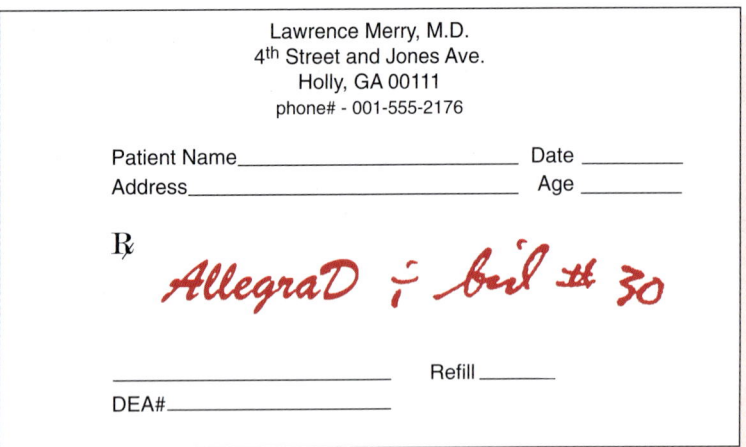

Write the directions as they should appear on the customer's bottle:
_____

3. A physician writes a prescription for minoxidil 10 mg tablets #40

Sig: 0.04 g po qd

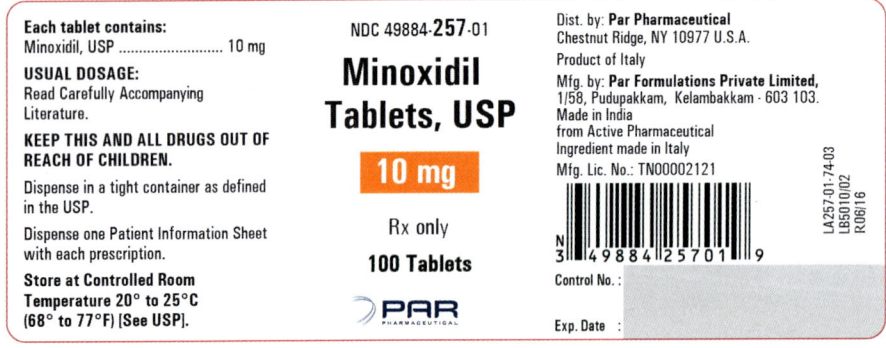

Reprinted with permission of Endo/Par Pharmaceutical

How many days would this prescription last?

How many tablets are needed for a 1-month supply?

Write the directions as they should appear on the customer's bottle:
_____

4. A physician writes a prescription for Lanoxin (digoxin) 0.125 mg tablets #40
Sig: 0.5 mg stat, 0.375 mg in a.m., then tab i qam.

How long would this prescription last after the two initial doses?

Write the directions as they should appear on the customer's bottle:
_____

5. What is the days' supply for the following prescription?

```
            Lawrence Merry, M.D.
           4th Street and Jones Ave.
                Holly, GA 00111
              phone# - 001-555-2176

Patient Name_____      Date _____
Address_____       Age _____

R    Biaxin XL 500
          # 20
     Ti po daily c food for
                sinus inf
     _____    Refill _____
     DEA#_____
```

Write the directions as they should appear on the customer's bottle:
_____

6. What is the days' supply for the following prescription of Altace (ramipril)?

```
              Lawrence Merry, M.D.
             4th Street and Jones Ave.
                  Holly, GA 00111
                phone# - 001-555-2176

  Patient Name_____  Date _____
  Address_____   Age _____

  Rx   Altace 5 mg
              # 62
         2 T b.i.d    BP
  _____  Refill _____
  DEA#_____
```

Interpret the prescription:

_____

7. A physician writes a prescription for 200 mL of erythromycin ethylsuccinate 200 mg tid.

Stock available: erythromycin ethylsuccinate for oral suspension 200 mg/5 mL when reconstituted/200-mL bottles

How many full days should the medication last?

How many doses of medication are available in the container?

Indicate the prescription label directions.

_____

Chapter 13 Interpreting Physicians' Orders for Dosages and Days' Supply   305

8. Interpret the following prescription:

_____

```
           Lawrence Merry, M.D.
          4th Street and Jones Ave.
               Holly, GA 00111
            phone# - 001-555-2176

Patient Name_____  Date _____
Address_____  Age _____

  Rx    Pepcid 20mg
        Sig: i po BID
        Dispn: #20
                                   Refill _____
  _____
  DEA#_____
```

What is the days' supply?

Write the directions as they should appear on the customer's bottle:
_____

9. What is the days' supply?

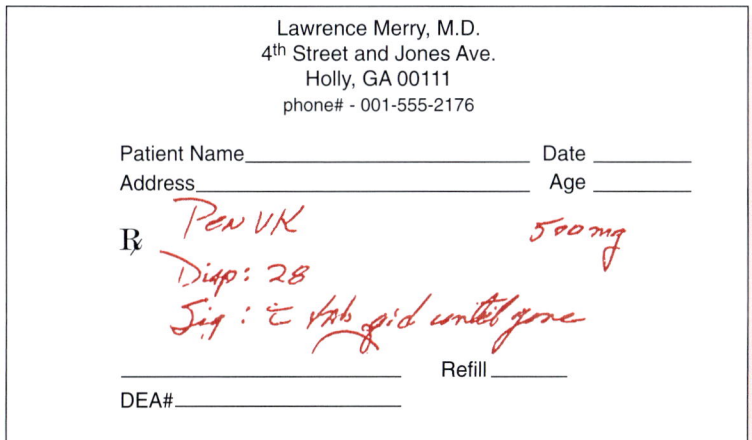

```
           Lawrence Merry, M.D.
          4th Street and Jones Ave.
               Holly, GA 00111
            phone# - 001-555-2176

Patient Name_____  Date _____
Address_____  Age _____

  Rx    Pen VK              500 mg
        Disp: 28
        Sig: i tab qid until gone
                                   Refill _____
  _____
  DEA#_____
```

Write the directions as they should appear on the customer's bottle:
_____

Copyright © 2019 by Elsevier, Inc. All rights reserved.

10. Interpret the following prescription:

_____

```
                Lawrence Merry, M.D.
              4th Street and Jones Ave.
                    Holly, GA 00111
                 phone# - 001-555-2176

     Patient Name_____   Date _____
     Address_____   Age _____

          ℞    Urocit. K        10 mEq
               #540             (1080 mg)

               Sig: ī po TID

               _____   Refill _____
               DEA#_____
```

What is the days' supply?

Write the directions as they should appear on the customer's bottle:

_____

11. A physician ordered pen G potassium 5,000,000 units in 1 L of fluid to be delivered over 12 hours (q12h) × 7 days. The vial has been reconstituted with 11.5 mL of diluent.

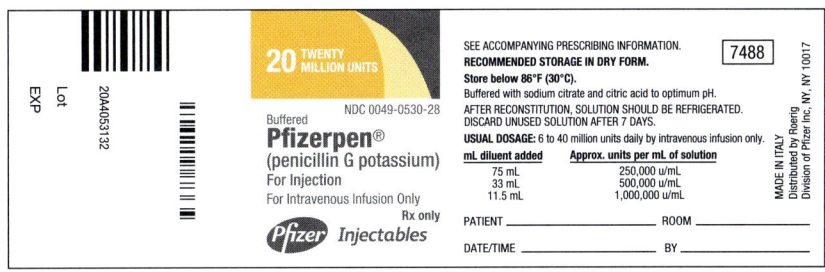

© Pfizer. Used with permission.

How many doses can be obtained from one vial of medication?

What is the days' supply from one vial?

What volume of medication should be added to each liter of fluid?

What three pieces of information should be written on the vial at the time of reconstitution if it is to be saved for future doses?

_____

_____

12. A physician prescribes 200 mg of Lorabid (loracarbef) po bid × 10 d

Stock available: loracarbef for oral suspension 100 mg/5 mL once reconstituted

How many full days would a 50-mL bottle last?

How many containers of Lorabid should be dispensed for a 10-day supply?

Indicate the prescription label directions:

_____

13. A physician prescribes Dilantin 300 mg po qam and Dilantin 100 mg po at bedtime for epilepsy.

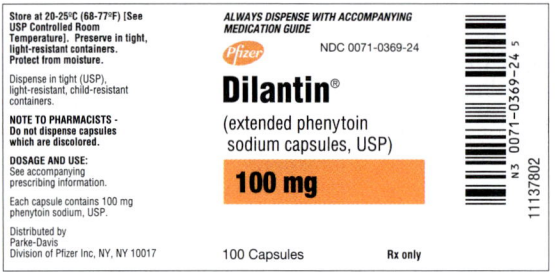

© Pfizer. Used with permission.

How many days would this container of medication last?

How many extra capsules are needed for a 1-month supply?

Write the directions as they should appear on the customer's bottle:

_____

_____

14. A physician prescribes Prozac (fluoxetine) Liquid 40 mg po qam.

Stock available: fluoxetine oral solution 20 mg/5 mL

How many days should 120 mL of medication last?

Write the directions as they should appear on the customer's bottle:

_____

15. A pediatrician prescribes diphenhydramine elixir 18.75 mg po q6h prn.

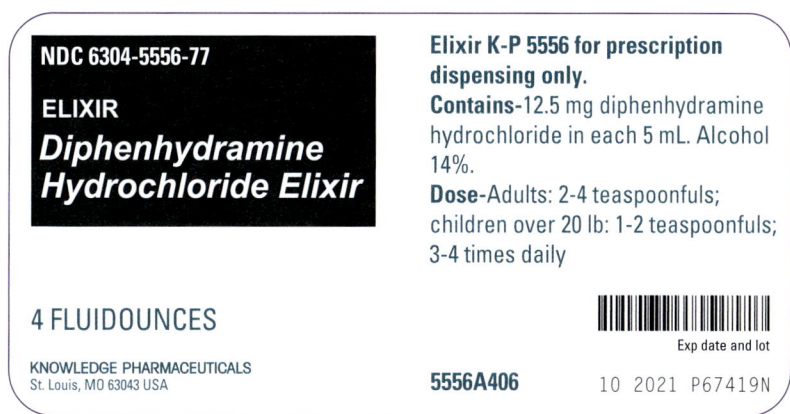

How many mL are needed for one dose?

How many doses are in this bottle?

What is the days' supply for insurance purposes?

16. A prescription reads as follows: Cortisporin Otic 2 gtt au tid × 10 d

What is the days' supply in a 10-mL bottle? (Remember to round down to a whole number.)

17. The physician ordered Xalatan 1 gtt ou qpm

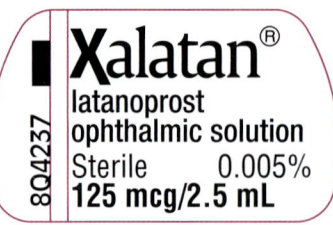

© Pfizer. Used with permission.

What is the days' supply using this 2.5-mL bottle?

Write the directions as they should appear on the customer's bottle:

18. A physician orders Lopid 600 mg qam and 300 mg qpm.

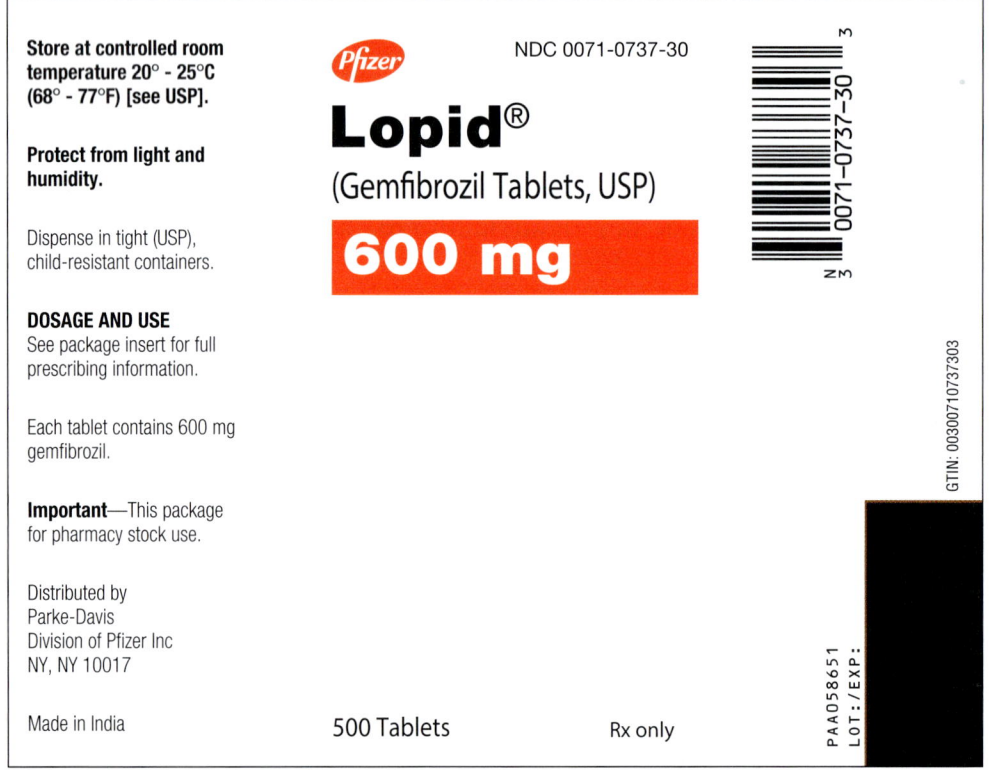

© Pfizer. Used with permission.

What is the days' supply if 135 tablets are dispensed?

If the insurance company only pays for a 30-day supply each time, how many should be dispensed?

Write the directions as they should appear on the customer's bottle:
_____

19. **ENDO** A physician provides a new prescription for Humulin R subcut 14 units tid 30 min ac

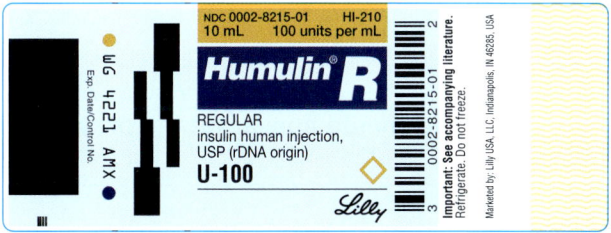

© Eli Lilly and Company. All Rights Reserved. Used with Permission.

What is the days' supply in one 10-mL vial? (Round down to the nearest whole number.)

How many vials of Humulin R are needed for a 90-day supply? (Round up to the nearest whole number.)

Write the directions as they should appear on the prescription label:
_____

20. **ENDO** A patient brings in a prescription for Humulin R 10 units tid pc and 25 units at bedtime.

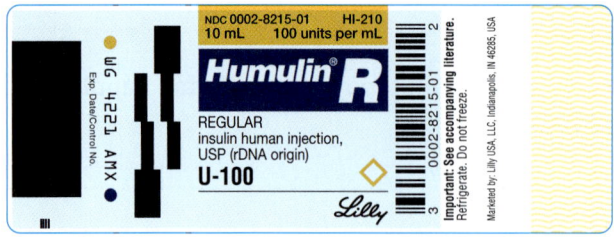

© Eli Lilly and Company. All Rights Reserved. Used with Permission.

What is the days' supply in one 10-mL vial?

How many vials of Humulin R are needed for a 30-day supply?

Write the directions as they should appear on the prescription label:
_____

REVIEW

In some cases, pharmacy technicians may be asked to calculate the amount of medication to be dispensed when the number of doses per day and the number of days for treatment is known. On other occasions, the calculation of the number of doses of medication in a container may be necessary to ensure the patient has adequate medication to complete the prescription or physician's order. Finally, for determining days' supply for insurance purposes, for monitoring refills to assess patient compliance, and for meeting insurance companies' regulations regarding restrictions on the amount of medication that can be dispensed at a given time, pharmacy staff will be required to determine how long the medication should last if taken according to the directions. All of these skills may be needed to accurately dispense medications.

Posttest

Complete the following calculations. A month is 30 days unless otherwise stated. Show your calculations. All calculations should be for full days.

1. Interpret the prescription.
   _____
   _____

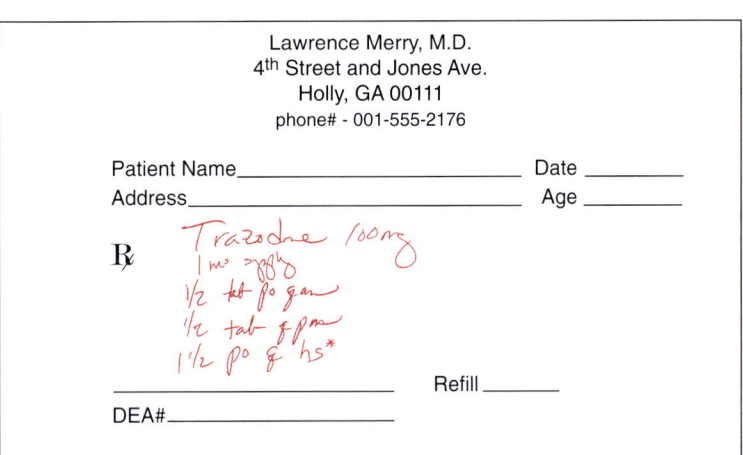

How many 100 mg tablets are needed to fill this prescription?

*Note: "hs" is an abbreviation found in the ISMP's List of Error-Prone Abbreviations, Symbols, and Dose Designations. It should never be used when communicating dose information but is still seen on some prescriptions. The phrase "at bedtime" is preferred.

Continued

Posttest, cont.

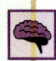

2. Interpret the following Neurontin (gabapentin) prescription.

   _____
   _____

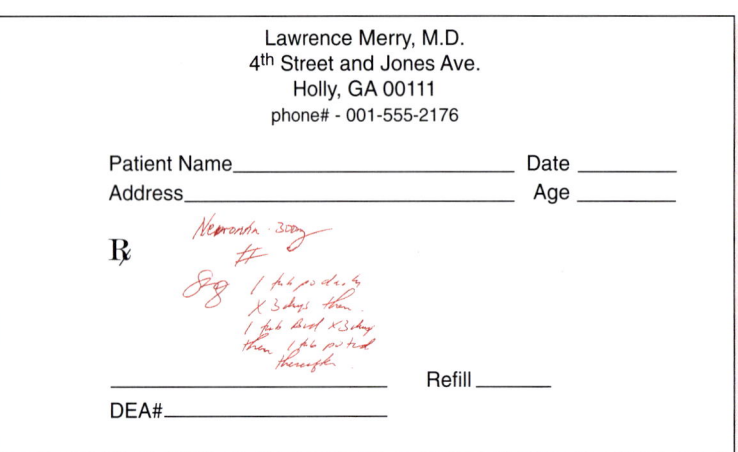

How many tablets are needed to fill this prescription for 30 days?

3. How many Alora (estradiol) patches are needed for a *28-day* supply?

Indicate the prescription label directions.

_____

Posttest, cont.

4. A physician writes a prescription for a 1:1:1 proportion of the following:

   Benadryl

   Lidocaine 1% viscous

   Maalox

   What is the amount of each component necessary to make 180 mL?

   How many doses of medication are available if the patient swishes and spits 5 mL q4h?

5. A physician writes a prescription for Decadron (dexamethasone) taper using 0.5 mg dexamethasone tablets: Sig: 1 po qid × 2 days, 1 tid × 2 days, 1 bid × 2 days, and 1 daily × 4 days.

   How many tablets are needed to fill this prescription?

   How many milligrams of dexamethasone would the patient receive on each day?

   Days 1 and 2:

   Days 3 and 4:

   Days 5 and 6:

   Days 7 to 10:

   Indicate the prescription label directions.

   _____
   _____
   _____

Continued

Posttest, cont.

6. Interpret the prescription.

   _____

   ```
   Lawrence Merry, M.D.
   4th Street and Jones Ave.
   Holly, GA 00111
   phone# - 001-555-2176
   ```

   Patient Name_____ Date _____
   Address_____ Age _____

   Rx Cipro 5w
        2u
        ¡ BId

   _____ Refill _____
   DEA#_____

   What is the days' supply of tablets?

7. A physician orders erythromycin ethylsuccinate 300 mg po tid for 10 days.
   Stock supply: 200 mL of erythromycin ethylsuccinate for oral suspension 200 mg/5 mL when reconstituted
   How many milliliters of medication are needed per dose?

   What total volume of medication is needed for the prescription as ordered?

   Is there sufficient medication in the container as shown on the label given?

   _____

Posttest, cont.

8. A physician writes the following prescription: Voltaren 50 mg bid with food for 7 days then decrease to qd

   How many Voltaren (diclofenac) 50 mg tablets are needed for the initial 30-day supply?

   Write the directions as they should appear on the customer's bottle:
   _____

9. The patient's instructions are as follows: Use 1 unit in jet nebulizer every 8 hours as needed for cough.

   ```
   Lawrence Merry, M.D.
   4th Street and Jones Ave.
   Holly, GA 00111
   phone# - 001-555-2176

   Patient Name_____   Date _____
   Address_____   Age _____

   Rx   Albuterol Unit Dose 2.5/3ml
        Disp 25
        Sig Use in Jet Neb Q8°
             prn cough
        _____   Refill _____
        DEA#_____
   ```

   What is the days' supply?

Continued

Posttest, cont.

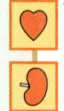

10. How many capsules are needed to provide a 3-month supply?

```
          Lawrence Merry, M.D.
         4th Street and Jones Ave.
              Holly, GA 00111
           phone# - 001-555-2176

   Patient Name_____      Date _____
   Address_____      Age _____

   ℞  HCTZ  12.5 mg  cap
       i po day

   _____       Refill _____
   DEA#_____
```

Interpret the order as written.
_____

11. A physician orders Coumadin (warfarin) 5 mg po on Sunday, Tuesday, Wednesday, Friday, and Saturday and Coumadin 7.5 mg po on the other days of the week. In order to use only one strength tablet, the doctor requests warfarin 2.5 mg tablets to fill this prescription.

How many tablets are needed for a 1-week supply?

What amount of Coumadin in milligrams would be taken in a week?

Write the directions as they should appear on the customer's bottle:
_____
_____

Posttest, cont.

12. What is the days' supply for this prescription?

```
          Lawrence Merry, M.D.
         4th Street and Jones Ave.
              Holly, GA 00111
           phone# - 001-555-2176

Patient Name_____   Date _____
Address_____   Age _____

 R  Amoxicillan 500mg #30
    mg. 1 BID for
    Infection

    _____   Refill _____
DEA#_____
```

13. The medication as prescribed is available in a 10-mL bottle filled with 5 mL of solution.

```
          Lawrence Merry, M.D.
         4th Street and Jones Ave.
              Holly, GA 00111
           phone# - 001-555-2176

Patient Name_____   Date _____
Address_____   Age _____

 R  Acular Opthalmic 0.5%
    1 drop left eye tid

    _____   Refill _____
DEA#_____
```

What is the calculated days' supply?

_____

Acular ophthalmic is only good for 4 weeks after opening, so it should be entered in the computer as a 28-day supply if the calculated value is greater than 28. Write the directions as they should appear on the customer's bottle:

_____

Continued

Posttest, cont.

14. How many doses of the medication are found in the ordered amount?

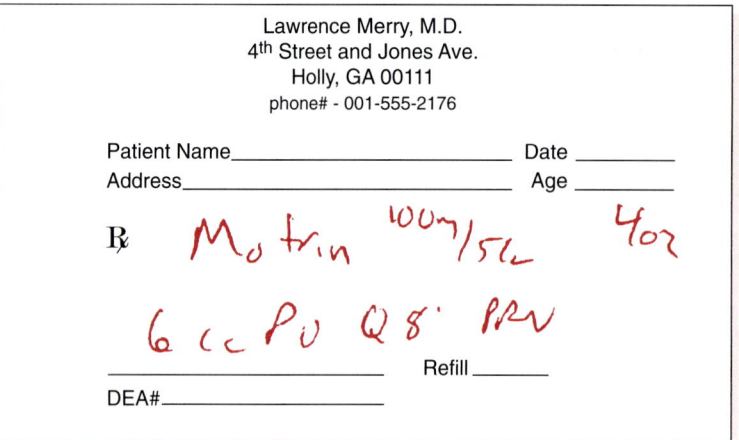

What weight in mg of Motrin (ibuprofen) is the patient receiving with each dose?

Interpret the prescription.
___
___

Write the directions as they should appear on the customer's bottle:
___

Posttest, cont.

15. A physician prescribes Dilantin 200 mg po bid for 14 days.

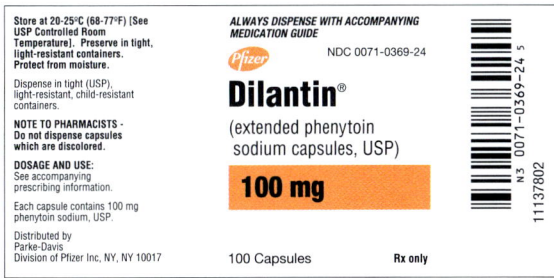

© Pfizer. Used with permission.

Using the provided label, how many capsules are needed to fill the prescription?

Write the directions as they should appear on the customer's bottle:
_____

16. A physician writes for Thorazine (chlorpromazine) 50 mg po qam and 75 mg po at bedtime.

Stock available: chlorpromazine 25 mg tablets

How many tablets are needed for a 30-day supply?

What is the total dosage per day of the medication?

Write the directions as they should appear on the customer's bottle:
_____

Continued

Posttest, cont.

17. Interpret the following prescription for Ceftin (cefuroxime).

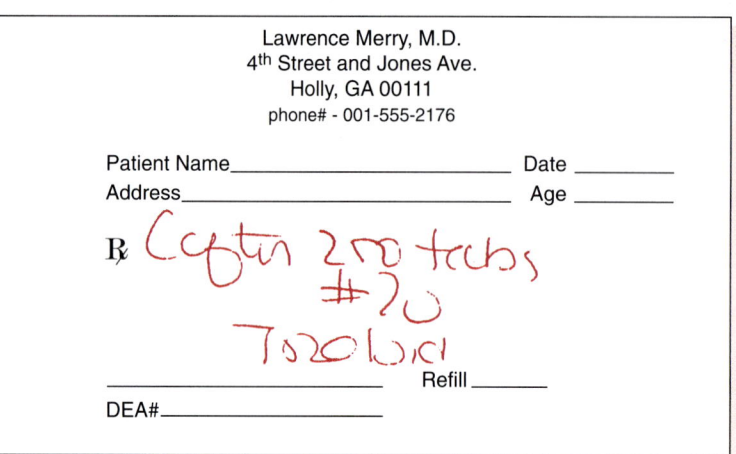

What is the days' supply?

18. A physician orders Mycostatin Oral Suspension 200,000 units divided in each side of the mouth qid. The available medication is Mycostatin Oral Suspension 100,000 units/mL.

How many milliliters are needed for a 30-day supply?

Posttest, cont.

19. Sig: Humulin R 25 units subcut ac breakfast and evening meal.

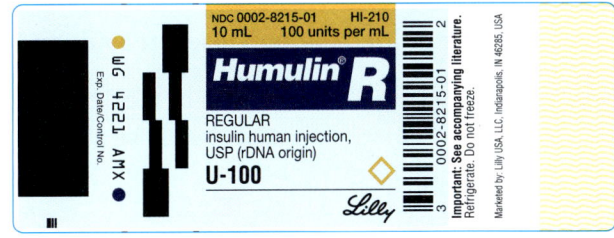

© Eli Lilly and Company. All Rights Reserved. Used with Permission.

What is the days' supply in one 10-mL vial?

How many vials of Humulin R should be dispensed for a 1-month supply?

Write the directions as they should appear on the prescription label:
_____
_____

20. A patient is to inject Lantus insulin 35 units subcut qam.
Stock strength: Lantus (insulin glargine) 100 units/mL, 10-mL vial
What is the days' supply in one 10-mL vial?

How many vials of Lantus are needed for a 1-month supply?

How many vials of medication would be needed for a 90-day supply?

Write the directions as they should appear on the prescription label:
_____

Continued

REVIEW OF RULES

- **Preparing Medications When the Quantity for Dispensing Is Unknown**

Total dosage necessary = Number of doses per day × Total number of days

- **Calculating the Number of Medication Doses in a Given Container**

$$\text{Number of doses in a container} = \frac{\text{Total amount of medication in container}}{\text{Dose size}}$$

- **Determining Days' Supply**

$$\text{Days' Supply} = \frac{\text{Total amount of medication}}{\text{Amount to be administered per day}}$$

IN SECTION IV

14 Calculations With Ratio and Percentage Strengths
15 Calculations for Simple Dilutions, Mixtures, and Compounding
16 Calculation of Medications Used Intravenously

SECTION IV
Special Medication Calculations

CHAPTER 14

Calculations With Ratio and Percentage Strengths

OBJECTIVES

1. Discuss the types of percentage strength.
2. Calculate the amount of solute in various premade intravenous preparations.
3. Calculate the amount of active ingredient expressed in percentage strength.
4. Discuss the types of ratio strengths.
5. Convert from ratio to percentage strength, and from percentage strength to ratio.

KEY WORDS

Medication strength Concentration of active ingredient in a medication
Percentage strength An amount of active ingredient per 100 parts total: $x/100 = x\%$
qs Quantity sufficient or required
qs ad Quantity sufficient to make
Ratio strength Expression of strength of weak solutions or liquid preparations; one part active ingredient in x parts total: (1:x)
Solute The smaller portion of a solution; the component to be dissolved in the solvent
Solvent The larger portion of a solution; the component doing the dissolving; aka **diluent**

Pretest

If you are comfortable with the subject matter, perform the following calculations to test your knowledge. If not, work your way through the chapter and return to them for extra practice. Show your calculations.

1. How many grams of sodium chloride are in 1,000 mL NS?

Continued

Copyright © 2019 by Elsevier, Inc. All rights reserved.

Pretest, cont.

2. How many grams of dextrose are in 500 mL of D5W?

3. A physician orders 250 mL D5W. How many grams of dextrose will the patient receive?

4. A physician orders 500 mL D5 ½ NS q8h as a continuous infusion. How many grams of dextrose will the patient receive in 8 hours?

How many grams of sodium chloride will the patient receive in 8 hours?

Pretest, cont.

 5. How many grams of sodium chloride are in the fluids shown in the following label?

```
LOT                EXP
                                    2B1313        1
                              NDC 0338-0043-03

              0.45% Sodium Chloride
              Injection USP                        2

              500 mL
              EACH 100 mL CONTAINS   450 mg SODIUM CHLORIDE USP
              pH 5.0 (4.5 TO 7.0)  mEq/L SODIUM 77  CHLORIDE 77   3
              HYPOTONIC OSMOLARITY 154 mOsmol/L (CALC)  STERILE
              NONPYROGENIC  SINGLE DOSE CONTAINER  ADDITIVES MAY BE
              INCOMPATIBLE  CONSULT WITH PHARMACIST IF AVAILABLE
              WHEN INTRODUCING ADDITIVES USE ASEPTIC TECHNIQUE  MIX
              THOROUGHLY  DO NOT STORE  DOSAGE INTRAVENOUSLY AS
              DIRECTED BY A PHYSICIAN  SEE DIRECTIONS  CAUTIONS
              SQUEEZE AND INSPECT INNER BAG WHICH MAINTAINS PRODUCT
              STERILITY  DISCARD IF LEAKS ARE FOUND  MUST NOT BE USED  4
              IN SERIES CONNECTIONS  DO NOT USE UNLESS SOLUTION IS
              CLEAR  Rx ONLY  STORE UNIT IN MOISTURE BARRIER
              OVERWRAP AT ROOM TEMPERATURE (25°C/77°F) UNTIL READY
              TO USE  AVOID EXCESSIVE HEAT  SEE INSERT
              VIAFLEX CONTAINER    PL 146 PLASTIC
              BAXTER VIAFLEX AND PL 146 ARE TRADEMARKS OF
              BAXTER INTERNATIONAL INC
              FOR PRODUCT INFORMATION 1-800-933-0303

              Baxter
              BAXTER HEALTHCARE CORPORATION
              DEERFIELD IL 60015 USA
              MADE IN USA
```

Courtesy of Baxter Healthcare Corporation. All rights reserved.

 6. A label reads Zephiran chloride 0.2%.

Interpret (w/v) _____

How many grams are in 500 mL?

Continued

Pretest, cont.

 7. A label reads sodium hypochlorite 10%.

   Interpret (w/v) _____

   How many grams are in 240 mL?

 8. How many grams of silver nitrate are in 250 mL of a 1:500 silver nitrate solution?

   How many milligrams of silver nitrate are necessary to prepare 250 mL of this solution?

   What is the percentage strength of this solution?

 9. A physician orders 5 mL of epinephrine 1% added to 45 mL of sterile water. What is the weight in milligrams of the epinephrine that has been added?

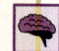 10. A physician orders Prostigmin 0.4 mg IM stat. How many milliliters of Prostigmin 1:2,000 are needed for this dose?

 11. A dentist orders an antiseptic mouthwash of sodium bicarbonate 1:40. How many grams of sodium bicarbonate are needed to make 6 oz of mouthwash?

 12. How many milliliters of boric acid solution are needed to prepare 500 mL of a 1:20 v/v solution?

INTRODUCTION

Percentage and ratio strengths are two additional methods for expressing **medication strength**, the amount or concentration of active ingredient present in medications. When the solute or active ingredient is described as part of the total amount of preparation, the resultant product may be expressed in **percentage strength** or **ratio strength**. Both express an amount of medication per unit of volume or weight of a total liquid or solid preparation. These medication labels express the percentage strength, such as Lidocaine 1%, or ratio strength, such as epinephrine 1:1,000. Many medications expressed as ratio or percentage strengths also list the total active ingredient amount, usually in the metric system, on the label. As with all medications, consider the total volume of medication in the container to determine the total amount of active ingredient found in a particular container.

Ratio strengths are usually used for liquid medications with a very low concentration of active ingredients. Percentage strengths are used to express some medications, as well as to express the amount of solutes in many premade intravenous solutions.

Types of Percentage Strength

Percentage strength is always interpreted as an amount out of 100. It is used to describe various solutions and topically applied drugs. There are three basic types:

1. weight in volume (w/v) = $\dfrac{x \text{ g}}{100 \text{ mL}}$

This is read as *x* grams of active ingredient in 100 milliliters of total solution.
For example, 10% calcium gluconate injection is 10 g of calcium gluconate in 100 mL of total solution and 5% dextrose in water (D5W) has 5 g of dextrose in 100 mL of total solution. Normal saline (NS; 0.9% sodium chloride) has 0.9 g of sodium chloride in 100 mL of total solution.

2. volume in volume (v/v) = $\dfrac{x \text{ mL}}{100 \text{ mL}}$

This is read as *x* milliliters of active ingredient in 100 milliliters of total solution.
For example, 5% hydrogen peroxide solution is 5 mL of hydrogen peroxide in 100 mL of total solution.

3. weight in weight (w/w) = $\dfrac{x \text{ g}}{100 \text{ g}}$

This is read as *x* grams active ingredient in 100 grams of total preparation.
For example, 1% hydrocortisone cream is 1 g hydrocortisone in 100 g of total cream.

Working with the last two types may get confusing because *both* the active ingredient and total preparation have the same unit. Label them with an *a* or a *t* to help identify the active ingredient measurement and the total preparation measurement. The total preparation value will *always* be 100 when interpreting percentage strengths.

$$\dfrac{x \text{ mL}_{(a)}}{100 \text{ mL}_{(t)}} \text{ or } \dfrac{x \text{ g}_{(a)}}{100 \text{ g}_{(t)}}$$

TECH NOTE
Percentage strength is always x/100.

TABLE 14.1 Abbreviations for Common Intravenous Solutions

ABBREVIATION	SOLUTION
NS	0.9% sodium chloride or normal saline
½ NS	0.45% sodium chloride or half-normal saline
D5W	Dextrose 5% in water
D10W	Dextrose 10% in water
D5LR	Dextrose 5% in lactated Ringer's
RL or LR	Ringer's lactate or lactated Ringer's
D5NS	Dextrose 5% in 0.9% sodium chloride
D5 ½ NS	Dextrose 5% in 0.45% sodium chloride

TECH NOTE

All w/v percentage or ratio strength preparations are g/mL, so any question involving milligrams requires the conversion factor of 1,000 mg = 1 g and any question involving liters requires the conversion factor of 1,000 mL = 1 L. These are multistep problems that are more easily solved using dimensional analysis (DA).

Calculating Amounts of Solutes in Intravenous Fluids

The ingredients found in prepared intravenous (IV) fluids, such as dextrose or sodium chloride, are expressed in percentage strengths. These fluids are labeled with the percentage of solute found in the total solution. D5W, or 5% dextrose in water, indicates that 5% dextrose is present in the total solution, with water as the solvent. Remember that percentage is always based on 100, so the percentage is shown per 100 mL of solution, indicating that 5 g of dextrose is found in 100 mL of fluid. However, if the solution is larger than 100 mL, the total weight of the solute must be calculated. The easiest method for calculating the weight of solute in this case is by ratio and proportion (R&P).

In most cases the physician will use common abbreviations for ordering IV fluids. These are shown in Table 14.1. Dextrose solutions are always ordered as a percentage. However, the two most commonly prescribed sodium chloride solutions are sometimes referred to as normal saline (NS), which is 0.9% sodium chloride (0.9% NaCl), and ½ normal saline (½ NS), which is 0.45% sodium chloride (0.45% NaCl). These solutions have 0.9 g of NaCl and 0.45 g of NaCl per 100 mL, respectively.

Always begin percentage strength calculations by identifying the known value. Whatever the percentage strength is, place that number over 100. Then set up your unknown equivalent. The easiest method for calculating the amount of solute is by using R&P.

EXAMPLE 14.1

A physician orders 500 mL D5W for a patient. What is the weight in grams of dextrose in this bag of fluids?

$$\frac{5 \text{ g dextrose}}{100 \text{ mL total solution}} = \frac{x}{500 \text{ mL total solution}}$$

$100x = 500$ g dextrose

$x = 25$ g dextrose

There are 25 g of dextrose in 500 mL of the above fluids.

EXAMPLE 14.2

How many *milligrams* of sodium chloride are in 250 mL of NS?

Normal saline is 0.9% sodium chloride, so the known information is 0.9 g NaCl/100 mL total solution. Because this is a multistep problem requiring the conversion from grams to milligrams, use DA.

$$mg = \frac{1{,}000 \text{ mg}}{1 \text{ g}} \cdot \frac{0.9 \text{ g}}{100 \text{ mL}} \cdot \frac{250 \text{ mL}}{1} = 2{,}250 \text{ mg}$$

There are 2,250 mg of NaCl in 250 mL of NS.

At this point in working with pharmaceutical calculations, some find it easy to convert between grams and milligrams mentally so that the calculation can be done with R&P as follows and then converted mentally to milligrams.

$$\frac{0.9 \text{ g}}{100 \text{ mL}} = \frac{x}{250 \text{ mL}}$$

$$100x = 225 \text{ g}$$

$x = 2.25$ g, which is then converted to 2,250 mg

TECH NOTE

Percentage is based on 100, so x% indicates that x (g or mL) is found in 100 (g or mL) of total product. When calculating combination products such as D5NS, there are 5 g of dextrose **and** 0.9 g of NaCl per 100 mL.

EXAMPLE 14.3

A physician orders 500 mL of 5.5% Travesol (amino acids) to be used in a total parenteral nutrition bag. How many grams of amino acids will be provided?

$$\frac{5.5 \text{ g amino acids}}{100 \text{ mL total solution}} = \frac{x}{500 \text{ mL}}$$

$$100x = 2{,}750 \text{ g}$$

$$x = 27.5 \text{ g}$$

Practice Problems A

Calculate the amount of solute found in the IV fluids. Show your work.

1. How many grams of dextrose are in 250 mL of D10W?

2. What is the weight in grams of dextrose in the IV?

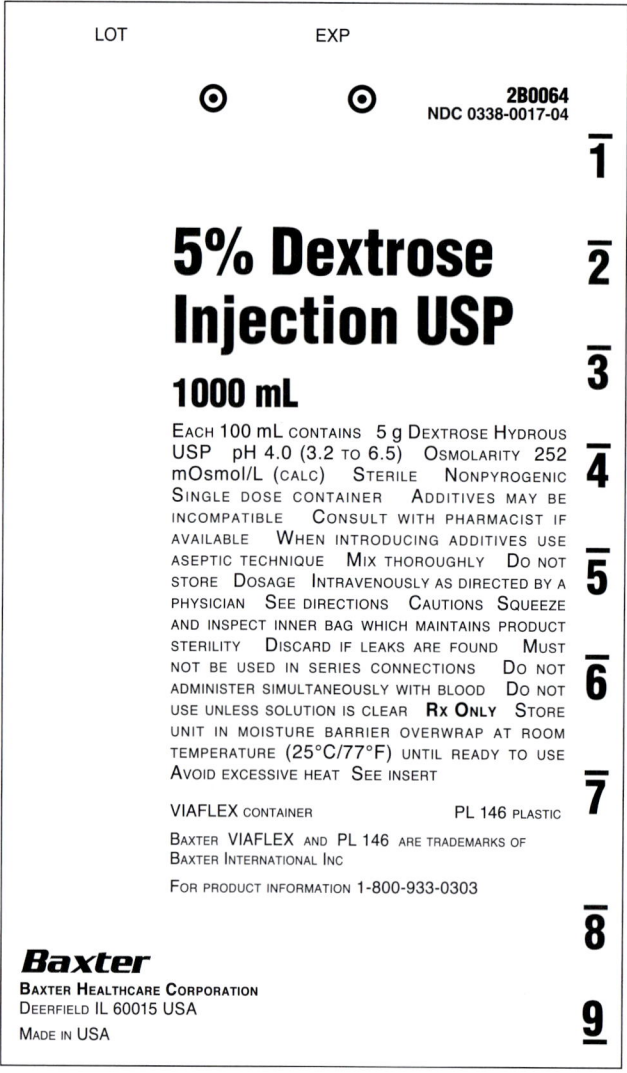

Courtesy of Baxter Healthcare Corporation. All rights reserved.

3. What is the weight in grams of sodium chloride in 500 mL of D5LR?

Note: Since the weight of sodium chloride in this IV is provided in milligrams/100 mL, change the weight of sodium chloride to g before using it in a R&P or use DA starting with "grams equals" and follow with the conversion factor.

What is the weight in grams of dextrose?

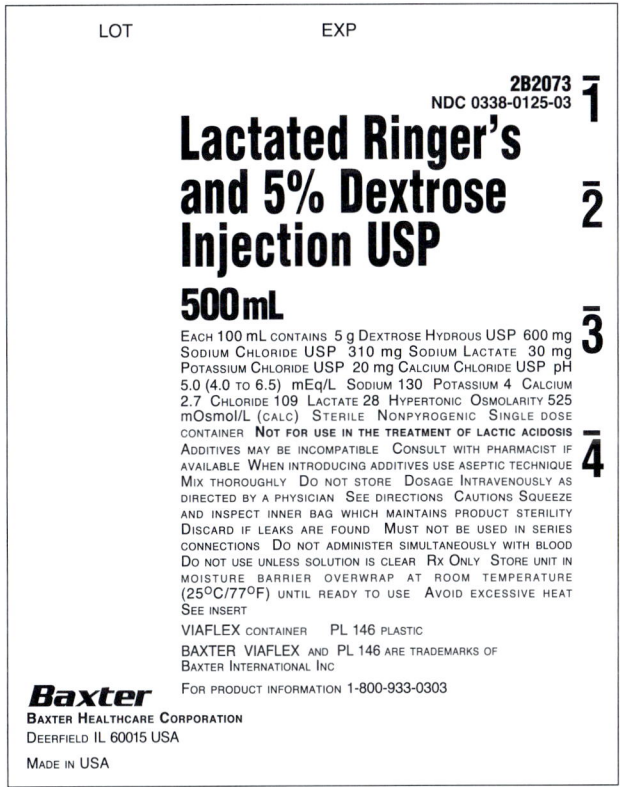

Courtesy of Baxter Healthcare Corporation. All rights reserved.

4. What is the weight of sodium chloride in grams in the fluids shown below?

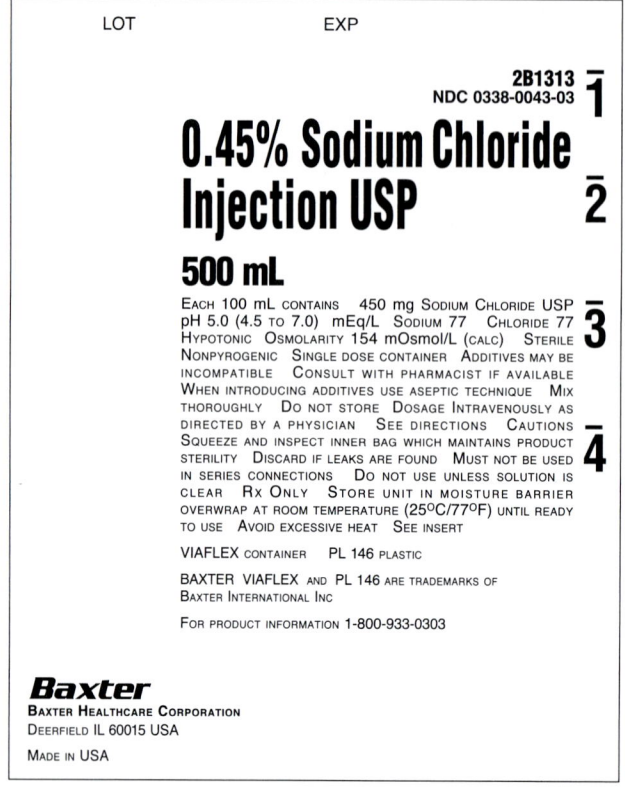

Courtesy of Baxter Healthcare Corporation. All rights reserved.

5. How many grams of dextrose are in 1 L of 3% dextrose?

If only 400 mL of the IV are administered, how many grams did the patient receive?

6. How many grams of dextrose are in 50 mL of D5W?

7. A physician orders 1 L of D10 ½ NS.

   How many grams of dextrose will the patient receive?

   How many grams of sodium chloride will the patient receive?

8. How many grams of dextrose are in 500 mL of D50W (50% dextrose solution)?

9. A physician orders 300 mL of 5.5% Travesol (amino acids) to be used in a total parenteral nutrition bag.

   How many grams of amino acids will be provided?

10. A physician orders 250 mL of 8.5% Travesol (amino acids) to be used in a total parenteral nutrition bag.

    How many grams of amino acids will be provided?

Determining the Amount of Active Ingredient With Percentage Strength

Percentages are also used for some liquid and semisolid medications to show different strengths, such as 1% lidocaine. As mentioned previously, when interpreting percentage labels, the amount of medication is expressed as either weight per volume (solid in liquid) such as 0.9% sodium chloride solution, weight per weight (solid in solid) such as 1% hydrocortisone cream, or volume per volume (liquid in liquid) such as 70% isopropyl alcohol, which is 70 mL of alcohol with enough sterile water to make 100 mL of total solution.

EXAMPLE 14.4

Interpret the following medication: 15% neomycin solution (w/v)

15 grams of neomycin in every 100 mL of total solution

How many grams of neomycin are in 200 mL of total solution?

$$\frac{15 \text{ g}}{100 \text{ mL}} = \frac{x}{200 \text{ mL}} \quad x = 30 \text{ g}$$

How many milligrams of neomycin are in 4 oz of 15% solution? *Use DA because this involves two conversion factors.*

$$mg = \frac{1,000 \text{ mg}}{1 \text{ g}} \cdot \frac{15 \text{ g}}{100 \text{ mL}} \cdot \frac{30 \text{ mL}}{1 \text{ oz}} \cdot \frac{4 \text{ oz}}{1} = 18,000 \text{ mg}$$

What is the strength in mg/mL? *Use DA because the answer has two units, mg and mL.*

$$\frac{mg}{mL} = \frac{1,000 \text{ mg}}{1 \text{ g}} \cdot \frac{15 \text{ g}}{100 \text{ mL}} = 150 \text{ mg/mL}$$

How much neomycin powder is needed to make 50 mL of 15% neomycin solution?

$$\frac{15 \text{ g}}{100 \text{ mL}} = \frac{x}{50 \text{ mL}}$$

$$x = 7.5 \text{ g}$$

A physician orders 3,000 mL of 15% Neomycin solution to use for irrigation of a wound. The available Neomycin is 0.5 g tablets.

How many grams of Neomycin are needed to fulfill the order?

$$\frac{15 \text{ g}}{100 \text{ mL}} = \frac{x}{3,000 \text{ mL}} \quad x = 450 \text{ g}$$

How many tablets of Neomycin are needed?

$$\frac{0.5 \text{ g}}{1 \text{ tab}} = \frac{450 \text{ g}}{x} \quad x = 900 \text{ tabs}$$

The answer to how many tablets are needed can be obtained in one step with DA.

$$tabs = \frac{1 \text{ tab}}{0.5 \text{ g}} \cdot \frac{15 \text{ g}}{100 \text{ mL}} \cdot \frac{3,000 \text{ mL}}{1} = 900 \text{ tabs}$$

Percentage strengths can also be used to determine how many milliliters contain a specific amount of medication, which is necessary when calculating a specific dosage that is needed. In these situations, with the desired answer in milliliters, the known percentage value may need to be inverted as follows:

EXAMPLE 14.5

How many milliliters of D50W (50% dextrose) should be administered to a hypoglycemic patient to provide 150 mg of dextrose?

Think of this as, "How much 50% dextrose contains 150 mg?"

$$mL = \frac{100 \text{ mL}}{50 \text{ g}} \cdot \frac{1 \text{ g}}{1,000 \text{ mg}} \cdot \frac{150 \text{ mg}}{1} = 0.3 \text{ mL}$$

TECH NOTE

Fractional values may be inverted as necessary as long as the units of the numerators and denominators of both fractions are in the same position with R & P and as long as the units are in the correct position to cancel with DA.

When making a specific quantity of a solution, there is no way to know exactly how much solvent is needed. The abbreviations **qs** or **qs ad** will be seen with many formulation instructions. These mean *quantity sufficient* and *quantity sufficient to make*, respectively. Once the amount of solute is calculated, the solvent is added in a quantity sufficient to make the total solution. For instance, in the previous example, the instructions would be as follows: 900 Neomycin 0.5 g tablets, qs ad 3,000 mL with sterile water.

Even v/v solutions do not always add up as expected. For example, making 100 mL of 70% alcohol requires 70 mL of 100% alcohol in 100 mL total solution. Adding 30 mL of water in this instance does not make 100 mL of total solution because the alcohol molecules fit in between the water molecules, resulting in a smaller total volume. Thus the instructions would read as follows: 70 mL 100% alcohol, qs to 100 mL with water.

EXAMPLE 14.6

How many milliliters of 15% neomycin solution can be made from 150 g neomycin?

$$\frac{15 \text{ g}}{100 \text{ mL}} = \frac{150 \text{ g}}{x}$$

$x = 1,000$ mL

How would the formulation instructions read for this preparation?

neomycin 150 g
qs ad sterile water 1,000 mL

Practice Problems B

Interpret the strengths of the medications shown, first as the number of g/100 mL, mL/100 mL, or g/100 g as indicated.

1. 7.5% magnesium sulfate solution (w/v)

   _____

   What is the strength in mg/mL?

2. 5% sodium chloride solution (w/v)

   _____

   What is the strength in mg/mL?

3. 0.5% glycerol solution (w/v)

___

What is the strength in mg/mL?

4. 5% formaldehyde solution (w/v)

___

What is the strength in mg/mL?

5. 1% hydrocortisone cream (w/w)

___

Interpret the strengths of the following medications in g/100 mL, and then determine the total weight of active ingredient in each container.

6. ciprofloxacin ophthalmic solution 0.3%

Interpret (w/v) ___
How many milligrams of active ingredient are in a 2.5-mL bottle?

7. Betadine Solution (10% povidone-iodine)

Interpret (w/v) ___
How many grams of povidone-iodine are present in a 3.78-L bottle?

8. Mucomyst-20 (20% acetylcysteine solution)

Interpret (w/v) ___
How many grams are present in a 10-mL container?

9.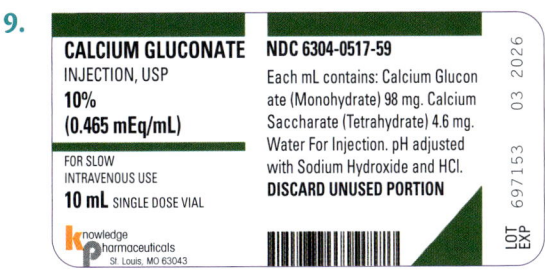

Interpret (w/v) _____

How many grams are present in the 10-mL vial?

How many milliequivalents are present in the 10-mL vial?

10.

Interpret (w/v) _____

How many grams are present in the entire container?

How many milliequivalents are present in the entire container?

What is the strength in milligrams per milliliter?

Indicate the amount of active ingredient needed to prepare the following solutions:

11. A physician orders 1 L of a 10% boric acid solution to be used for compresses.

    How many grams of boric acid are needed for this order?

12. How many grams of sucrose are needed to make 500 mL of a 75% solution?

    How many grams are needed to make 1,000 mL?

    How many grams are needed to make 250 mL?

13. How many milliliters of 10% solution can be made from 750 g of active ingredient?

    How many liters is this?

14. A 20-mL vial contains 50 mg/mL.

    What is the total weight of the medication in the vial in grams?

    What is the percentage strength of the medication?

15. How many grams of boric acid are needed to make 60 mL of a 5% solution?

16. What total volume of 2.5% solution can be prepared from 75 g of sucrose?

    How would the formula instructions for this solution be written?

17. How many mL of D50W (50% dextrose) should be administered to a hypoglycemic patient to provide 300 mg of dextrose? *Hint: How much 50% dextrose contains 300 mg?*

18. How many grams of dextrose are needed to prepare 3 L of a 10% solution?

19. How many 650 mg tablets of sodium bicarbonate are needed to prepare 325 mL of a 1% sodium bicarbonate solution? *Hint: Use DA starting with tabs = 1 tab/650 mg.*

    How much solvent is needed?

20. How many milliliters of 10% silver nitrate solution are needed to provide 150 mg of silver nitrate? *Hint: How much 10% silver nitrate contains 150 mg?*

Types of Ratio Strengths

The numerical amount of active ingredient in ratio strengths is *always* 1. Ratio strength is expressed as 1:*x*, with *x* representing the total amount of product. It is frequently used to describe solutions with a very small amount of active ingredient. The three types are as follows:

1. weight: volume   1 g : *x* mL

    This is read as 1 gram of active ingredient in *x* milliliters of total solution.
    For example, epinephrine 1:1,000 is 1 g of epinephrine in 1,000 mL of total solution.

2. volume: volume   1 mL : x mL

   This is read as 1 milliliter of active ingredient in x milliliters of total solution.
   For example, 1:15 sodium hypochlorite solution is 1 mL sodium hypochlorite in 15 mL of total solution.

3. weight: weight   1 g : x g

   This is read as 1 gram of active ingredient in x grams of total preparation
   For example, a 1:500 hydrocortisone cream contains 1 g of hydrocortisone in 500 g of total product.
   Performing calculations with the last two types may be confusing because *both* the active ingredient and total preparations have the same unit. Label them as follows to help identify the active ingredient measurement and the total preparation measurement:

   $1 \text{ mL}_{(a)} : x \text{ mL}_{(t)}$ or $1 \text{ g}_{(a)} : x \text{ g}_{(t)}$

TECH NOTE
Ratio strength is always in the form of 1:x.

TECH NOTE
Ratio strength is typically used to describe liquid medications with very low concentrations.

Determining the Amount of Medication with Ratio Strength

EXAMPLE 14.7

Interpret the following: 1:1,000 sodium bicarbonate solution

1 g of sodium bicarbonate in each 1,000 mL of total solution

How many grams of sodium bicarbonate are in 300 mL of 1:1,000 sodium bicarbonate solution?

$$\frac{1 \text{ g sodium bicarbonate}}{1,000 \text{ mL total solution}} = \frac{x}{300 \text{ mL}} \quad x = 0.3 \text{ g}$$

What is the strength in mg/mL?

$$\frac{\text{mg}}{\text{mL}} = \frac{1,000 \text{ mg}}{1 \text{ g}} \cdot \frac{1 \text{ g}}{1,000 \text{ mL}} = 1 \text{ mg/mL}$$

EXAMPLE 14.8

A physician orders 75 mL of a 1:15 sodium hypochlorite solution to be used in the office.

How many grams of sodium hypochlorite are needed to prepare the solution?

$$\frac{1 \text{ g}}{15 \text{ mL}} = \frac{x}{75 \text{ mL}} \quad x = 5 \text{ g}$$

How many milliliters of solvent are needed? qs to 75 mL

EXAMPLE 14.9

How many milliliters of epinephrine 1:1,000 solution are need to provide a 0.5-mg IM dose?

$$mL = \frac{1,000 \text{ mL}}{1 \text{ g}} \cdot \frac{1 \text{ g}}{1,000 \text{ mg}} \cdot \frac{0.5 \text{ mg}}{1} = 0.5 \text{ mL}$$

EXAMPLE 14.10

What ratio strength solution is made by dissolving Benadryl 50 mg in a lotion to make 150 mL?

Begin by changing 50 mg to 0.05 g:

$$\frac{0.05 \text{ g}}{150 \text{ mL}} = \frac{1 \text{ g}}{x} \quad 0.05x = 150 \text{ mL} \quad x = 3,000$$

Ratio strength = 1 : 3000

Practice Problems C

Interpret the meaning of the medication in 1 through 4, and answer the following questions. Show all work.

1. epinephrine solution 1:10,000 (w/v)

    _____

    How many grams are in 100 mL of solution?

2. 1:100 potassium permanganate solution (w/v)

    _____

    How many grams are in 200 mL of solution?

3. 1:50,000 lidocaine solution (w/v)

   How many grams are in 20 mL of solution?

   How many micrograms are in 20 mL of solution?

   What is the strength in milligrams per milliliter?

4. 1:1,000 Zephiran chloride solution

   How many grams are in 100 mL of solution?

5. How many grams of sodium perborate are in 200 mL of 1:50 solution? How many grams are in 100 mL of solution?

6. How many grams of epinephrine are in 1 mL of epinephrine 1:1,000? What is the strength in milligrams per milliliter?

7. How many grams of epinephrine are in 1 mL of epinephrine 1:10,000? What is the strength in milligrams per milliliter?

8. How many grams of active ingredient are in 400 g of a 1:2,500 w/w ointment?

9. A physician orders epinephrine 4 mg to be added to 500 mL of D5W. The available strength is 1:1,000 injectable.

   How many milliliters of epinephrine need to be added to the IV fluids?

10. How many grams of NaCl are needed to make 500 mL of a 1:5,000 solution?

11. How many milliliters of a 1:500 strength medication provides 750 mg?

12. How many milliliters of epinephrine 1:10,000 are needed to provide 2.5 mg?

13. How many grams of Neosporin are needed to prepare 1,500 mL of 1:1,000 Neosporin irrigation?

14. How many milliliters of Neostigmine 1:1,000 strength are needed to provide 16 mg?

15. A medication contains 4 mg/mL of solution. What is the ratio strength of the solution? *Hint: Ratio strength is expressed as 1 g per x mL, so a conversion from milligrams to grams must be calculated.*

Changing From Ratio to Percentage Strength

Set up an R&P that asks the question, "If there is 1 part active ingredient in x parts total preparation, how many parts of active ingredient would be in 100 parts total preparation?"

EXAMPLE 14.11

What is the percentage strength of a 1:10,000 w/v solution?

If there is 1 g active ingredient in 10,000 mL, how many grams would be in 100 mL?

$$\frac{1\ g}{10{,}000\ mL} = \frac{x}{100\ mL}$$ 1 times 100 equals 100, divided by 10,000 equals 0.01

This means there are 0.01 g in 100 mL: $\frac{0.01\ g}{100\ mL}$

Answer: 0.01%

EXAMPLE 14.12

What is the percentage strength of a 1:200 w/w ointment?

If there is 1 g active ingredient in 200 g total, how many $g_{(a)}$ would be in $100 g_{(t)}$?

$$\frac{1\ g_{(a)}}{200\ g_{(t)}} = \frac{x}{100\ g_{(t)}}$$ 1 times 100 equals 100, divided by 200 equals 0.5

This means that there are 0.5 g in 100 g: $\frac{0.5\ g_{(a)}}{100\ g_{(t)}}$

Answer: 0.5%

A shortcut for changing ratio strength to percentage strength is to express the ratio as a fraction and multiply it by 100. That is essentially what is being done with the R&P method.

EXAMPLE 14.13

What is the percentage strength of a 1:5,000 preparation?

$$\frac{1}{5{,}000} \cdot 100 = 0.02\%$$

Practice Problems D

Change the following ratio strengths to percentage strengths.

1. 1:100 potassium permanganate solution (w/v)

2. 1:50 Chloraseptic solution (w/v)

3. 1:1,000 Zephiran chloride solution (w/v)

4. 1:2,000 (w/v)

5. 1:100,000 (w/v)

6. What is the percentage strength of 1:500 silver nitrate solution?

How many milligrams of silver nitrate are in 250 mL?

Changing From Percentage to Ratio Strength

Set up an R&P that asks the question, "If there are x parts active ingredient in 100 parts total preparation, 1 part active ingredient would be in how much total preparation?"

EXAMPLE 14.14

What is the ratio strength of a 0.04% w/v solution?

$$\frac{0.04 \text{ g}}{100 \text{ mL}} = \frac{1 \text{ g}}{x} \quad \text{1 times 100 divided by } 0.04 = 2{,}500$$

This means that there is 1 g in 2,500 mL, so the answer is 1:2,500.

EXAMPLE 14.15

What is the ratio strength of a 0.01% w/v solution?

$$\frac{0.01 \text{ g}}{100 \text{ mL}} = \frac{1 \text{ g}}{x} \quad \text{1 times 100 divided by } 0.01 = 10{,}000\text{, so the answer is 1:10,000.}$$

Practice Problems E

Change the following percentage strengths to ratio strengths.

1. 5% formaldehyde solution

2. 0.01% epinephrine solution

3. 1% lidocaine solution

4. 0.025% solution

5. 0.5% hydrocortisone cream

REVIEW

Percentage and ratio strengths represent the amount of solute in a total amount of product. Percentage strength depicts the amount of active ingredient (solute) in 100 parts of total product. Ratio strength depicts one part of active ingredient (solute) in a total amount of product. Ratio strength is most commonly used for weak solutions. Percentage is expressed using % as an indication of the amount of active ingredient in a medication. The ratio is divided by a colon (:) to separate the solute and the solution.

Posttest

Show all calculations.

1. A. B.

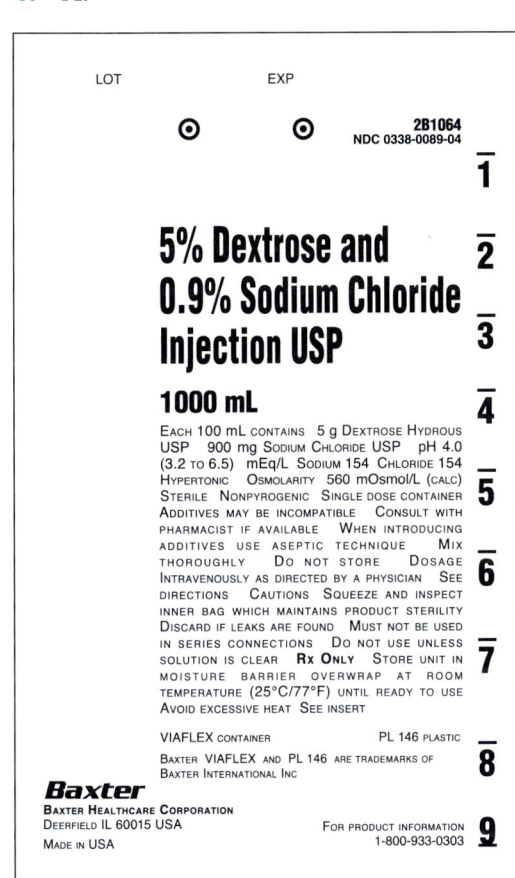

Courtesy of Baxter Healthcare Corporation. All rights reserved.

Courtesy of Baxter Healthcare Corporation. All rights reserved.

How many grams of NaCl are in the IV labeled A?

How many grams of dextrose are in the IV labeled A?

If a patient receives 400 mL of IV B, how much dextrose has been administered?

Continued

Posttest, cont.

2. A label for isopropyl alcohol reads "70% isopropyl alcohol in water."
   Interpret (v/v) _____
   How many milliliters of alcohol are in a pint of 70% alcohol?

3. A label reads "epinephrine 2.25% nebulizer."
   Interpret (w/v) _____
   How many milligrams are in a 0.5 mL vial?

   What is the strength in milligrams per milliliter?

4. The available medication is 1% lidocaine for injection.
   How many milligrams of lidocaine are in each milliliter of fluids?

5. If 15 mg of amoxicillin is added to 100 mL of sterile water, what is the percentage strength of the total volume of prepared medication? *(Do not round.)*

6. The label on a 25-mL saline vial shows a 1:25 solution.
   How many grams of NaCl are in the 25-mL vial?

Posttest, cont.

7. A Burow's solution 100-mL label reads 1:7.5 v/v.
   What is the volume of Burow's solution in the total volume? *(Round to tenths.)*

   What is the volume of *solvent* in the mixture?

8. How many milliliters of vinegar are in 500 mL of a 1:200 (v/v) vinegar solution?

   What is the percentage strength of this solution?

9. How many grams of silver nitrate are in 1 L of 1:25,000 silver nitrate solution to be used by a urologist?

   What is the percentage strength of silver nitrate?

10. How many milligrams of a drug are in 1.5 mL of a 1:5,000 solution?

11. How many milligrams of a drug are found in 1,500 mL of a 1:750 solution?

12. Tylenol with codeine elixir is approximately 0.25% codeine. What is the ratio strength?

Continued

Posttest, cont.

13. A physician asks for 0.4 g of potassium permanganate qs ad 1 pint of solution. *(Round to hundredths)*

    What is the percentage strength of the solution?

    What is the ratio strength of the solution?

14. A physician orders a 1-L solution of sodium chloride 1:200.

    How many grams of sodium chloride would be necessary to complete this order?

15. How many milliliters of a 10% solution of boric acid can be prepared from 20 g of boric acid?

16. If 15 mL of peppermint oil is in 500 mL of a solution, what is the percentage strength of the fluids?

17. A physician orders a 2% vinegar solution as a douche. How many milliliters of vinegar should be used to make 1 pint of solution?

    How could the patient approximate this in household measurements?

18. What volume of 1:5,000 solution can be made from 0.1 g NaCl?

Posttest, cont.

19. If a medication is available in 1:500 concentration, how many milliliters are needed to provide 750 mg?

20. How many milliliters of 40% boric acid solution are needed to prepare 1 L of 10% boric acid solution? *Hint: Calculate how many grams are needed for the new solution, then how many milliliters of stock are needed to provide that amount.*

REVIEW OF RULES

- To calculate the amount of drug in a specific amount of preparation using R & P, write the percentage or ratio strength as a fraction to show the amount of medication found in the total amount (known value) and set up an equivalent fraction to solve for the unknown value.
- To change from ratio strength to percentage strength, write the ratio as a fraction and set it equal to $x/100$.
- To change from percentage to ratio strength, write the percentage as a fraction and set it equal to $1/x$.
- To calculate milligrams per milliliter, use the known strength with the conversion factor 1,000 mg = 1 g in a DA equation, cancel units, and solve.

CHAPTER 15

Calculations for Simple Dilutions, Mixtures, and Compounding

OBJECTIVES

1. Dilute stock medications to the required strength.
2. Use alligation to calculate the weight/volume of stock medications needed to prepare a desired strength.
3. Interpret formulations for compounded preparations.
4. Enlarge and decrease compounding formulations as necessary.

KEY WORDS

aa Abbreviation meaning *of each*

Alligation alternate Mathematical method for determining the amount of *two* preparations of different strengths needed to prepare a required strength in between the two; aka **tic-tac-toe**

Alligation medial Calculation method by which the weighted average strength of a mixture of *two or more* preparations of known quantity and concentration may be determined

Component Any of the ingredients used to compound a product

Compound A product prepared in a pharmacy to fill a prescription for a product that is *not* commercially available in the ordered dose or dosage form

Compounding formulation Similar to a recipe; list of all components needed for a particular compound

Diluent An inert component in which other components (such as the active ingredient) are mixed or dissolved (e.g., water, elixir, cream, or ointment bases); aka **base or solvent**

Dilution Process of making a more concentrated preparation less concentrated by adding a diluent containing no active ingredient such as water or white petrolatum

Nonsterile compounding The mixing of two or more components that does not require a sterile environment

qs Abbreviation meaning quantity sufficient or required

qs ad Abbreviation meaning quantity sufficient to make

Stock medication Medication provided by a manufacturer and kept on hand for use in preparing medication orders or prescriptions

Pretest

Interpret the following labels to show the weight/volume of solute in the total amount of preparation. Round answers to tenths. Show calculations.

1. An order is to supply 10 mL of a drug at 50 mg/mL. The stock supply is 2.5 g/10 mL.

    How many milliliters of stock solution (solute) are needed? _____

    How many milliliters of solvent (diluent) are needed? _____

2. A physician asks that 500 mL of 10% solution of a medication be prepared. The stock supply of the solution is 75%.

    How many milliliters of stock solution (solute) are needed? _____

    How many milliliters of solvent (diluent) are needed? _____

3. A physician asks the pharmacy to prepare 1 L of 1:2,000 silver nitrate solution to be used for an irrigation solution. The stock solution is 1% silver nitrate solution.

    How many milliliters of silver nitrate stock solution are needed? _____

    How many milliliters of solvent are needed? _____

Continued

Pretest, cont.

4. Prepare 250 mL of 0.02% benzalkonium chloride solution to be used for cleansing skin before surgery. Stock strength of the solute is 1%.

   How many milliliters of stock solution (solute) are needed? _____

   How many milliliters of solvent (diluent) are needed? _____

   How many milliliters of solute would be needed to prepare 500 mL of solution? _____

   How many milliliters of solvent would be needed to prepare 500 mL of solution? _____

5. A medical office needs 0.25 L of 10% Lysol solution for disinfecting the office.

   How many milliliters of 25% Lysol are needed to prepare the solution? _____

   How many milliliters of water (solvent) are needed? _____

Pretest, cont.

6. A physician orders 100 mL of 50% creosol solution prepared from a 1:2 creosol solution.

   How many milliliters of 1:2 creosol solution are needed to prepare this order?
   _____

   How many milliliters of solvent should be added for the order as above?
   _____

7. How many milliliters of 10% methyl salicylate are needed to prepare 3 pints of 4% lotion? *Hint: Remember that the units must be in the same measurements.*

8. Epinephrine is available as a 5% solution.

   How many milliliters are needed to prepare 10 mL of 2.5% solution of epinephrine?

Continued

Pretest, cont.

9. On hand is a 15% solution of sodium hypochlorite. The physician wants 1 L of 0.15% solution.

   How many milliliters of sodium hypochlorite are needed? _____

   How many milliliters of solvent should be added? _____

10. A stock liter contains 50% sodium bicarbonate. A physician desires 2 L of 6% solution.

    How many milliliters of 50% sodium bicarbonate are needed to fill this order? _____

    How many milliliters of solvent are needed? _____

11. A physician orders 20% KCl solution, and there are only 10% and 50% solutions in stock. How much of each are needed to prepare 100 mL of 20% solution?

Pretest, cont.

12. Prepare 750 mL of 0.75% sodium chloride solution from 0.9% NaCl and 0.45% NaCl. How many milliliters of each solution need to be combined to fill this order?

13. A physician orders 50 g of 1.5% hydrocortisone ointment. Available in stock is 100 g of 5% ointment and 100 g of petrolatum ointment base. *Hint: Just because 100 g of 5% hydrocortisone ointment and 100 g of petrolatum are available does not mean that the entire amount will necessarily be used.*

How many g of each are needed?

Continued

Pretest, cont.

14. How much of each ingredient is needed to make 4 oz of the following formulation?

<u>Meloxicam 3 mg/mL Gel[1]</u>

meloxicam	300 mg
triethanolamine	2 g
carbomer (Carbopol 940)	1.6 g
water, purified	qs 100 mL

How many mg of meloxicam are needed to make 4 oz?

How many g of triethanolamine are needed to make 4 oz?

How many g of carbomer are needed to make 4 oz?

How many mL of purified water are needed to make 4 oz?

15. A physician orders 30 g of ointment containing 3% of Drug A and 7% of Drug B. Both are available as pure powders. How many grams of each are needed?

Drug A

Drug B

Ointment base

INTRODUCTION

This chapter covers simple dilution, mixtures, and basic compounding calculations. Dilution may be necessary to compound a lesser strength ordered by a physician. Stock medications may be ordered from manufacturers in concentrated strengths for storage and economic reasons and diluted later with a specific volume or weight of diluent. By using stock solutions that are purer and stronger forms of a drug, larger amounts of medication may be prepared from small quantities. The solute and solvent (aka diluent) may be in solid form, as well as liquid. A solid diluent is frequently referred to as a base. The pharmacy staff is responsible for diluting to fill prescriptions and medication orders.

A solution is made of a solute (the drug dissolved) and a solvent or diluent (the substance in which the solute is dissolved). Various methods may be used to determine the amount of concentrated medication and diluent needed to compound an ordered strength. Simple dilution is used when *one* product concentration is combined with a diluent that has zero concentration of active ingredient, thus making a more concentrated product less concentrated. Alligation alternate is a mathematical calculation that determines the necessary amount of *two* different concentrations required to compound a concentration in between the two. Alligation medial can be used to calculate the concentration of a mixture of *two or more* different concentrations of medications.

The following procedures will make these calculations easier:

1. Convert all strengths to percents before performing calculations.
2. Convert all amounts to metric measurements before performing calculations.

Compounding is considered to be preparing medications according to prescription orders for medications that are not commercially available in the desired strength or dosage form. Whereas many solutions are prepared for use in an inpatient setting, other compounded prescriptions are intended for dispensing to a consumer. Compounding medications in specially ordered doses has become very popular, giving rise to compounding pharmacies. Special populations such as geriatric or pediatric patients often require different medication strengths than those found in stock medications from the manufacturer. Individualized hormone replacement therapy, as well as other medication, requires specialty compounding. Specific requirements governing the process of nonsterile compounding are found in USP <795>. Pharmacy technicians can earn special certification in compounding.

TECH NOTE
All compounding calculations should be performed using the metric system.

Simple Dilution of Stock Medications

With simple dilution, the amount of active ingredient or solute remains the same and the solvent amount is increased, thus reducing the strength of the stock solution. Simple dilution is the process of making a more concentrated product less concentrated by adding a diluent with no active ingredient. Common diluents with no active ingredient (0% medication strength) include sterile water (SW) for liquid solutions and petrolatum (ointment base) for solid solutions. Various cream bases are also available.

The following method can be used to solve dilution problems as long as they involve only *one* stock strength solution to be diluted with a diluent containing no active ingredient—for example, a 50% solution diluted with water to a 40% solution or a 1% ointment diluted to a 0.25% ointment with petrolatum. The most important thing to remember with this method is that the volume units of the stock and desired product should be milliliters, the weight units must be the same, and the strength units of the stock and desired product must be the same; usually both are changed to percentages.

Equation for Diluting Stock Liquids

Volume units must be the same! Strength units must be the same!

$SV \cdot SS = DV \cdot DS$

SV = stock volume   SS = stock strength

DV = desired volume   DS = desired strength

Equation for Diluting Stock Solids

Weight units must be the same! Strength units must be the same!

$SW \cdot SS = DW \cdot DS$

SW = stock weight   SS = stock strength

DW = desired weight   DS = desired strength

Solute—substance being dissolved; the stock strength that is being diluted
Solvent—substance doing the dissolving; diluent or base with 0% active ingredient

To determine the amount of solvent needed, use one of the following:

Solvent volume = DV − SV

Solvent weight = DW − SW

Follow these steps to solve simple dilution problems:

1. Identify the *three known variables,* and use a question mark to identify the unknown variable.
2. Make certain that the units of volume or weight are the same and the units of strength are the same.
   a. Calculations for compounding and diluting are always performed in the metric system, so change all weight and volume measurements to the metric system before placing them in the formula.
   b. It is easiest to work with percentage strengths so convert all strengths to percentages. (The formula will work no matter what strength designation is used as long as both the SS and DS are the *exact* same unit. If using both in ratio strength, write them as fractions and solve. As long as both values are in mg/1 mL, that value can be used also.)
3. Write the equation.
4. Fill in the variables, and solve for the unknown value.
5. Round to the nearest whole number if dealing with large quantities, tenths if dealing with small quantities, and hundredths if dealing with answers less than zero.

EXAMPLE 15.1

A physician orders 250 mL of a 15% solution to be prepared from a stock supply of 80% solution.

How many milliliters of stock solution and solvent are needed?

SV = ?   SS = 80%   DV = 250 mL   DS = 15%

SV · SS = DV · DS

SV · 80% = 250 mL · 15%

SV • 80 = 3,750 mL divide both sides by 80

SV = 46.9 mL = 47 mL

How many milliliters of the solvent/diluent (sterile water) are needed?

Solvent volume = DV – SV

Solvent volume = 250 mL – 47 mL = 203 mL

Directions: Combine 47 mL of 80% solution and 203 mL of sterile water to make 250 mL of 15% solution.

EXAMPLE 15.2

An order is received for 10 g of petrolatum to be combined with 25 g of 0.2% hydrocortisone ointment. This example deals with weight in grams and the unknown value is the desired strength.

What is the strength of the final product?

SW = 25 g   SS = 0.2%   DW = 35 g (10 g + 25 g)   DS = ?

SW • SS = DW • DS

25 g • 0.2% = 35 g • DS

5% = 35 • DS

5% = 35 • DS   divide both sides by 35

0.14% = DS

TECH NOTE
It is always important to identify your variables so that you can identify the unknown value. Any time a question states, "A physician orders" or "prepare," what follows will be the desired values.

EXAMPLE 15.3

Prepare 500 mL 5% creosol solution from a stock solution of creosol 1:10.

How many milliliters of stock solution and solvent are needed?

SV = ?   SS = 1:10   DV = 500 mL   DS = 5%

The first step is to convert the 1:10 strength to a percent so that it can be used in the formula.

$$\frac{1\,g}{10\,mL} = \frac{x}{100\,mL} \quad x = 10\,g \quad 1:10 = 10\%$$

SV = ?   SS = 10%   DV = 500 mL   DS = 5%

SV • SS = DV • DS

SV • 10% = 500 mL • 5%

SV • 10 = 2,500 mL divide both sides by 10

SV = 250 mL

Solvent volume = DV − SV

Solvent volume = 500 mL − 250 mL = 250 mL

Directions: Combine 250 mL of 5% creosol solution and 250 mL of sterile water to make 250 mL of 1:10 solution.

> **TECH NOTE**
> When diluting a product to exactly half the original strength, equal parts of solute and solvent will be used.

EXAMPLE 15.4

 Prepare 1 oz of a 0.002% solution of merthiolate from a 1% stock solution.

How many milliliters of stock solution and solvent are needed?

SV = ?   SS = 1%   DV = 1 oz   DS = 0.002%

The first step is to convert ounces to milliliters so that the calculations can be performed in the metric system. 1 oz = 30 mL is one of the common conversion factors:

SV = ?   SS = 1%   DV = 30 mL   DS = 0.002%

SV · SS = DV · DS

SV · 1% = 30 mL · 0.002%

SV = 0.06 mL   Such a small volume of stock *should* not be rounded.

Solvent volume = DV − SV

Solvent volume = 30 mL − 0.06 mL = 29.94 mL

Directions: Combine 0.06 mL of 1% solution and 29.94 mL of sterile water to make 30 mL of 0.002% solution.

EXAMPLE 15.5

A physician orders 15 mL of a 10 mcg/mL dilution of a drug for a child. The stock medication is 40 mcg/mL.

How many milliliters of stock solution and solvent are needed?

SV = ?   SS = 40 mcg/mL   DV = 15 mL   DS = 10 mcg/mL

Because both strengths are in the *exact* same unit (mcg/1 mL), they can be used in this formula:

SV · SS = DV · DS

SV · 40 mcg/mL = 15 mL · 10 mcg/mL

SV · 40 = 150 mL   Divide both sides by 40.

SV = 3.75 mL = 3.8 mL

Solvent volume = DV − SV

Solvent volume = 15 mL − 3.8 mL = 11.2 mL

Directions: Combine 3.8 mL of 40 mcg/mL solution and 11.2 mL of sterile water to make 15 mL of 10 mcg/mL strength solution.

Other variables are sometimes used to represent this equation such as IV or IW and IS for initial volume or weight and initial strength and FV or FW and FS for final volume or weight and final strength. The concept is the same no matter what variables are used to represent the equation.

Practice Problems A

Calculate the following problems. Show your work.

1. Prepare 1 L of Lysol 3% from a stock solution of Lysol 10%.

    How many milliliters of stock solution (solute) are needed? _____

    How many milliliters of solvent are needed? _____

2. Prepare 8 oz of 40% solution of isopropyl alcohol from a 70% stock solution.

    How many milliliters of stock solution (solute) are needed? _____

    How many milliliters of solvent are needed? _____

3. Prepare 1.5 L of creosol 1:200 from a 2% stock solution.

How many milliliters of stock solution (solute) are needed? _____

How many milliliters of solvent are needed? _____

4. A physician orders 250 mL of 15% glycerin solution as an enema. The available stock solution is glycerin 25%.

How many milliliters of stock solution (solute) are needed? _____

How many milliliters of solvent are needed? _____

5. A physician orders 1 pint of 7.5% dextrose in water. The stock solution is 50%.

   How many milliliters of stock solution (solute) are needed? _____

   How many milliliters of solvent are needed? _____

6. How many milliliters of 20% Zephiran chloride are necessary to prepare 8 oz of a 7.5% solution?

   How many milliliters of stock solution (solute) are needed? _____

   How many milliliters of solvent are needed? _____

7. A physician orders 1.5 L of potassium chloride 15% to be made from a 20% stock solution.

How many milliliters of stock solution (solute) are needed? _____

How many milliliters of solvent are needed? _____

8. A medical office needs 3 L of a 1:10 solution of hypochlorous acid. The stock solution is 25% hypochlorous acid.

How many milliliters of stock solution (solute) are needed? _____

How many milliliters of solvent are needed? _____

9. A physician orders 8 oz of Betadine solution 2%. The stock solution is Betadine 10%.

How many milliliters of stock solution (solute) are needed? _____

How many milliliters of solvent are needed? _____

10. Prepare 3 L of hydrogen peroxide 1:40. The stock solution is hydrogen peroxide 5%.

How many milliliters of stock solution (solute) are needed? _____

How many milliliters of solvent are needed? _____

11. Prepare 600 mL of a 2.5% solution from a 10% hydrogen peroxide solution.

   How many milliliters of stock solution (solute) are needed? _____

   How many milliliters of solvent are needed? _____

12. Prepare 4 L of a 1:50 solution of potassium permanganate from a 5% potassium permanganate stock solution.

   How many milliliters of stock solution (solute) are needed? _____

   How many milliliters of solvent are needed? _____

13. Prepare 10 mL of 0.01% adrenaline solution for injection from a 2% adrenaline ampule. *Do not round answers!*

How many milliliters of stock solution (solute) are needed? _____

How many milliliters of solvent are needed? _____

14. A physician orders 500 mL of 2% calcium chloride solution to be given IV. The stock solution is calcium chloride 10%.

How many milliliters of stock solution (solute) are needed? _____

How many milliliters of solvent are needed? _____

If the calcium chloride is available in 5-mL ampules, how many ampules are needed to prepare the solution? _____

15. How many milliliters of a 6% solution can be made from 30 mL of a 36% solution?

    Hint: Take care when identifying the three known variables.

16. A stock solution of 1:50 of mercuric chloride is available to prepare 250 mL of 0.02% solution.

    How many milliliters of stock solution (solute) are needed? _____

    How many milliliters of solvent are needed? _____

17. If 300 mL of a 20% stock solution is added to 2.7 L of sterile water, what is the percent strength of the final solution? *Hint: See example 15.2*

18. A physician orders 80 mL of a 1:1,000 solution. In stock is a 1:250 solution.

How many milliliters of stock solution (solute) are needed? _____

How many milliliters of solvent are needed? _____

CALCULATIONS USING ALLIGATION

Alligation is a mathematical method of solving questions involving the mixing of solutions or compounds possessing different percentage strengths. The process is the same whether dealing with weight or volume solutions.

Alligation Alternate

Alligation alternate, also known as *tic-tac-toe*, is a method that is used to calculate the number of parts of two different percentage strengths of medication that can be mixed together to prepare a third strength that is not available. If a physician orders 20% KCl solution and only 10% and 50% KCl solutions are in stock, the amount of each solution needed to prepare the prescribed amount of the 20% solution can be calculated. This can only be achieved when the strength desired is *in between* the two strengths being mixed. Mixing a 5% and a 10% solution cannot result in a 15% solution, but mixing a 5% and a 15% solution can result in a 10% solution.

All strengths must be converted to percentages before performing alligation alternate. As mentioned, the final strength of the mixture must lie somewhere between the strengths of the component parts. This means that the prepared mixture must be stronger than its weakest component and weaker than its strongest component. If the mixture contains more of the weaker component, the prepared mixture will be closer to the strength of the weaker component. If the mixture contains more of the stronger component, the mixture will be closer to the strength of the stronger component.

Alligation alternate:

Step 1—Prepare a graph, similar to a box for tic-tac-toe.
Step 2—Place the strength to be calculated in the center box.
Step 3—Place the highest percentage concentration in the left upper corner.
Step 4—Place the lowest percentage concentration in the lower left corner.
Step 5—Subtract the center square amount from the left upper corner amount, and place the answer in the lower right corner to determine the number of parts of the lowest percentage concentration to be used in the mixture.
Step 6—Subtract the lower left corner amount from the center square amount, and place the answer in the upper right corner to reveal the number of parts of the highest percentage concentration to be used in the mixture.
Step 7—Add the two calculated parts in the far right column to find the total parts of the two ingredients in the compound.
Step 8—When a specific quantity is included in the order, the two parts of the mixture are written as fractions of the whole, and each is multiplied by the total amount needed to calculate the exact amount of each ingredient needed.

EXAMPLE 15.6

Prepare 1,000 mL of 70% w/v solution from a 50% solution and a 95% solution.

Step 1—Draw a graph.

Step 2—Place the desired strength in the center box.

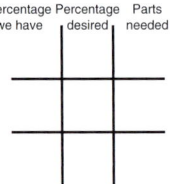

Step 3—Place the highest percentage concentration in the left upper corner.

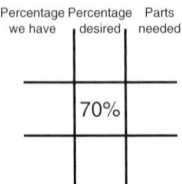

Step 4—Place the lowest percentage concentration in the lower left corner.

Step 5—Subtract the center square amount from the left upper corner amount, and place the answer in the lower right corner to determine the parts of the lowest percentage concentration needed.

> **! TECH ALERT**
>
> Notice that the answers are in parts, not unit values.

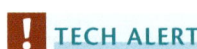

Step 6—Subtract the lower left corner amount from the center box amount, and place the answer in the upper right corner to reveal the parts of the highest percentage concentration needed.

Percentage we have	Percentage desired	Parts needed
95%		20 parts
	70%	
50%		25 parts

Step 7—Add both parts to obtain the total parts in the compound.

Percentage we have	Percentage desired	Parts needed
95%		20 parts
	70%	
50%		25 parts
		45 parts

To prepare this solution, mix 20 parts of 95% with 25 parts of 50%. Specifically, $20/45$ of the desired amount will need to be the 95% solution, which can be written to the right of the top row of the graph; $25/45$ of the desired amount will need to be the 50% solution, which can be written to the right of the bottom row of the graph. These are the fractional parts that are used to find the exact amounts to be mixed when the total weight or volume of the compound is indicated.

Step 8—The total desired amount of the 70% solution is 1,000 mL.

$$\frac{20 \text{ parts}}{45 \text{ parts}} \times 1{,}000 \text{ mL} = 444.4 \text{ mL} = 444 \text{ mL of } 95\% \text{ solution}$$

$$\frac{25 \text{ parts}}{45 \text{ parts}} \times 1{,}000 \text{ mL} = 555.6 \text{ mL} = 556 \text{ mL of } 50\% \text{ solution}$$

Adding the two amounts should equal 1,000 mL:

444 mL of 95% solution + 556 mL of 50% solution = 1,000 mL of 70% solution

TECH NOTE
Always check your calculations to be sure the total volume/weight of the calculated compound equals the desired prescription weight/volume.

Steps 1 to 7 determine the *parts* of each stock medication needed for the compound. Step 8 is to find the volume/weight of each stock medication needed to prepare a *specific* amount.

If one component has a zero percent strength, such as water or petrolatum, the alligation method can still be used by placing a zero in the bottom left square and proceeding in the same manner. The other choice is to use the equation from the dilution section because this would be a simple dilution.

Alligation Medial

Alligation medial is a method of calculation that may be used to determine the total percentage strength when *two or more* substances with known quantities and strengths are mixed. This method allows for the rapid calculation of final strengths. The quantities must be expressed in common measurements such as the same weight or volume.

Steps

Step 1—Add the number of milliliters or grams being mixed to obtain the total volume or weight that is being prepared.

Step 2—Multiply the percentage strength of each component, written in decimal form, by the total number of grams or milliliters being used in the preparation, to obtain the total number of g or mL of active ingredient that component will add to the total product as shown in the following equation:

Decimal form of percentage strength times g or mL used
   = g or mL provided by that component

Step 3—Add the amounts of active ingredient provided by each component.

Step 4—Place the total amount of active ingredient over the total amount of milliliters or grams and multiply by 100 to determine the percent strength of the new product.

EXAMPLE 15.7

What is the final percentage strength of a w/v solution when 300 mL of 95%, 1,000 mL of 70%, and 200 mL of 50% solutions are combined?

Step 1—Add the number of milliliters being mixed to obtain the total volume being prepared.

$$300 \text{ mL} + 1{,}000 \text{ mL} + 200 \text{ mL} = 1{,}500 \text{ mL}$$

Step 2—Determine how many grams of medication are in each quantity to be mixed.

How many grams of active ingredient are in 300 mL of 95% solution?

$$0.95 \times 300 = 285 \text{ g}$$

This calculation is actually a shortcut of the following calculation that was covered in Chapter 14. The shortcut from step 2 can be used in place of the following:

$$\frac{95 \text{ g}}{100 \text{ mL}} = \frac{x}{300 \text{ mL}} \quad 100x = 95 \text{ g} \cdot 300$$

$$x = 285 \text{ g}$$

300 mL of 95% solution contains 285 g of medication

How many grams of active ingredient are in 1,000 mL of 70% solution?

$$0.7 \times 1{,}000 = 700 \text{ g}$$

How many grams of active ingredient are in 200 mL of 50% solution?

$$0.5 \times 200 = 100 \text{ g}$$

Step 3—Add all three amounts.

$$285 \text{ g} + 700 \text{ g} + 100 \text{ g} = 1{,}085 \text{ g}$$

Step 4—Place total number of grams over the total milliliters and multiply by 100.

$$\text{Total number of } \frac{\text{grams}}{\text{milliliters}} \times 100$$

$$\frac{1{,}085 \text{ g}}{1{,}500 \text{ mL}} \times 100 = 72.3\%$$

This is actually a shortcut for solving a ratio and proportion between the fraction in step 4 and $\frac{x}{100}$ to determine the percent strength of the total mixture.

$$\frac{1{,}085 \text{ g}}{1{,}500 \text{ mL}} = \frac{x}{100 \text{ mL}} \quad 1{,}500x = 108{,}500 \text{ g} \quad x = 72.3 \text{ g}$$

By definition, $\frac{72.3 \text{ g}}{100 \text{ mL}} = 72.3\%$.

What is the ratio strength of the final answer?

$$\frac{72.3 \text{ g}}{100 \text{ mL}} = \frac{1 \text{ g}}{x} \quad 72.3x = 100 \text{ mL} \quad x = 1.4$$

The ratio strength is $1:1.4$.

> **TECH NOTE**
> If the original strengths are provided as ratios, step 1 will be to change the ratio strengths to percentages.

Alligation medial can also be used as a quick means of verifying alligation alternate results. The following example uses the answers from Example 16.6 in an alligation medial process as a check.

EXAMPLE 15.8

To verify the results of Example 16.6, what is the final percentage strength of a solution when 444 mL of 95% solution is mixed with 556 mL of 50% solution? (It should be 70%.)

Step 1: $444 \text{ mL} + 556 \text{ mL} = 1{,}000 \text{ mL}$

Step 2: $444 \text{ mL} \times 0.95 = 421.8 = 422 \text{ g}$ of active ingredient

$556 \text{ mL} \times 0.5 = 278 \text{ g}$ of active ingredient

Step 3: $422 \text{ g} + 278 \text{ g} = 700 \text{ g}$ of active ingredient

Step 4: $\frac{700 \text{ g}}{1{,}000 \text{ mL}} \times 100 = 70\%$

This shows that the calculations using alligation alternate are correct.

When performing calculations with v/v or w/w solutions, it may help to label which portion is the active ingredient and which part is the total product because both the amount of active ingredient and the total amount of preparation will have the same unit.

Practice Problems B

Complete these problems using alligation. Round to tenths unless otherwise indicated. Label answers as grams or milliliters and the appropriate percentage strength of each. Show your work.

1. How many *milliliters* of 6% and 15% sodium hypochlorite solution are needed to prepare 500 mL of a 10% solution?

2. In stock are two ointment strengths containing 5% and 20% boric acid. How many grams of each are needed to prepare 1 g of a 12.5% ointment?

3. A physician orders 20 g of a 15% tannic acid ointment. How many grams of 12% and 25% tannic acids are needed? Use alligation medial to verify your answers.

4. Prepare 500 mL of 15% potassium chloride solution using 20% potassium chloride and 5% potassium chloride solution.

   How many milliliters of each solution need to be combined to fill this order?

5. Prepare 500 mL of 0.9% sodium chloride solution from a 10% sodium chloride solution.

   How many mL of each solution need to be combined to fill this order? *Hint: The diluent of sterile water necessary for this calculation has 0% sodium chloride. Use alligation alternate and SV · SS = DV · DS and compare your answers.*

6. Prepare 750 mL of 3% sodium bicarbonate solution from a 15% solution and 1% solution. How many milliliters of each solution need to be combined to fill this order?

7. Prepare 200 mL of 10% dextrose solution using 5% dextrose solution and 50% dextrose solution. How many milliliters of each solution need to be combined to fill this order?

8. Prepare 3 L of 3% Lysol solution using 1.5% Lysol and 5% Lysol solutions. How many milliliters of each solution need to be combined to fill this order? *(Round to whole numbers.)*

9. A physician orders 50 g of a 7.5% ointment. The available ointments are 2.5% and 15%.

   How many grams of each need to be combined to fill this order?

10. Prepare 1,800 mL of 40% alcohol from 10% alcohol and 55% alcohol.

   How many milliliters of each solution need to be combined to fill this order?

11. Prepare 500 mL of 4% potassium permanganate solution using 1:10 potassium permanganate solution and 1:50 potassium permanganate solution.

   How many milliliters of each solution need to be combined to fill this order? *Hint: Change ratio strengths to percentage strengths first.*

12. Prepare 250 mL of 8% dextrose solution. The available dextrose solutions are D5W and D10W.

   How many milliliters of each solution need to be combined to fill this order?

13. A physician orders 50 mL dextrose 7.5% to be administered IV stat. The available strengths are D5W and D50W. How many milliliters of each solution are needed?

14. Prepare 200 mL of 5% potassium chloride. The available potassium chloride is 20%.

    How many milliliters of 20% KCl and sterile water need to be combined to fill this order?

15. Prepare 50 mL of 1.8% sodium chloride solution. The available sodium chloride solutions are 0.9% and 5%. How many milliliters of each solution are needed?

16. Prepare 2.5 g of hydrocortisone ointment 7.6%. The available hydrocortisone ointments are in strengths of 2.5% and 10%.

    How many grams of each strength need to be combined to fill this order?

17. A physician orders 1.5 L of a 12% Burow's solution. The available Burow's solutions are 5% and 25%. How many milliliters of each solution need to be combined to fill this order?

18. A patient needs epinephrine for an acute asthma attack. The physician orders 100 mL of epinephrine 4%. The available epinephrine is 1:10 and 1:100.

    How many milliliters of each solution need to be combined to fill this order?

COMPOUNDING

Developing a Medication Formula From a Prescription

Sometimes physicians will order a particular strength and amount of medication that they want to be dispensed. In these cases, pharmacy personnel need to calculate the formula to use. Once this is done, a compounding pharmacy may maintain a book, similar to a recipe book, containing frequently prescribed formulations of medications. Calculations to determine formulas can be performed using the following methods.

EXAMPLE 15.9

  How much hydrocortisone (solute) and how much Eucerin cream (commercially prepared base/solvent) should be combined to prepare the following prescription:

hydrocortisone 2.5% cream 30 g

Amount of hydrocortisone needed:

$$\frac{2.5\ g_{(a)}}{100\ g_{(t)}} = \frac{x}{30\ g_{(t)}} \quad x = 0.75\ g$$

Amount of Eucerin cream needed:

$$30\ g_{(t)} - 0.75\ g_{(a)} = 29.25\ g$$

This question can also be thought of as follows: How much hydrocortisone (100% powder) and how much Eucerin cream are needed to prepare 30 g of hydrocortisone 2.5% cream?

Amount of hydrocortisone needed:

$$SW = ? \quad SS = 100\% \quad DW = 30\ g \quad DS = 2.5\%$$

$$SW \cdot SS = DW \cdot DS$$

$$SW \cdot 100\% = 30\ g \cdot 2.5\%$$

$$SW \cdot 100 = 75\ g$$

$$SW = 0.75\ g$$

Amount of Eucerin cream needed: 30 g − 0.75 g = 29.25 g

If more than one active ingredient is to be added to a compound, the strength or amount of each is calculated according to the total amount to be prepared.

EXAMPLE 15.10

 Prepare 1 g of 0.25% menthol and 0.5% phenol in petrolatum. *Use dimensional analysis because the answer is requested in mg requiring a conversion factor.*

How many milligrams of menthol are needed?

$$mg = \frac{1{,}000\ mg}{1\ g} \times \frac{0.25\ g_{(a)}}{100\ g_{(t)}} \times \frac{1\ g_{(t)}}{1} = 2.5\ mg$$

How many milligrams of phenol are needed?

$$mg = \frac{1{,}000\ mg}{1\ g} \times \frac{0.5\ g_{(a)}}{100\ g_{(t)}} \times \frac{1\ g_{(t)}}{1} = 5\ mg$$

How many milligrams of petrolatum are needed?

1 g total product is equal to 1,000 mg.

$$1{,}000\ mg - 2.5\ mg - 5\ mg = 992.5\ mg\ petrolatum$$

Sometimes a compound must be prepared using another strength of commercially prepared product. This can be calculated using strategies from Chapter 14 or simple dilution.

EXAMPLE 15.11

  A physician orders 200 g of 2.5% hydrocortisone cream. The stock medication on hand is 10% hydrocortisone cream.

How many grams of hydrocortisone are needed to prepare 200 g of 2.5% cream?

$$\frac{2.5 \text{ g}_{(a)}}{100 \text{ g}_{(t)}} = \frac{x}{200 \text{ g}_{(t)}} \quad x = 5 \text{ g of hydrocortisone}$$

How many g of 10% hydrocortisone cream contain 5 g of hydrocortisone?

$$\frac{10 \text{ g}_{(a)}}{100 \text{ g}_{(t)}} = \frac{5 \text{ g}_{(a)}}{x} \quad x = 50 \text{ g of 10\% cream provide 5 g of hydrocortisone}$$

To compound 200 g of 2.5% hydrocortisone cream from 10% hydrocortisone cream and a base cream, measure 50 g of 10% cream and add 150 g base.

This question can be approached as a simple dilution.

How many grams of 10% hydrocortisone cream are needed to prepare 200 g of 2.5% cream?

$$SW = ? \quad SS = 10\% \quad DW = 200 \text{ g} \quad DS = 2.5\%$$

$$SW \cdot SS = DW \cdot DS$$

$$SW \cdot 10\% = 200 \text{ g} \cdot 2.5\%$$

$$SW \cdot 10 = 500 \text{ g}$$

$$SW = 50 \text{ g of 10\% hydrocortisone cream}$$

How many grams of base cream are needed?

$$200 \text{ g} - 50 \text{ g} = 150 \text{ g base}$$

Practice Problems C

Calculate the following problems. Show your calculations.

1. A prescription is written to prepare 30 g of 0.05% triamcinolone ointment using Aristocort A Ointment (0.1% triamcinolone) and white petrolatum. How much of each is needed?

2. How many grams of 100% zinc oxide and white petrolatum are needed to prepare 4 oz of a 10% ointment? *Hint: Convert ounces to grams first.*

3. A dermatologist writes a prescription for 0.5% menthol and 0.6% phenol in petrolatum to make 30 g of ointment.

   How many grams of menthol are needed?

   How many grams of phenol are needed?

   How many grams of petrolatum are needed?

4. Prepare 30 mL of 5 mg/mL tadalafil suspension.

   How many milligrams of tadalafil are needed?

   How many tadalafil 20 mg tablets are needed?

   How much suspending vehicle is needed?

5. Prepare 5 mL of ceftazadime fortified eye drops 50 mg/mL. *This would be compounded in a hood for sterility purposes.*

   How many total milligrams of cetazadime are needed?

   How many milliliters of cetazadime 1 g/10 mL sterile injection are needed?

   How much sterile water is needed?

Preparing a Compounded Prescription From a Formula

If the compounding formulation is written, the instructions need to be followed exactly to prepare the prescription correctly. The abbreviations qs, meaning quantity required, and qs ad, meaning quantity sufficient to make, are frequently found in compounding formulations.

The following example illustrates some of the information that can be calculated from a formula.

EXAMPLE 15.12

Mouthwash	
tetracycline	*1 g*
nystatin suspension	*60 mL*
diphenhydramine	*48 mL*
dexamethasone	*qs to 240 mL*

What is the percentage of tetracycline (w/v) in the final compound?

The known information is that there is 1 g of tetracycline in 240 mL, so the question is, "How many grams would be in 100 mL?"

$$\frac{1\,g}{240\,mL} = \frac{x}{100\,mL} \quad x = 0.42\,g \text{ (rounded to the hundredths place)}$$

Therefore the strength of tetracycline is 0.42%.

What is the percentage of nystatin (v/v) suspension in the final mixture?

$$\frac{60\,mL}{240\,mL} = \frac{x}{100\,mL} \quad x = 25\,mL$$

Therefore the strength of nystatin is 25%.

What is the percentage of diphenhydramine (v/v) in the final mixture?

$$\frac{48\,mL}{240\,mL} = \frac{x}{100\,mL} \quad 240x = 4,800\,mL \quad x = 20\,mL$$

Therefore the strength of diphenhydramine is 20%.

What volume of dexamethasone is needed to prepare the desired volume?

This cannot be determined exactly because it is not known how much volume 1 g of tetracycline will displace, so the answer is qs ad 240 mL.

TECH NOTE
When compounding, it can be helpful to know that 1 mL of water weighs 1 g.

In addition to the abbreviations qs and qs ad, the abbreviation $\overline{aa}$, meaning *of each*, is frequently found in compounding formulations. When used in a formulation, it means to use equal amounts of each component listed as follows:

EXAMPLE 15.13

A dentist sends a prescription for a mouthwash to swish and spit for pain.

> *Lidocaine 0.5%*
>
> *Benadryl*
>
> *Maalox*
>
> *Sig: $\overline{aa}$ qs 120 mL*

What volume of each medication is needed to prepare this prescription?

Because there are three parts to the formulation and there is to be an equal amount of each used, divide 120 mL by 3 to get 40 mL of each component.

Lidocaine	*40 mL*
Benadryl	*40 mL*
Maalox	*40 mL*
Total	*120 mL*

What would be the percentage (v/v) strength of each?

Each one is one-third of the total, so each would be 33.3%.

Use ratio and proportion to prove this:

$$\frac{40 \text{ mL}}{120 \text{ mL}} = \frac{x}{100 \text{ mL}} \quad 120x = 4{,}000 \text{ mL} \quad x = 33.3 \text{ mL}$$

33.3 mL/100 mL is 33.3%

A compounding prescription may also be written in parts.

EXAMPLE 15.14

Calculate the amounts required to make 2 oz (60 g) of the following formula:

coal tar	*1 part*
zinc oxide	*5 parts*
wool fat	*10 parts*
white paraffin	*20 parts*

Step 1—Find the total of all of the parts: 1 + 5 + 10 + 20 = 36.

Step 2—Determine how much of each ingredient is needed:

Coal tar:

$$\frac{1 \text{ part}}{36 \text{ parts}} = \frac{x}{60} \quad 36x = 60 \quad x = 1.7 \text{ g}$$

Zinc oxide (g):

$$\frac{5 \text{ parts}}{36 \text{ parts}} = \frac{x}{60} \quad 36x = 300 \quad x = 8.3 \text{ g}$$

Wool fat (g):

$$\frac{10 \text{ parts}}{36 \text{ parts}} = \frac{x}{60} \quad 36x = 600 \quad x = 16.7 \text{ g}$$

White paraffin:

$$\frac{20 \text{ parts}}{36 \text{ parts}} = \frac{x}{60} \quad 36x = 1{,}200 \quad x = 33.3 \text{ g}$$

Step 3—Check your calculations.

If the calculations are correct, adding all of the parts will equal 60 g.

1.7 g + 8.3 g + 16.7 g + 33.3 g = 60 g

Practice Problems D

1. Calculate the amount of grams of each required to make 30 g of the following:

drug B	*1 part*
lanolin	*1 part*
petrolatum	*8 parts*

   drug B

   lanolin

   petrolatum

2. Calculate the amounts needed to prepare 30 g of the following prescription:

salacylic acid	0.9%
menthol	0.4%
1% triamcinolone cream	qs ad 30 g

   salicylic acid (mg)

   menthol (mg)

   1% triamcinolone cream (g)

3. Prepare a solution containing:

hydrochlorothiazide 50 mg tablets	24
purified water	qs ad 120 mL

   What is the strength of the resulting solution in milligrams per milliliter?

4. Prepare a cream from the following formula:

hydrocortisone	600 mg
cream base	29.4 g

   What is the percent strength of the cream? (Round to a whole number.)

5. Calculate the amount needed to make 120 g of the following ointment:

coal tar	1 part
starch	5 parts
zinc oxide	3 parts
petrolatum	7 parts

   coal tar

   starch

   zinc oxide

   petrolatum

6. How much of the following ingredients are needed to prepare 44 g of the following:

   All-Purpose Nipple Ointment[2]

Stock*	Final Concentration
Bactroban (mupirocin) 2% Ointment	1%
betamethasone diproprionate	0.05%
miconazole	2%
Yellow color 2% solution	1 drop
Aquaphor Ointment	qs 44 g

   *If the stock strength is not listed, it is 100% as with betamethasone and miconazole.

   mupirocin

   betamethasone dipropionate *(Do not round.)*

   miconazole

Reducing and Enlarging Compounded Prescriptions

When an amount of a compounding formulation requires reducing or enlarging to meet a physician's order, the original amounts in the formulation are used to calculate the new formulation by ratio and proportion.

EXAMPLE 15.15

Decreasing the amount of product

Formulation: 3% ibuprofen gel

ibuprofen	3 g
base	97 g

Prepare 30 g

Ibuprofen:

$$\frac{3 \text{ g}}{100 \text{ g}} = \frac{x}{30 \text{ g}} \quad 100x = 90 \text{ g} \quad x = 0.9 \text{ g ibuprofen}$$

Base:

$$\frac{97 \text{ g}}{100 \text{ g}} = \frac{x}{30 \text{ g}} \quad 100x = 2{,}910 \text{ g} \quad x = 29.1 \text{ g base}$$

EXAMPLE 15.16

Increasing the amount of product

Formulation: 3% ibuprofen gel

ibuprofen	3 g
base	97 g

Prepare 120 g

Ibuprofen:

$$\frac{3\text{ g}}{100\text{ g}} = \frac{x}{120\text{ g}} \quad 100x = 360\text{ g} \quad x = 3.6\text{ g ibuprofen}$$

Base:

$$\frac{97\text{ g}}{100\text{ g}} = \frac{x}{120\text{ g}} \quad 100x = 11,640\text{ g} \quad x = 116.4\text{ g base}$$

TECH NOTE

The amounts calculated when reducing or increasing a formulation must add up to the new amount required.

EXAMPLE 15.17

The following recipe is for 10 mg/mL of drug A:

Drug A 100 mg	#10
Sterile water	18 mL
Cherry flavoring	3 mL
Simple syrup	qs as 100 mL

Prepare 4 oz.

First change 4 oz to 120 mL because compounding calculations are always performed in the metric system.

Set up a ratio and proportion: If 10 tablets are needed to make 100 mL, how many are needed to make 120 mL?

Drug A:

$$\frac{10\text{ tabs}}{100\text{ mL}} = \frac{x}{120\text{ mL}} \quad 100x = 1,200\text{ tabs} \quad x = 12\text{ tabs}$$

Follow the same process with the other ingredients.

Sterile water: (This will be used to dissolve the crushed tablets.)

$$\frac{18\text{ mL water}}{100\text{ mL}} = \frac{x}{120\text{ mL}} \quad 100x = 2,160\text{ mL water} \quad x = 21.6\text{ mL water}$$

Cherry flavoring:

$$\frac{5\text{ mL flavoring}}{100\text{ mL}} = \frac{x}{120\text{ mL}} \quad 100x = 600\text{ mL flavoring} \quad x = 6\text{ mL flavoring}$$

Simple syrup qs ad 120 mL

Practice Problems E

1. A prescription is written for a mouthwash:

tetracycline	800 mg
nystatin suspension	40 mL
diphenhydramine elixir	60 mL
qs ad dexamethasone elixir	240 mL

   How much of each ingredient is needed to prepare 90 mL?

   tetracycline (mg)

   nystatin suspension

   diphenhydramine elixir

   dexamethasone elixir

2. A prescription is received for a hydrocortisone enema to be prepared from the following formulation:

hydrocortisone	4.5 g
emulsifier	5 mL
methylcellulose 1%	240 mL
normal saline	qs ad 500 mL

   How much of each ingredient is needed to prepare 30 mL?

   hydrocortisone (mg)

   emulsifier

   methylcellulose 1%

   normal saline

3. How much of each of the following is needed to make 60 suppositories?

   Glycerin suppositories #20

glycerin	36 g
sodium stearate	3.6 g
water	1.8 g

   glycerin

   sodium stearate

   water

4. How much of each is needed to prepare 45 mL of mouthwash?

lidocaine 0.5%	1 part
diphenhydramine	1 part
Maalox	1 part

   Sig: $\overline{aa}$ qs 120 mL

   lidocaine

   diphenhydramine

   Maalox

REVIEW

Stock supplies in concentrated strengths are often used to prepare compounds that are less concentrated. To prepare the correct strength of medication for a physician's order or to administer a more accurate dose of medication, the stock medication may need dilution. Simple dilution involves adding more solvent to prepare a weaker product. This can be calculated using the following formulas: SV · SS = DV · DS or SW · SS = DW · DS. When two or more medications are combined, alligation is used. Alligation alternate can be used when combining two strengths of medications. However, if the "weighted average" percentage strength is necessary for mixture of two or more substances with a known quantity and concentration, alligation medial is used. As a pharmacy technician, you must know how to calculate the strength and must also know the correct method for calculation on the basis of the information given.

Although dilution and alligation calculations are frequently used in inpatient settings, compounding pharmacies may also use these calculations for filling outpatient prescription orders. The pharmacy personnel may need to formulate a prescription, interpret a compounding prescription, or increase or decrease the amount of a compounding prescription.

Posttest

Calculate the following problems using the appropriate method for each. Show your work. Round to tenths, unless otherwise indicated.

1. How many milliliters of 1:10 boric acid solution are needed to prepare 100 mL of a 5% solution?

2. An order is written for 1,500 mL of a 1:10 antiseptic solution. The stock solution is 1:5.

    How many milliliters of stock solution (solute) are needed? _____

    How many milliliters of solvent (diluent) are needed? _____

3. A lotion of 5% methyl salicylate is to be prepared for a patient with allergic dermatitis.

    What amount of a 10% methyl salicylate lotion is needed to prepare 240 mL?

Continued

Posttest, cont.

4. A lotion of 250 mL of 3% calamine lotion is to be prepared from a 7.5% calamine lotion.

   How many milliliters of stock solution (solute) are needed? _____

   How many milliliters of solvent are needed? _____

5. A stock pint of sodium bicarbonate contains 60% solution. The physician prescribes 1.5 L of 15% sodium bicarbonate solution. *Hint: Just because the stock is provided in a pint bottle does not mean the whole pint will be used.*

   How many milliliters of stock solution (solute) are needed? _____

   How many milliliters of solvent are needed? _____

6. A boric acid solution of 1:5 is available as a stock solution. A physician asks that you prepare 300 mL of 15% solution.

   How many milliliters of 1:5 strength boric acid are needed? _____

   How many milliliters of solvent (sterile water) are needed? _____

Posttest, cont.

7. A boric acid solution of 1:5 is available as a stock solution. A physician asks that you prepare 300 mL of 2% solution.

How many milliliters of 1:5 strength boric acid are needed? _____

How many milliliters of solvent (sterile water) are needed? _____

8. A liquid is available in a 1:350 concentration. Prepare a pint of 1:500 solution.

How many milliliters of stock solution (solute) are needed? _____

How many milliliters of solvent are needed? _____

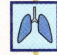
9. A physician orders 250 mL 0.05% epinephrine solution. The available epinephrine is 1:500 in 10-mL vials.

How many mL of 1:500 epinephrine are needed? _____

How many mL of sterile water are needed as a solvent? _____

How many vials of medication are needed to complete the order? _____

Continued

Posttest, cont.

10. A physician orders 250 mL of 15% dextrose in water. The stock solution is 50% dextrose in 10-mL ampules.

    How many milliliters of stock solution are needed? _____

    How many milliliters of sterile water are needed? _____

    How many ampules of dextrose are needed to complete the order? _____

11. A physician orders 4 oz of glycerin solution 7.5% to be used as a retention enema. The available stock glycerin solution is 25%.

    How many milliliters of stock solution are needed? _____

    How many milliliters of solvent are needed? _____

12. Prepare 250 mL of 3% hydrogen peroxide solution from 12% hydrogen peroxide solution.

    How many milliliters of stock solution (solute) are needed? _____

    How many milliliters of solvent are needed? _____

Posttest, cont.

 13. How many milliliters of 2.5% hydrogen peroxide solution can be prepared from 1 pint of 15% hydrogen peroxide stock solution?

14. On hand are 5% sodium hypochlorite solution and 20% sodium hypochlorite solution.

How many milliliters of each solution need to be combined to prepare 1 L of 12% sodium hypochlorite solution? *(Round to whole numbers and label your answers.)*

15. Prepare 500 mL of a 12.5% dextrose solution. Available are D5W and D50W. How many milliliters of each solution need to be combined to fill this order?

Continued

Posttest, cont.

 16. Prepare 1.5 L of 6% Lysol solution using 5% Lysol and 8% Lysol. How many milliliters of each solution need to be combined to fill this order? *Check your answers using alligation medial.*

17. How much of the following ingredients are needed to make 120 mL?

Bromhexine Hydrochloride 0.8-mg/mL Syrup[3]

bromhexine hydrochloride	80 mg
glycerin	20 mL
sodium benzoate	240 mg
fruit flavor	qs
tartaric acid	340 mg
Sorbitol 70% solution	45 mL
sodium carboxymethylcellulose	200 mg
purified water	qs 100 mL

bromhexine HCl

glycerin

sodium benzoate

Posttest, cont.

tartaric acid

70% Sorbital

sodium carboxymethylcellulose

purified water

What is the percentage of sorbital in the final preparation?

18. How much capsaicin (mg) is needed to prepare the following?
    capsaicin 0.05% clear Medication Stick[4] – #20 tubes

capsaicin	?
sodium stearate	7 g
alcohol	65 g
propylene glycol	25 g
cyclomethicone	3 g

REVIEW OF RULES

- Simple dilution: diluting one strength

    SV • SS = DV • DS

    SW • SS = DW • DS

- Alligation alternate: diluting one strength or combining two strengths

- Alligation medial: combining two or more strengths

REFERENCES

1. Int J Pharm Compd. 2010;14(6):482.
2. Int J Pharm Compd. 2010;14(6):485.
3. Int J Pharm Compd. 2010;14(6):516.
4. Int J Pharm Compd. 2010;14(6):517.

CHAPTER 16

Calculation of Medications Used Intravenously

OBJECTIVES

1. Define important terms such as *intravenous, continuous infusion, piggyback,* and *parenteral nutrition.*
2. Calculate intravenous infusion rates, and calculate the amount of medication a patient has received.
3. Calculate intravenous flow rates in drops per minute.
4. Calculate time needed to infuse an ordered volume of IV fluids.
5. Calculate parenteral nutrition formulations.

KEY WORDS

Additives Medications added to IVs, in particular to total parenteral nutrition (TPN) solutions and peripheral parenteral nutrition (PPN) solutions; electrolytes, multiple vitamins, trace elements, regular insulin, and other medications

Base solution Solution for a TPN or PPN that contains carbohydrates (dextrose), protein (amino acids), and sometimes lipids (fatty acids)

Continuous infusion Introduction of IV fluids without interruption of therapy

Conversion factor, time Factor needed to change from one unit of time to another such as hours to minutes; 1 hr = 60 min

Conversion factor, volume Factor needed to change from one unit of volume to another without changing the value, such as liters to milliliters; 1 L = 1,000 mL

Dose time Amount of time needed to administer the medication dose

Dose volume Volume of medication administered per dose

Drip rate Specific type of flow rate calculated in drops per minute; gtt/min

Drop factor Size of drop from the drip chamber; found on IV tubing (gtt/mL)

Flow rate Speed at which IV medications are infused into the body; aka **infusion rate**

Intravenous Into or within a vein (IV)

Macrodrip infusion sets Infusion sets used for measuring rate of IV fluids; macrodrip sets provide large drops of fluid called *macrodrops*

Microdrip infusion sets Infusion sets used for measuring rate of IV fluids; microdrip sets supply small drops called *microdrops*

Parenteral nutrition IV solution used to provide nutrition to a patient; aka **hyperalimentation**

Peripheral parenteral nutrition (PPN) IV containing a low concentration of amino acids, dextrose, electrolytes, and sometimes lipids, which is administered through a peripheral vessel

Piggyback A small-volume IV (50 to 250 mL) with added medication administered through an established IV line that is kept patent (open) by a continuous IV solution or by flushing

Total parenteral nutrition (TPN) IV containing a high concentration of amino acids, dextrose, and sometimes lipids with electrolytes and other medications, which is administered through a large central vessel

Copyright © 2019 by Elsevier, Inc. All rights reserved.

Pretest

If you are already comfortable with the subject matter, perform the following calculations to test your knowledge. If not, work your way through the chapter and return to them for extra practice. Round final answers to the nearest drop or nearest milliliter (if less than 1, round to the nearest tenth). When adding medication to fluids, the volume of medication(s) added should be included when calculating the total volume of fluids.

1. A physician orders a continuous infusion of 1,000 mL D5W with 20 mEq KCl q8h.

   How many milliliters will the patient receive per hour?

   How many milliequivalents of KCl will the patient receive each hour?

2. A physician orders 1 L of D5NS to be infused over 8 hours.

   What is the flow rate in milliliters per hour?

   How many milliliters per minute will the patient receive?

   Using a drop factor of 20 gtt/mL, how many drops per minute should be administered?

Pretest, cont.

3. A physician orders 3,000 mL lactated Ringer's solution to infuse over 16 hours. How many milliliters per hour should be administered?

   How many milliliters per minute should be administered?

   Using a drop factor of 10 gtt/mL, how many drops per minute should be administered?

4. A physician orders Ancef (cefazolin) 1 g in 100 mL D5W IVPB to be infused over 1 hour.
   If the tubing drop factor is 20 gtt/mL, how many drops per minute should the patient receive?

5. A 250 mL IV is to be administered over 45 minutes using a 20 gtt/mL infusion set. How many drops per minute should be administered?

Continued

Pretest, cont.

6. A physician orders 1,500 mL 0.45% NaCl IV over 24 hours. The drop factor on the infusion set is 20 gtt/mL.

   What is the weight in grams of sodium chloride in the total solution?

   How many milliliters of solution should be administered to the patient in 8 hours?

   How many drops per minute should the patient receive?

7. One liter of D10W is to be administered over 6 hours with a drop factor of 10 gtt/mL.

   What is the total number of drops in the solution using the given infusion set?

   What drip rate is needed?

8. A physician orders lactated Ringer's solution to be administered with a 20 gtt/min infusion set. Calculate the amount of fluid needed for 24 hours if administered at 2 mL/min.

Pretest, cont.

 9. A physician orders D5NS q24h with a flow rate of 50 mL/hr. How many milliliters will the patient receive in 1 day?

 10. What total amount of D5NS will be administered over 24 hours at 40 mL/hr? How many liter bags of fluids are needed for 24 hours?

How many drops per minute should be administered using tubing with a drop factor of 20 gtt/mL?

Continued

Pretest, cont.

11. How many grams of dextrose are in the fluid for the label shown?

How many minutes will it take to infuse at 2 mL/min?

How many drops per minute should be administered with a drop factor of 15 gtt/mL?

Lactated Ringer's and 5% Dextrose Injection USP
500 mL

Each 100 mL contains 5 g Dextrose Hydrous USP 600 mg Sodium Chloride USP 310 mg Sodium Lactate 30 mg Potassium Chloride USP 20 mg Calcium Chloride USP pH 5.0 (4.0 to 6.5) mEq/L Sodium 130 Potassium 4 Calcium 2.7 Chloride 109 Lactate 28 Hypertonic Osmolarity 525 mOsmol/L (calc) Sterile Nonpyrogenic Single dose container Not for use in the treatment of lactic acidosis

Courtesy of Baxter Healthcare Corporation. All rights reserved.

Pretest, cont.

12. One liter of D5NS is to infuse at 8 mL/min with a drop factor of 20 gtt/mL.

How minutes would it take to infuse?

How many drops per minute should the patient receive?

13. A physician orders Kefzol (cefazolin) 1 g IVPB in 100 mL D5W to infuse over 1 hour. The drop factor is 50 gtt/mL.

What is the rate in drops per minute?

How many milliliters will be infused within 30 minutes?

How many milligrams of Kefzol will be administered in 15 minutes?

Continued

Pretest, cont.

14. If 3 L of D10W are to infuse over a 24-hour period, what is the infusion rate in milliliters per hour?

    How many milliliters per minute will the patient receive?

    If the drop factor is 10 gtt/mL, how many drops per minute will the patient receive?

15. One liter of D5NS is infusing at the rate of 45 gtt/min. The drop factor is 15 gtt/mL.

    How many milliliters per hour will the patient receive?

16. A physician orders Pepcid (famotidine) 20 mg in 100 mL lactated Ringer's solution IVPB to infuse over 30 minutes q12h. The medication is available in 10 mg/mL vials.

    How many milliliters of famotidine should be added to each 100 mL PB?

    If the drop factor is 20 gtt/mL, how many drops per minute are infused?

Pretest, cont.

17. A physician orders amphotericin B 40 mg IV in 500 mL D5W infused over 12 hours. After reconstitution, the medication strength is 50 mg/10 mL.

How many milliliters of amphotericin B would be added to 500 mL of fluids?

How many milliliters should be administered per hour?

If the drop factor is 25 gtt/mL, how many drops per minute should be administered?

18. A physician orders ampicillin 2 g IVPB. After adding to 500 mL of D5 ½ NS, it will be administered over 2 hours using a drop factor of 10 gtt/mL.

ampicillin is available in 1-g vials to be reconstituted with 2.5 mL NS for a total of 3 mL. How many milliliters need to be added to the 500 mL IV?

How many milliliters per hour should be given to the patient?

How many drops per minute should be administered?

Continued

Pretest, cont.

19. Prepare a 3 L TPN solution containing 20% dextrose and 4.25% amino acids. How many milliliters of 50% dextrose injection are needed?

How many milliliters of 8.5% amino acids injection are needed?

How many milliliters of sterile water for injection are needed?

20. An order is received for the following to be added to a standard TPN solution containing 50% dextrose, 10% amino acids, and 20% lipids. Calculate the amount of each additive to be included in the final compounded TPN solution.

TOTAL PARENTERAL NUTRITION ADDITIVE ORDERS	ADDITIVE STOCK STRENGTHS
sodium chloride 15 mEq	50 mEq/20 mL vial
magnesium sulfate 16 mEq	40.6 mEq/10 mL vial
potassium chloride 8 mEq	40 mEq/20 mL vial
MVI 10 mL	10 mL two-chambered single-dose vial

sodium chloride

magnesium sulfate

potassium chloride

MVI

INTRODUCTION

Intravenous (IV) medications require precise measurements because the medication immediately enters the bloodstream with 100% bioavailability. Hospital pharmacy technicians usually prepare and deliver a 24-hour supply of intravenous solutions to nursing stations. Large-volume parenterals (LVPs) contain more than 250 mL of solution, whereas small-volume parenterals (SVPs) contain 250 mL or less. LVPs for continuous infusion, with or without added medications, may drip slowly into a vein either by gravity or through a pump. An IV infusion set includes tubing for carrying fluid from the container to the patient. Medications may be added to small volumes of fluids for administration on an intermittent basis either through an injection port in the tubing or a secondary line called an **IV piggyback** (IVPB). See Fig. 16.1. Most IVPBs are SVPs that are delivered over 30 to 60 minutes. The physician determines the type and volume of fluid, whether medications are added to the fluid, and the amount of time over which it should be administered.

Parenteral nutrition (PN) is delivery of a patient's nutritional needs via IV infusion. It is generally prescribed when a patient is unable to ingest and process nutrients orally. It can be used to maintain nutritional needs on a short- or long-term basis. Standardized parenteral solutions are available, but they can also be customized to meet individualized

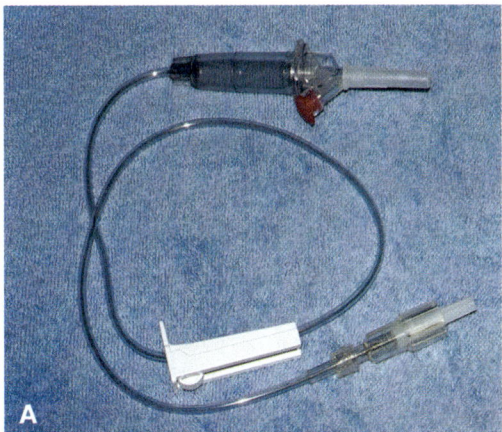
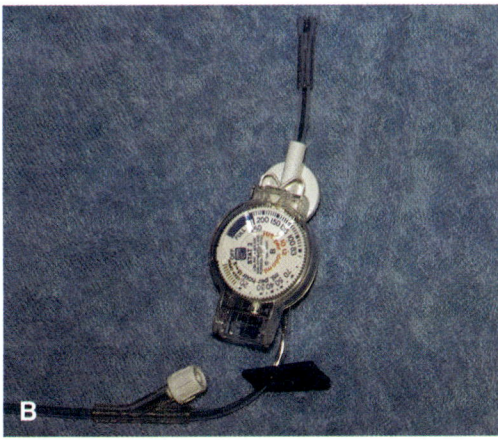
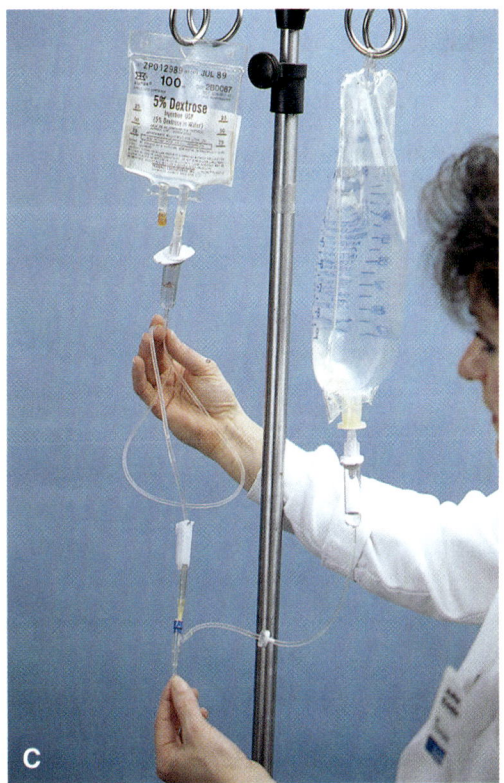

FIGURE 16.1 **A,** Primary infusion set showing drip chamber, tubing, and roller clamp. **B,** Primary infusion set for IVPB additions. **C,** IVPB being added to a primary line. (*A* and *B*, From Brown M, Mulholland JM: *Drug calculations: process and problems for clinical practice,* ed 8, St. Louis, MO, Mosby, 2008. C, From Potter P, Perry A: *Fundamentals of nursing,* ed 8, St. Louis, MO, Mosby, 2013.)

nutritional requirements. Because of the regulations that surround the compounding of parenteral solutions, many pharmacies and hospitals contract out their parenteral nutrition orders to compounding companies that specialize in this area. Familiarization with the basic calculations necessary to fill such an order is still important.

CALCULATING INTRAVENOUS INFUSION RATES

A rate is a value per unit of time. An **infusion** or **flow rate** refers to the amount of IV fluid entering the body over a specific amount of time. It may be expressed in terms of milliliters per minute, milliliters per hour, an amount of drug (mcg, mg, g, units, or mEq) per minute or hour, or drops per minute. The reason for therapy dictates the type of fluid and rate of infusion ordered. Fluids given to keep a vein open (KVO) are given slowly, whereas replacement fluids are given at a rate that will provide the necessary fluids while preventing an overload on the vascular system. The pharmacy technician must be able to calculate how long a particular volume of fluid will run in order to calculate how much longer a currently hanging intravenous solution will last and when the next IV is due. This ultimately will determine the amount of IV solution to be prepared for a 24-hour period. Calculations with IV infusion rates can be used to determine the following:

1. The amount of medication delivered (mg, g, mEq, or units) over a specific period of time
2. The volume of medication delivered (gtt, mL, or L) over a specific period of time – **dose volume**
3. The volume of medication needed to last a specific amount of time
4. The length of time a medication dose will last – **dose time**

Each of these problems can be solved using dimensional analysis (DA) or ratio and proportion (R&P). The following examples are shown using the simplest method for solving each one.

EXAMPLE 16.1

How much fluid will a patient receive in 5 hours at an infusion rate of 125 mL/hr?

$$\frac{125 \text{ mL}}{1 \text{ hr}} = \frac{x}{5 \text{ hr}} \quad x = 625 \text{ mL}$$

What is the infusion rate in milliliters per hour of a 1,000-mL IV to run over 8 hours?

This can be thought of as simply reducing the fraction $\frac{1,000 \text{ mL}}{8 \text{ hr}}$ to 125 mL/hr

What is the infusion rate in milliliters per minute of a 1,500-mL IV to run over 12 hours?

$$\frac{\text{mL}}{\text{min}} = \frac{1,500 \text{ mL}}{12 \text{ hr}} \cdot \frac{1 \text{ hr}}{60 \text{ min}} = 2 \text{ mL/min}$$

How long would a 1,000-mL IV last at 50 mL/hr?

$$\frac{50 \text{ mL}}{1 \text{ hr}} = \frac{1,000 \text{ mL}}{x} \quad x = 20 \text{ hr}$$

Rates can also be presented as amount of medication delivered per hour or minute.

EXAMPLE 16.2

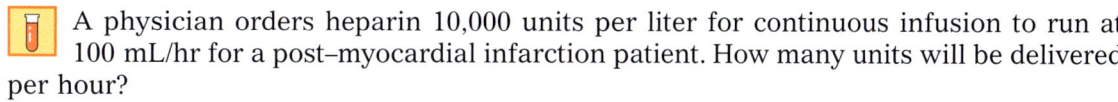 A physician orders heparin 10,000 units per liter for continuous infusion to run at 100 mL/hr for a post–myocardial infarction patient. How many units will be delivered per hour?

$$\frac{\text{units}}{\text{hr}} = \frac{10{,}000 \text{ units}}{1 \text{ L}} \cdot \frac{1 \text{ L}}{1{,}000 \text{ mL}} \cdot \frac{100 \text{ mL}}{\text{hr}}$$

$$= \frac{1{,}000 \text{ units}}{\text{mL}} = 1{,}000 \text{ units/mL}$$

One more step is needed to get to units per minute.

$$\frac{\text{units}}{\text{min}} = \frac{10{,}000 \text{ units}}{1 \text{ L}} \cdot \frac{1 \text{ L}}{1{,}000 \text{ mL}} \cdot \frac{100 \text{ mL}}{\text{hr}} \cdot \frac{1 \text{ hr}}{60 \text{ min}}$$

$$= 16.7 \text{ units/min}$$

This would be rounded to 17 units per minute.

Practice Problems A

Answer the following questions based on the previous examples. Show your work.

1. What is the infusion rate of 1 L (1,000 mL) D5W given over 10 hours?

2. What is the infusion rate of 500 mL of NS administered over 10 hours?

3. How many milliliters of fluid will a patient receive in 3 hours if the infusion rate is 125 mL/hr?

4. How much fluid will a patient receive in 10 hours if the order is for 50 mL/hr?

5. How long will 500 mL of D5NS last at an infusion rate of 25 mL/hr?

6. How long will a 50 mL piggyback last if the infusion rate is 100 mL/hr?

7. A physician orders an IV of 40 mEq of potassium chloride in 1,000 mL NS to run at 125 mL/hr. How many milliequivalents will be delivered per hour?

8. A 1,000 mL solution of NS is to run over 24 hours. How many milliliters are delivered per minute?

TECH NOTE
A large-volume IV bag can hang for a maximum of 24 hours before it must be changed, according to the USP.

CALCULATIONS OF AMOUNTS OF MEDICATION

Calculations can also be made to determine how much medication a patient has received at a particular point in their therapy in case the IV is discontinued or infiltrates and must be stopped before it is completely finished.

EXAMPLE 16.3

A 1 L IV of D5W contains 80 mEq of potassium chloride. The IV was discontinued after 650 mL of the fluid infused. How many milliequivalents of KCl did the patient receive?

(If there are 80 mEq of KCl in 1,000 mL, how many milliequivalents of KCl are in 650 mL?)

$$\frac{80 \text{ mEq KCl}}{1{,}000 \text{ mL}} = \frac{x}{650 \text{ mL}} \quad 1{,}000x = 52{,}000 \text{ mEq}$$

$$x = 52 \text{ mEq}$$

Practice Problems B

Calculate the amounts of medication received. Round to tenths if necessary. Show your work.

1. A 200 mL IV contains furosemide 100 mg. The patient received 150 mL. What amount of furosemide did the patient receive?

2. An IV contains Sublimaze (fentanyl) 50 mcg in D5W 500 mL. The patient only received 400 mL.

   How many grams of dextrose did the patient receive?

   How many milligrams of fentanyl did the patient receive? *(Do not round.)*

3. A physician orders 1 L of 3% dextrose to be administered over 6 hours.

   If the complete bag of fluids is administered, how many grams of dextrose will the patient receive?

   If the fluids run for 5 hours only and the patient is discharged, how many grams of dextrose did the patient receive?

4. A physician writes a medication order for lidocaine 150 mg to be added to 200 mL of D5W. The available strength of medication to add is 1% lidocaine for injection. How many mL of lidocaine 1% should be added to the 200 mL of D5W?

How many milligrams of lidocaine are in each milliliter of fluid? Hint: Use the total volume after adding the lidocaine to determine this answer.

If the patient receives only 65 mL of the IV fluids, how many milligrams of LIDOCAINE will the patient receive?

5. A 50-mL container of NS contains penicillin 1.5 million units (1,500,000 units) to be infused over 30 minutes.

If the patient receives the medication for 25 minutes, how many units of penicillin are delivered?

6. A physician orders aminophylline as a loading dose of 5 mg/kg to be administered IVPB over 1 hour for a patient who weighs 154 lb. The available medication is aminophylline 250 mg/10 mL.

How many milligrams of medication will the patient receive?

How many milligrams of medication will the patient receive per hour if the IVPB is to be infused over 2 hours?

7. A physician orders Pitocin (oxytocin) 2 units in 1 L of D5W.

   How many units are in 100 mL of the solution?

   What is the dose of Pitocin if the patient only receives 750 mL of the IV fluids?

8. A physician orders magnesium sulfate 10 g added to 1 L of LR. The available strength is 50% magnesium sulfate solution for injection.

   What is the concentration of 50% magnesium sulfate in milligrams per milliliter?

   How much magnesium sulfate solution should be added to the LR solution?

   If this is infused over 5 hours, how many milligrams of magnesium sulfate will the patient receive per hour?

CALCULATING INTRAVENOUS FLOW RATES IN DROPS PER MINUTE

A **drip rate** (DR), sometimes called a **drop rate**, represents the number of drops (gtt) administered over a specific time via IV infusion. It is a specific type of infusion or flow rate, measured in drops per minute. The calculation of drip rate is affected by the size of the tubing used to deliver the medication. A **drop factor** (gtt/mL) is found on each tubing package. Various drop factors are available: 10, 15, and 20 gtt/mL are **macrodrip tubing sets**, whereas 60 gtt/mL is considered a **microdrip tubing set** because the drops are much smaller (think of 60 drops being 1 mL) (Fig. 16.2).

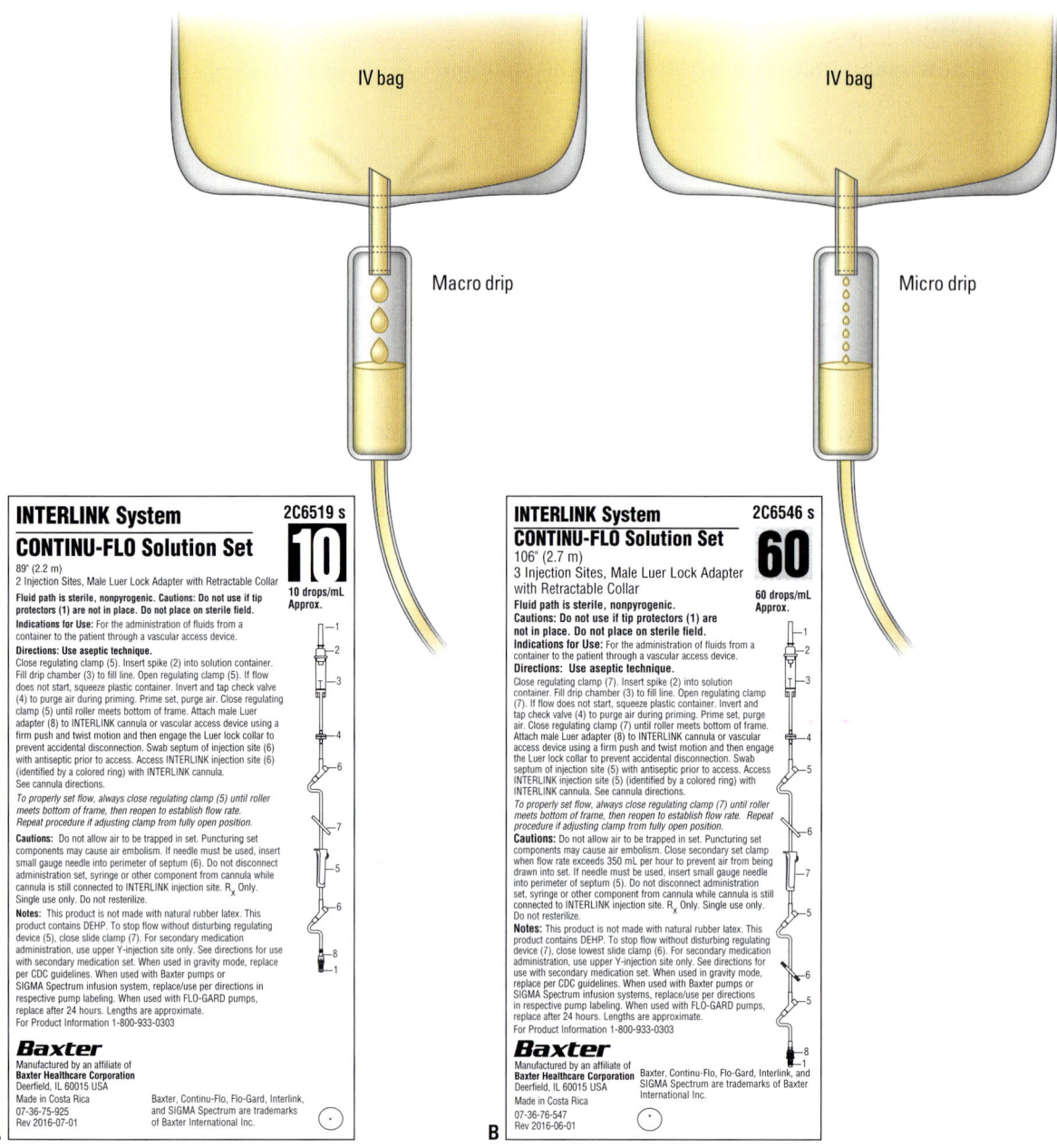

FIGURE 16.2 Infusion sets for administration of IV fluids. **A,** Macrodrip set shows 10 gtt/mL. (Labels courtesy of Baxter Healthcare Corporation. All rights reserved.)

> **! TECH ALERT**
>
> The number of drops per milliliter for the infusion set is found on the tubing box. Tubing is not interchangeable! This information is essential for proper fluid administration time and calculation of IV flow rates.

The rate of infusion for IV fluids must be calculated to complete the physician's order, which provides the type and amount of fluids and usually a desired infusion rate or infusion time. The proper infusion set must be chosen to supply the fluids as ordered. Therefore the four factors to be considered with administration are as follows:

- The total amount of fluids to be administered in *milliliters (mL)*
- The calibration of the administration (infusion) set in *drops per milliliter (gtt/mL)*
- The flow rate of the fluids in *drops per minute (gtt/min)*
- The time for the fluids to infuse in *minutes (min)*

Calculating flow rates for IV fluids is accomplished most easily by using DA. You do not need to learn a specific formula as long as you follow the rules for DA to achieve your desired answer. *Always* round drip rates measured in drops per milliliter to the nearest whole number.

EXAMPLE 16.4

 A physician orders Pepcid (famotidine) 20 mg in a total of 50 mL NS to run over 25 minutes. Calculate the drops per minute if the drop factor is 20 gtt/mL.

First, start with the units of your desired answer followed by an equal sign:

$$\frac{gtt}{min} =$$

Next, place the information containing the desired unit of the numerator in the numerator position of the first fraction:

$$\frac{gtt}{min} = \frac{20\ gtt}{mL}.$$

Then place the information containing the unit you want to cancel with the first denominator in the numerator position of the next fraction:

$$\frac{gtt}{min} = \frac{20\ gtt}{mL} \cdot \frac{50\ mL}{25\ min}$$

Continue this process until you only have the units of the desired answer left. In this example, the desired unit is drops per minute, so the only step left is to solve the equation.

$$\frac{gtt}{min} = \frac{20\ gtt}{mL} \cdot \frac{50\ mL}{25\ min} = \frac{40\ gtt}{min}$$

This same pattern can be repeated for any infusion or drip rate problem. Sometimes these calculations will require the use of the **conversion factor for volume,** 1 L = 1,000 mL and/or **the conversion factor for time,** 1 hr = 60 min.

EXAMPLE 16.5

A physician orders 3 L of D5W to run over 24 hours. If the drop factor is 20 gtt/mL, what is the drip rate?

$$\frac{gtt}{min} = \frac{20\ gtt}{mL} \cdot \frac{1{,}000\ mL}{1\ L} \cdot \frac{3\ L}{24\ hr} \cdot \frac{1\ hr}{60\ min}$$
$$= 41.6 = 42\ gtt/min$$

TECH NOTE
Remember that with DA, you are completing the entire problem in one step.

Practice Problems C

Calculate the flow rate in drops per minute. Round answers for medication weight/volume to the nearest tenth and for drops per minute to the nearest whole number.

1. A physician orders 2 L of lactated Ringer's solution over 12 hours. The drop factor is 20 gtt/mL.

   How many drops per minute should be infused?

2. A physician orders D5W 100 mL IV over 2 hours. The drop factor is 50 gtt/mL.

   How many drops per minute should be infused?

3. A physician orders 250 mL D5NS to be administered over 16 hours to keep a vein open. The drop factor is 60 gtt/mL.

   How many drops per minute should be administered?

   How many milliliters will be administered per hour?

4. A physician orders 1,000 mL D5NS to be administered over 12 hours. The drop factor is 10 gtt/mL.

   How many drops per minute should be infused?

5. A physician orders 150 mL of D5NS to be infused over 40 minutes. The drop factor is 15 gtt/mL.

   How many drops per minute should be infused?

6. A physician orders a piggyback infusion of ampicillin 250 mg in 75 mL of NS to infuse over 1 hour using an infusion set labeled 50 gtt/mL.

   How many drops per minute will be infused?

   What weight (in mg) of ampicillin will be infused in 45 minutes?

7. A physician orders oxytocin 10 units in 500 mL of NS to be infused over 30 minutes. The drop factor is 20 gtt/mL.

   How many drops per minute should be infused?

8. A physician orders Zantac (ranitidine) 50 mg in 100 mL NS to infuse over 15 minutes. The drop factor is 15 gtt/mL.

   How many drops per minute should be infused?

   How many milligrams of Zantac will the patient receive in 12 minutes?

9. **ENDO** A physician orders Solu-Medrol (methylprednisolone sodium succinate) 500 mg in 150 mL NS to infuse over 2 hours. The drop factor is 20 gtt/mL.

   How many drops per minute should be infused?

   How many milligrams of methylprednisolone sodium succinate will be administered to the patient in 1 hour and 15 minutes?

10. A physician orders nafcillin 1 g to be added to 100 mL D5W to run over 1 hour. The drop factor is 15 gtt/mL.

    How many drops per minute should be infused?

11. **ENDO** A physician orders Novolin R 60 units to infuse in 500 mL NS over 4½ hours. The drop factor is 15 gtt/mL.

    How many drops per minute will be infused?

    How many units of regular insulin will infuse in 1 hour?

12. A physician orders tobramycin 1 mg/kg in LR 50 mL IVPB to run for 50 minutes. The patient weighs 178 lb. The drop factor is 10 gtt/mL.

    What dose (in mg) of tobramycin should be prepared for the infusion?

    How many drops per minute should be set for the infusion to meet the physician's order?

    How many milligrams of tobramycin will be infused in 45 minutes?

13. A physician orders Premarin (conjugated estrogens) 25 mg in 50 mL D5W to run over 15 minutes. The drop factor is 15 gtt/mL.

    How many drops per minute should be infused?

    How many milligrams of estrogens will be infused in 6 minutes?

14. A physician orders 2,000 mL of ½ NS to run for 16 hours. The drop factor is 50 gtt/mL.

    How many drops per minute should be infused?

    How many total grams of NaCl will the patient receive?

15. A physician orders Garamycin (gentamicin) 0.02 g in 50 mL NS for infusion over 45 minutes. The drop factor is 20 gtt/mL.

    How many drops per minute should be infused?

    How many milligrams of gentamicin would be added to the fluids?

CALCULATING INTRAVENOUS INFUSION TIMES

In some instances the physician will provide an order for the amount of fluids to be infused and the milliliters per hour without providing the specific infusion time. The problem then becomes a question of how long it will take for each volume of fluid to be infused using the rate ordered by the physician. As the pharmacy technician, you have a responsibility to ensure that fluids are available for the next dose as ordered. Therefore when the time is not designated but the amount is designated, the necessary calculation may include deciding how long the ordered fluids will take to infuse when the infusion rate and/or drop factor is provided.

EXAMPLE 16.6

 A physician orders LR in 250 mL to be infused at 50 gtt/min with an infusion set of 10 gtt/mL.

What will be the infusion time in minutes?

$$\text{min} = \frac{1 \text{ min}}{50 \text{ gtt}} \cdot \frac{10 \text{ gtt}}{\text{mL}} \cdot \frac{250 \text{ mL}}{1} = 50 \text{ min}$$

EXAMPLE 16.7

 A physician orders 2,500 mL of D5NS to infuse at 30 gtt/min with an infusion set of 10 gtt/mL.

How many minutes will it take for these fluids to infuse?

$$\text{min} = \frac{1 \text{ min}}{30 \text{ gtt}} \cdot \frac{10 \text{ gtt}}{\text{mL}} \cdot \frac{2,500 \text{ mL}}{1} = 833 \text{ min}$$

What is the infusion time in hours and minutes?

$$\text{hr} = \frac{1 \text{ hr}}{60 \text{ min}} \cdot \frac{1 \text{ min}}{30 \text{ gtt}} \cdot \frac{10 \text{ gtt}}{\text{mL}} \cdot \frac{2,500 \text{ mL}}{1} = 13.9 \text{ hr}$$

Because there are 60 minutes in 1 hour, multiply 0.9×60 to change to minutes.

$$\text{min} = \frac{60 \text{ min}}{1 \text{ hr}} \cdot \frac{0.9 \text{ hr}}{1} = 54 \text{ min}$$

The answer is 13 hours and 54 minutes.

EXAMPLE 16.8

 A physician orders amphotericin B 40 mg IVPB to be administered in D5W 250 mL to be infused at a rate of 20 gtt/min with a drop factor of 60 gtt/mL.

How many milliliters should be added to the fluids if the amphotericin B is reconstituted to 50 mg/10 mL?

$$\frac{50 \text{ mg}}{10 \text{ mL}} = \frac{40 \text{ mg}}{x} \quad 50x = 400 \text{ mL} \quad x = 8 \text{ mL}$$

What is the total volume to be infused?   250 mL + 8 mL = 258 mL

How many minutes will the IV take to infuse?

$$\text{min} = \frac{1 \text{ min}}{20 \text{ gtt}} \cdot \frac{60 \text{ gtt}}{\text{mL}} \cdot \frac{258 \text{ mL}}{1} = 774 \text{ min}$$

EXAMPLE 16.9

 A physician orders a piggyback of Vancocin (vancomycin) 1 g in 100 mL D5W. The drop factor is 20 gtt/mL and the infusion rate is 1.5 mL/min.

After reconstitution to 500 mg/10 mL, how many milliliters of Vancocin solution must be added to the 100-mL piggyback fluid?

$$mL = \frac{10\ mL}{500\ mg} \cdot \frac{1{,}000\ mg}{1\ g} \cdot \frac{1\ g}{1} = 20\ mL$$

What is the total volume to be infused?   100 mL + 20 mL = 120 mL

How many minutes will it take for the Vancocin order to infuse?

$$min = \frac{1\ min}{1.5\ mL} \cdot \frac{120\ mL}{1} = 80\ min$$

How many drops per minute would be infused?

$$\frac{gtt}{min} = \frac{20\ gtt}{mL} \cdot \frac{120\ mL}{80\ min} = 30\ gtt/min$$

TECH NOTE
When using DA, always start with the unit of the answer desired followed by an equal sign.

Practice Problems D

Complete the following problems. Round all answers to whole numbers. Show your work.

1. A physician orders 500 mL D5NS to be infused at 15 gtt/min. The drop factor is 10 gtt/mL.

   How many minutes will it take to infuse?

2. A physician orders Amikin (amikacin) 1 g in 100 mL D5W to infuse at 25 gtt/min using an infusion set delivering 60 gtt/mL.

   What is the running time for the infusion in minutes?

   What is the running time for the infusion in hours?

   If the drug has a recommended infusion time of at least 1 hour, is this order safe? _____

   How many milligrams of Amikin will the patient receive in 10 minutes?

3. A physician orders 2 L of D5W to be infused at 25 gtt/min. The drop factor is 10 gtt/mL.

   How many minutes will the infusion last?

4. A physician orders gentamicin 1.5 mg/kg/dose to be given q8h IVPB in 150 mL NS for a patient who weighs 148 lb. The infusion rate is 25 gtt/min. The drop factor is 20 gtt/mL.

   How many milligrams of gentamicin should the patient receive per dose?

   How long will it take for this medication to be infused in hours?

   How many milligrams will the patient receive in 45 minutes?

5. A physician orders 500 mL of D5 ½ NS to be administered at 30 gtt/min with a drop factor of 60 gtt/mL.

   How long will this infusion last in hours and minutes?

6. A patient is to receive 1.5 L of D5 ½ NS at the rate of 100 gtt/min using an administration set with a drop factor of 10 gtt/mL.

   How long will it take for these fluids to infuse in minutes?

   How long will it take in hours and minutes?

7. A physician orders ampicillin 250 mg in 50 mL NS IVPB to be infused at 30 gtt/min. The drop factor is 10 gtt/mL.

   If the volume of medication added to NS is 8 mL, how long will it take for the entire piggyback to infuse in minutes?

8. A physician orders aminophylline 750 mg to be added to a 100-mL piggyback of fluids for a patient with severe asthma. The medication is available as aminophylline 500 mg/25 mL. The drop factor is 60 gtt/mL, and the rate of infusion is 10 gtt/min.

   What volume of medication should be added to the IVPB?

   How long in minutes will it take for the entire bag of fluids to infuse?

   How long is this in hours and minutes?

9. A physician orders erythromycin 200 mg in 250 mL D5W. The medication is available as 400 mg/5 mL after reconstitution. The drop factor is 30 gtt/mL, and the rate of infusion is 20 gtt/min.

   How many milliliters of erythromycin should be added to the bag of fluids?

   How many minutes will it take for the piggyback to infuse?

10. A physician orders 1,000 mL LR with 20 mEq KCl. The drop factor is 10 gtt/mL. The infusion rate is 20 gtt/min.

    How long will it take for this order to infuse in minutes?

    How long will it take in hours and minutes?

11. A physician orders heparin sodium 3,500 units from the following vial to be added to 100 mL of NS for IV infusion. The drop factor is 60 gtt/mL, and the infusion rate is 20 gtt/min.

    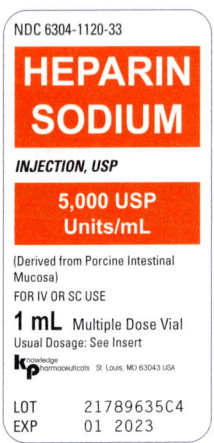

    How many milliliters of heparin should be added to the fluids?

    How many minutes will it take for these fluids to infuse?

12. A physician orders 150 mL D5W. The drop factor is 60 gtt/mL, and the infusion rate is 0.5 mL/min.

    How long in hours will it take for the fluids to be infused?

    How many drops per minute will be infused?

CALCULATIONS WITH PARENTERAL NUTRITION

Traditional 2-in-1 parenteral nutrition (PN) supplementation includes **base solutions** of two essential macronutrients, dextrose (carbohydrates) and amino acids (protein), along with electrolytes, vitamins, trace elements, and water. A stable IV lipid (fat) emulsion, IVFE, is included in some formulations, resulting in what is called a 3-in-1 formulation, which includes three macronutrients: carbohydrates, protein, and fats. In addition, parenteral nutrition solutions can contain medications such as regular insulin and others as needed and indicated given the patient's clinical situation.

Parenteral nutrition can be administered via either central or peripheral lines, with central lines often placed in the superior vena cava and peripheral lines inserted into the veins of the arm or hand. **Peripheral parental nutrition** (PPN) must be *lower* in strength than **total parenteral nutrition** (TPN). TPN is administered through larger central lines where the solution is diluted in the bloodstream quickly. Peripheral vessels are smaller so the solution is not diluted in the bloodstream as quickly. Chronic parenteral nutrition can even be administered and managed by patients in the ambulatory setting.

Parenteral Nutrition Calculations

Two types of calculations are used to determine the contents of a parenteral nutrition solution. The first involves determination of the amount of base solutions: dextrose, amino acids, and lipids. The second involves calculation of the amount of additives, such as electrolytes and medications, to be included. When calculating the amount of stock solutions to use to obtain the appropriate strength of base solution ordered, the dilution equation, $SV \cdot SS = DV \cdot DS$, may be used.

EXAMPLE 16.10

A medication order calls for 1 L of TPN solution containing 2.125% amino acids and 25% dextrose. In stock are 8.5% amino acids, 50% dextrose, and sterile water for injection.

Calculate the volumes of 8.5% amino acids injection and 50% dextrose injection needed to prepare the desired concentration of each ingredient, then qs with sterile water for injection to 1,000 mL.

The final 1,000 mL solution is to contain 2.125% amino acids. The stock solution is 8.5%.

$SV \cdot SS = DV \cdot DS$

$SV \cdot 8.5\% = 1,000 \text{ mL} \cdot 2.125\%$

$SV \cdot 8.5 = 2,125 \text{ mL}$

$SV = 250 \text{ mL of } 8.5\%$ amino acids needed

The final 1,000 mL solution is to contain 25% dextrose. The stock solution is 50%.

SV · SS = DV · DS

SV · 50% = 1,000 mL · 25%

SV · 50 = 25,000 mL

SV = 500 mL of 50% dextrose needed

To calculate the volume of sterile water for injection needed to bring the solution to a final volume of 1 L, subtract the volumes calculated above from the final volume desired:

1,000 mL (1 L) − 250 mL − 500 mL
= 250 mL of sterile water for injection needed

> **TECH NOTE**
> If electrolytes and other medications are added before bringing the volume up to the total desired, their total volume will also be subtracted before determining the amount of sterile water needed.

EXAMPLE 16.11

An order calls for the following to be added to a standard 1 L TPN solution that contains 50% dextrose, 10% amino acids, and 20% fat. Calculate the amount of each additive needed.

TPN ADDITIVE ORDERS	ADDITIVE STOCK STRENGTHS
sodium chloride 30 mEq	50 mEq/20 mL vial
potassium acetate 15 mEq	40 mEq/20 mL vial
potassium chloride 25 mEq	30 mEq/15 mL vial
calcium gluconate 9.4 mEq	4.7 mEq/10 mL vial
regular insulin 10 units	U-100 (1,000 units/10 mL vial)

Calculate each additive individually to determine the amount to be added to the 1 L solution.

Sodium chloride: When the stock strength is presented as the entire vial, it can be reduced before making calculations, so 50 mEq/20 mL can be reduced to 5 mEq/2 mL.

$$\frac{5 \text{ mEq}}{2 \text{ ml}} = \frac{30 \text{ mEq}}{x}$$

Cross multiply and divide. $5x = 60$ mL $x = 12$ mL

Potassium acetate: 40 mEq/20 mL can be reduced to 2 mEq/mL.

$$\frac{2 \text{ mEq}}{1 \text{ mL}} = \frac{15 \text{ mEq}}{x}$$ $2x = 15$ mL $x = 7.5$ mL

Potassium chloride: 30 mEq/15 mL can be reduced to 2 mEq/mL.

$$\frac{2 \text{ mEq}}{1 \text{ mL}} = \frac{25 \text{ mEq}}{x}$$ $2x = 25$ mL $x = 12.5$ mL

Calcium gluconate:

$$\frac{4.7 \text{ mEq}}{10 \text{ mL}} = \frac{9.4 \text{ mEq}}{x} \quad 4.7x = 94 \text{ mL} \quad x = 20 \text{ mL}$$

Regular insulin:

$$\frac{100 \text{ units}}{1 \text{ mL}} = \frac{10 \text{ units}}{x} \quad 100x = 10 \quad x = 0.1 \text{ mL}$$

What is the total amount of additives? 12 mL + 7.5 mL + 12.5 mL + 20 mL + 0.1 mL = 52.1 mL

If the TPN is hung at 0800 and is to run at 75 mL/hr, when will the next bag be due?

$$\frac{75 \text{ mL}}{1 \text{ hr}} = \frac{1{,}052.1 \text{ mL}}{x} \quad 75x = 1{,}052.1 \text{ hr} \quad x = 14 \text{ hr}$$

14 hours after 0800 is 2200.

Practice Problems E

Perform the following PN calculations showing all of your work.

1. A physician writes an order for a 1 L TPN containing 4.25% amino acids and 20% dextrose. Available stock is 8.5% amino acids injection, 50% dextrose injection, and sterile water for injection.

   How many milliliters of 8.5% amino acids injection are needed?

   How many milliliters of 50% dextrose injection are needed?

   How many milliliters of sterile water for injection are needed to reach the desired volume?

2. Prepare a 1.5 L TPN solution containing 2.125% amino acids, 10% dextrose, and 3% lipids.

   How many milliliters of 8.5% amino acids injection are needed?

   How many milliliters of 50% dextrose injection are needed?

   How many milliliters of 20% lipids are needed?

   How many milliliters of sterile water for injection are needed to reach the desired volume of 1.5 L?

3. An order is received for the following to be added to a standard TPN solution containing 10% amino acids, 50% dextrose, and 20% fat.

TPN ADDITIVE ORDERS	ADDITIVE STOCK STRENGTHS
sodium chloride 25 mEq	50 mEq/20 mL vial
potassium acetate 15 mEq	40 mEq/20 mL vial
calcium gluconate 4.7 mEq	4.7 mEq/10 mL vial
MVI-12 (multivitamin injection) 10 mL	10 mL (two-chambered single-dose vial)
regular insulin 25 units	U-100 vial

Calculate the amount of each additive to be included in the TPN solution.

Sodium chloride:

Potassium acetate:

Calcium gluconate:

MVI-12:

Regular insulin:

What is the total of all of the additives?

4. Perform the following TPN calculations for each of the additives and the base solutions.

TPN ADDITIVES	ADDITIVE STOCK STRENGTHS AVAILABLE	
potassium chloride	2 mEq/ mL	
sodium chloride	14.6%	2.5 mEq/ mL
calcium gluconate	10%	4.65 mEq/10 mL
magnesium sulfate	50%	40.6 mEq/10 mL
sodium acetate	2 mEq/mL	
sodium phosphate	45 mM/15 mL	60 mEq/15 mL
potassium acetate	19.6%	2 mEq/mL
potassium phosphate	15 mM/5 mL	4.4 mEq/mL
Humulin R insulin	100 units/mL	
vitamin C	250 mg/2 mL	
folic acid	5 mg/mL	

Notice that some strengths are listed in two different ways. Use the one that is in the order. Remember that 50% magnesium sulfate means 50 g/100 mL.

Calculate the following amounts needed for each additive. Show all work.

Potassium chloride 15 mEq

Sodium chloride 10 mEq

Magnesium sulfate 250 mg

Sodium acetate 4 mEq

Sodium phosphate 20 mEq

Humulin R insulin 50 units

Vitamin C 500 mg

Folic acid 10 mg

Trace elements   5 mL

MVI-12   5 mL

What is the total amount of all of the additives?

Base Solutions

Travesol (amino acids) 7.5%   400 mL
Dextrose 50%   400 mL
Sterile water for injection   qs ad 1,000 mL

What is the final concentration of Travesol (amino acids)

What is the final concentration of dextrose?

How much sterile water for injection is needed to reach 1,000 mL? *Be sure to account for the total amount of additives.*

How many grams of amino acids are in this TPN?

How many g of dextrose are in this TPN?

If it is hung at 0600 and run at 75 mL/hr, when will the next bag be due?

REVIEW

The pharmacy is responsible for providing the medications and fluids to fill physicians' medication orders. In addition, the pharmacy is responsible for ensuring that adequate amounts of fluids are provided for the desired length of therapy. Furthermore, you may be asked to calculate the amount of time that a container of fluids will last, the necessary volume of fluids, or the rate of infusion per minute or hour to provide the medication as ordered. Patient safety is ensured when the correct fluids ordered by the physician are calculated for the correct infusion rate. Because of the immediate action of medications administered through an IV route, the pharmacy must take extreme care with these calculations. As the pharmacy technician, you must be sure the correct fluids are chosen, along with the correct medications. Rechecking calculations always enhances patient safety.

Posttest

Calculate the following using the method most comfortable for you. Use total volume after addition of additives for calculations. Round to the nearest whole number for minutes and drip rates. Show your calculations.

1. A physician orders furosemide 60 mg in 500 mL of D5W. The drop factor is 20 gtt/mL, and the drop rate is 60 gtt/min. Use the following label for your calculations.

   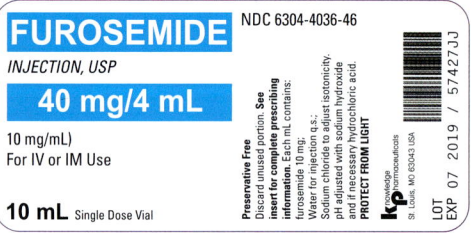

   How much furosemide should be added to the fluids?

   How long in minutes will the fluids take to infuse?

Posttest, cont.

 2. A physician orders Humulin R 60 units added to NS 100 mL as an IVPB. The drop factor is 60 gtt/mL. The physician wants the insulin to infuse at 2.5 units/hr. Use the following label for your calculations.

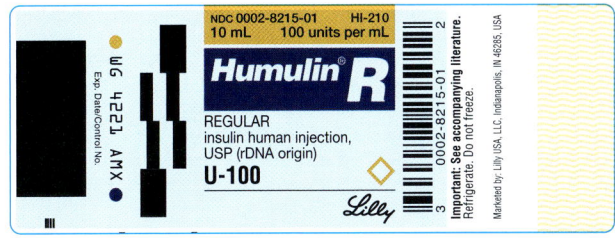

© Eli Lilly and Company. All Rights Reserved. Used with Permission.

How many milliliters of insulin should be added to the fluids?

How many milliliters per hour will be infused?

How long will the fluids take to infuse?

Continued

Posttest, cont.

3. A physician orders ampicillin sodium 1 g to be added to lactated ringer's solution 100 mL. The drop factor is 60 gtt/mL. The medication must be given over a 2-hour time period. Use the directions on the following label for reconstitution with 1.8 mL of diluent.

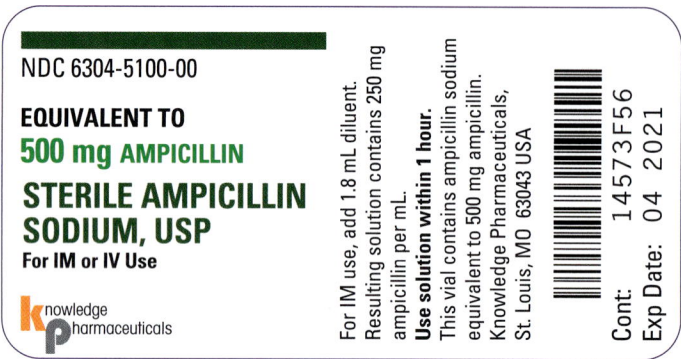

How many milliliters of ampicillin should be added to the fluids?

What is the flow rate in milliliters per minute?

How many drops per minute will the patient receive?

How many milligrams of medication will be administered in 45 minutes?

If the order is for q6h, how many vials of medication will be needed per day?

What will be the total daily dose of medication in milligrams?

Posttest, cont.

4. A physician orders nitroglycerin 50 mg in D5W 250 mL to be infused at the rate of 50 mcg/min. The drop factor is 60 gtt/mL.

How many micrograms are in 1 mL of solution?

What is the flow rate in milliliters per minute?

How long will it take these fluids to infuse in hours and minutes?

How many milliliters provide 5 mg of nitroglycerin?

Continued

Posttest, cont.

5. A physician orders D5NS 3,000 mL over 24 hours. The drop factor is 15 gtt/mL.

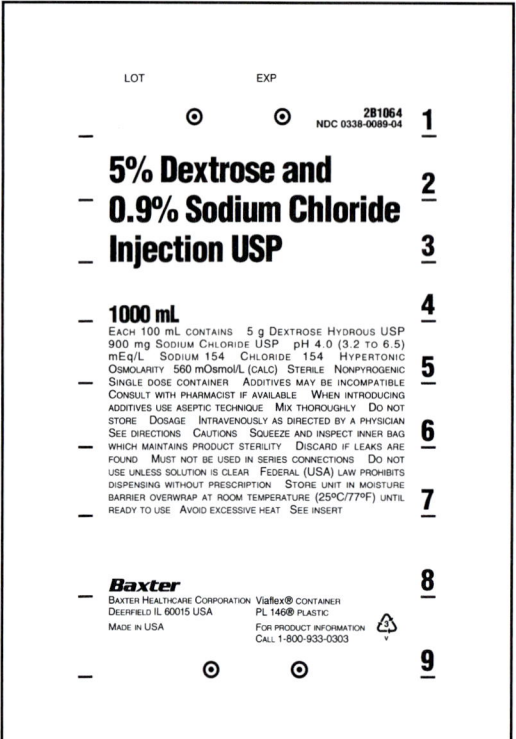

Courtesy of Baxter Healthcare Corporation. All rights reserved.

How many milliliters of fluids should be supplied for each 8-hour shift?

How many 1-L containers of solution should be provided for the physician's order?

How many milliliters per hour should be infused?

Posttest, cont.

How many milliliters will the patient receive in 5 hours?

How many grams of dextrose will the patient receive after 5 hours?

6. A physician orders Amikin 5 mg/kg q8h in 100 mL of fluids IVPB. The patient weighs 176 lb. The drop factor is 20 gtt/mL. The time of infusion is 2 hours.
How many milligrams of medication should be added to the fluids?

If the medication is available as amikacin 50 mg/mL, how many milliliters should be added?

What is the flow rate in drops per minute?

7. How many minutes will it take to infuse 1 L of D5W at 3 mL/min?

How many total milliliters of fluids are required for 24 hours?

How many grams of dextrose will the patient receive in a 24-hour period?

Continued

Posttest, cont.

8. A physician orders 500 mL D5LR to be infused over 12 hours. The drop factor for the infusion set is 60 gtt/mL.

   What is the flow rate in milliliters per minute?

   How many milliliters of IV fluid will be infused in an hour?

   How many drops per minute should be infused?

9. A physician orders D5NS 1,000 mL for a child who is dehydrated. The physician wants the patient to receive 90 mL the first hour and the remainder over 12 hours. The drop factor is 60 gtt/mL.

   What is the flow rate in milliliters per minute for the first hour?

   What is the flow rate in milliliters per minute for the remaining 12 hours?

10. A physician orders Rocephin (ceftriaxone) 25 mg/kg IVPB in 100 mL NS to run over 1 hour q12h. The patient weighs 176 lb. The drop factor is 15 gtt/mL. The available medication is 2 g/vial.

    How many grams of Rocephin are administered every 12 hours?

    What is the infusion rate in milliliters per minute?

Posttest, cont.

11. A physician orders potassium chloride 30 mEq added to D5W 150 mL IVPB to infuse over 2½ hours with a drop factor is 20 gtt/mL.

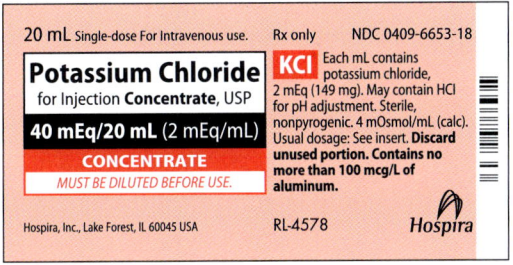

© Pfizer. Used with permission.

How many milliliters of KCl should be added to the IVPB fluids?

How many milliliters of fluids will be infused in a minute?

How many milliliters of fluids will be infused in an hour?

What is the infusion rate in drops per minute?

Continued

Posttest, cont.

12. A physician orders doxycycline 150 mg IVPB in LR 85 mL to be administered over 1½ hours. Doxycycline is available as 100 mg/10 mL. The drop factor is 20 gtt/mL.

How many milliliters of doxycycline should be added to the fluids?

What is the flow rate in milliliters per minute for this order?

What would the flow rate be in milliliters per minute if the physician wanted the fluid to be infused over 1 hour?

13. A physician orders Retrovir (zidovudine) 2 mg/kg/dose IVPB for a 165-lb patient. The dose is to be placed in 100 mL D5W and infused over 1 hour with a drop factor of 15 gtt/mL q4h × 24 hours.

The 20-mL single-use vial of Retrovir for IV infusion 10 mg/mL must be further diluted in 5% dextrose injection to no greater than 4 mg/mL before being infused. How many mL of the reconstituted medication should be added to the D5W per dose?

What is the infusion rate in milliliters per minute?

How many mg of zidovudine will the patient receive in a 24-hour period?

How many drops per minute will the patient receive with each dose?

Posttest, cont.

What is the final concentration of zidovudine in each bag?

Is this within the allowable concentration?
_____

 14. A physician orders heparin sodium 20,000 units in NS 500 mL to run over 24 hours. The administration set delivers 60 gtt/mL.

What is the flow rate in drops per minute?

How many units of heparin will the patient receive each hour?

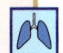 15. A physician orders epinephrine 3 mg added to D5W 250 mL to be infused at 10 mL/hr. The administration set delivers 60 gtt/mL.

How many milligrams of epinephrine will the patient receive in an hour? *(Do not round.)*

How many micrograms will the patient receive in a minute?

What volume will have infused in 24 hours?

How many drops per minute will the patient receive?

Continued

Posttest, cont.

16. A physician orders lidocaine 100 mg in D5W 250 mL to be infused over an hour. The lidocaine is available in 10 mg/mL. The drop factor is 40 gtt/mL.

What volume of lidocaine should be added to the fluids?

What is the flow rate in milliliters per minute that the patient will receive?

How many milligrams of lidocaine will the patient receive per minute?

How many drops per minute will be administered?

17. A physician orders epinephrine 50 mcg/min to be administered from fluids that contain epinephrine 5 mg in D5LR 500 mL. The drop factor is 20 gtt/mL.

How many minutes will it take for the fluids to infuse?

What is the rate of infusion in drops per minute?

What is the flow rate in milliliters per hour?

How many milligrams of epinephrine did the patient receive if the IV was stopped after 300 mL had infused?

Posttest, cont.

18. A physician orders amphotericin B 200 mg added to D5W 500 mL to infuse over 6 hours with a drop factor of 15 gtt/mL. The medication is available in a 100 mg/20 mL vial.

How many milliliters of amphotericin should be added to the fluids?

How many vials of medication are needed to complete the order?

What is the flow rate in drops per minute?

What is the flow rate in milliliters per hour?

If the fluids infused for 4 hours, how many milligrams of amphotericin B were received?

19. The following solutions are ordered for a TPN:

Travesol (amino acids) 7.5%	500 mL
dextrose 70%	300 mL
sterile water for injection	200 mL

What is the final concentration of Travesol?

What is the final concentration of dextrose?

If the TPN is hung at 0200 and run at 50 mL/hr, when will the next bag be due?

Continued

Posttest, cont.

20. Perform the following TPN calculations.

TPN ADDITIVES	ADDITIVE STOCK STRENGTHS AVAILABLE	
potassium chloride	2 mEq/mL	
sodium chloride	14.6%	2.5 mEq/mL
calcium gluconate	10%	4.65 mEq/10 mL
magnesium sulfate	50%	40.6 mEq/10 mL
sodium acetate	2 mEq/mL	
sodium phosphate	45 mM/15 mL	60 mEq/15 mL
potassium acetate	19.6%	2 mEq/mL
potassium phosphate	15 mM/5 mL	4.4 mEq/mL
Humulin R insulin	100 units/mL	
vitamin C	250 mg/2 mL	
folic acid	5 mg/mL	

Calculate amounts needed for each additive. Show your work.

Potassium chloride 10 mEq

Sodium chloride 15 mEq

Calcium gluconate 7.5 mEq

Magnesium sulfate 2 mEq

Sodium acetate 3 mEq

Sodium phosphate 12 mEq

Humulin R insulin 40 units

Vitamin C 500 mg

Folic acid 10 mg

Posttest, cont.

| MVI-12 | 10 mL |

What is the total amount of all of the additives?

Base Solutions

Travesol 10%	300 mL
dextrose 50%	400 mL
lipids 20%	100 mL
sterile water for injection	qs ad 1,000 mL

What is the final concentration of Travesol?

What is the final concentration of dextrose?

What is the final concentration of lipids?

How much sterile water for injection is needed to reach 1,000 mL? *Be sure to account for the total amount of additives.*

If it is hung at 0400 and run at 100 mL/hr, when will the next bag be due?

REVIEW OF RULES

IV calculations involve determination of the:

- amount of medication delivered (mg, g, mEq, or units) over a specific period of time
- volume of medication delivered (gtt, mL, or L) over a specific period of time – *dose volume*
- volume of medication needed to last a specific amount of time
- length of time a medication dose will last – *dose time*

Equations used:

Flow rate = dose volume/dose time

Specific type of flow rate:

Drip rate = gtt/min

Factors to be considered with IV administration are as follows:

- Total amount of fluids to be administered in *milliliters – dose volume (mL)*
- Calibration of the administration (infusion) set in *drops per milliliter – drop factor (gtt/mL)*
- Flow rate of the fluids in *drops per minute – drip rate (gtt/min)*
- Time for the fluids to infuse in *minutes (min)* or *hours (h or hr)*

IN SECTION V

17 Business Math for Pharmacy Technicians

SECTION V
Business Math

CHAPTER 17

Business Math for Pharmacy Technicians

OBJECTIVES

1. Calculate overhead expenses.
2. Calculate depreciation.
3. Calculate prescription markup.
4. Calculate discounts on merchandise.
5. Calculate net and gross income/profit.
6. Calculate insurance reimbursement using average wholesale prices, dispensing fees, and capitation.
7. Manage inventory, including par levels and inventory turnover rate.
8. Perform a daily cash report.

KEY WORDS

Adjudication Electronic process by which insurance companies evaluate prescriptions to determine their validity and the price to charge the patient

Assets Any property owned by a business

Average wholesale price (AWP) Price that a pharmacy theoretically pays for medication; this price is theoretical because discounts, sales, and special deals may affect the actual wholesale price; this is the price basis used for insurance reimbursement

Capitation fee Set amount of third-party money paid monthly to the pharmacy for a specific patient regardless of the number of prescriptions filled

Cash flow Receipts and expenses for a business

Cost of inventory List of the quantity and respective cost of merchandise in stock

Daily cash or sales report Report made at the end of each day that summarizes the sales, discounts, and amount of cash, checks, refunds, and credit card charges that have occurred during the day's operations

Depreciation Decrease in value of an asset based on total value of the asset, its estimated length of use, and its value at disposal; part of overhead

Discount percentage A percentage amount to be subtracted from the markup price of an item to lower the selling price

Discount Reduction in the price of an item; offered to customers by the pharmacy (**markdown**) or offered to the pharmacy from wholesalers when a bill is paid by a certain date

Dispensing fee Amount of money added to the cost of a prescription; intended to cover various aspects of preparing and dispensing; often a set price determined by insurance companies

Gross income/gross profit Sales price of merchandise minus its purchase cost; usually refers to total income for a business

Inventory All of the merchandise in stock

Markup Amount of money added to the cost of the product

Markup amount Difference between the selling price and the purchase cost of an item; also purchase cost times markup percentage

Markup percentage or gross margin A percentage amount added to the purchase cost of merchandise to ensure a profit; markup amount divided by the cost times 100

Markup price Purchase cost plus markup amount; becomes the selling/retail price

Net income/net profit Gross profit minus overhead; usually refers to total income for a business

Overhead Expenses of a business, *not including cost of inventory*, such as rent, wages, utilities, insurance, license fees, depreciation, taxes paid, and other costs of doing business

PAR level (periodic automatic replenishment) Predetermined point for automatic inventory reordering of items used in a pharmacy ; **par level** is also used to indicate a specific quantity to be kept in stock

Purchase cost Price paid by a business to obtain items for sale; also referred to as **wholesale**, **acquisition**, or **inventory cost**

Selling price Price at which items are offered for sale to customers; also referred to as **retail price**

Turnover rate Rate at which the inventory is sold over a specified period of time

Pretest

If you are already comfortable with the subject matter, perform the following business math calculations to test your knowledge. If not, work your way through the chapter and return to them for extra practice. Round answers to the nearest tenth or dollars and cents as appropriate.

1. A pharmacy sells a prescription for $43.50. The medication costs the pharmacy $22.65.

    What is the markup?

2. A pharmacy buys a medication at a discount rate of $555 for 1,000 tablets. The selling price for the medication is $45.50 for 50 tablets.

    What is the markup on the prescription?

Pretest, cont.

3. A customer brings in a discount coupon for 25% off her first prescription and 10% off her second prescription. One prescription costs $15 and the other costs $24.50. The pharmacist tells you to take the 25% off the most expensive prescription.

    What will the first prescription cost the patient?

    What will the second prescription cost the patient?

    What is the total cost for both prescriptions?

4. A pharmacy has a monthly income of $535,356 with inventory purchases of $456,980, salaries and wages of $76,000, and maintenance costs of $1,567.50.

    What is the net income of the pharmacy for the month?

5. What is the percentage markup of a prescription that has an inventory cost of $14.50 and is sold for $21?

6. A pharmacy buys a new computer program for $9,500 in January. The expected time of use is 3 years, and it will be discarded at the end of 3 years.

    What will be the amount of depreciation for this equipment for a year?

Continued

Copyright © 2019 by Elsevier, Inc. All rights reserved.

Pretest, cont.

7. A pharmacy has a reorder level of 2,500 capsules for antibiotic during the winter influenza season. The pharmacy technician counts 950 capsules still in inventory. The wholesaler has a deal for 5,000 capsules for $1,500 with a 10% discount. The average use of the capsules is 3,000 capsules per week.

   How many capsules need to be ordered to maintain the PAR level?

   Would it be appropriate for the pharmacy technician to ask the pharmacist if she desires to take advantage of the discounted medication? _____ Explain your answer. _____

   What is the discounted price for 5,000 capsules?

8. A pharmacy is contracted with an insurance company for a reimbursement of AWP plus 15% and a dispensing fee. The prescription costs the pharmacy $12.50. The dispensing fee is $7.50.

   What is the amount to be charged to the insurance company?

9. A pharmacy is contracted with an insurance company for reimbursement based on a capitation fee of $55 per month for a patient. The patient received prescriptions for $16.50 and $12.00.

   What is the balance available for additional prescriptions?

   If the patient brings in other prescriptions totaling $27.50 before the end of the month, what would the pharmacy lose from capitation reimbursement?

10. A pharmacy has an opening cash drawer of $150. At the end of the day the purchases are $1,895.67. The drawer contains $14.50 in coupons, discounts of $12.50, refunds of $13.50, and credit card purchases of $45.60. *Hint: None of these amounts are included in the ending balance for deposit the same day.*

    What is the ending balance for deposit if the cash drawer beginning balance should remain the same for each day?

    If checks are for $25.60, $111.47, $268.15, and $46.18, what is the cash amount to be deposited?

INTRODUCTION

Pharmacy technicians in retail settings, as well as in hospital settings, may be involved with business calculations. For a business to remain profitable, the **net income**, or **net profit**, from the sales of medications must exceed the cost of doing business. Mathematical calculations include using percentages to determine **discounts** and **markups**, as well as addition and subtraction to maintain the necessary inventory **PAR levels**. An adequate markup must be in place so the receipts of the business are in excess of the expenses and the supply of **inventory** must be adequate to cover demand but not so excessive that it ties up the **cash flow** of the business. Monitoring of pricing and inventory, as well as obtaining necessary inventory levels, may be a task of the pharmacy technician. The cash flow of the pharmacy is directly related to the mathematical calculations performed for inventory and **profit** (or loss) that are calculated routinely. Therefore costs of new inventory must be carefully checked each time new stock arrives to be sure they have not changed since the last order. If inventory prices change and the prices for sales are not changed simultaneously, profits will be affected. A pharmacy technician may have a major role in inventory control and reordering, which affects **turnover rate** and **gross and net income or profit**.

OVERHEAD EXPENSES

Overhead is the actual cost of doing business. It includes all costs for the pharmacy, such as salaries, licenses, equipment purchases and repairs, depreciation, utilities, telephone, insurance, taxes paid (e.g., employer's payroll taxes), and rent. Overhead does *not* include the cost of inventory.

Depreciation

Depreciation is a rate representing the decrease in value of an **asset** (equipment, building, computer, printer) over time. For example, consider a computer purchased for $1,000, which is intended to be useful for 5 years. The amount to depreciate is $1,000 taken over 5 years. If the depreciation were taken as an equal value over all 5 years, the amount would be $200 per year.

Annual depreciation = Cost ÷ Estimated time of use in years

To calculate overhead, total all business expenses (*excluding* inventory).

EXAMPLE 17.1

A pharmacy spends $12,585 for inventory for a week; the salaries for all persons involved are $12,500. The rent is $1,600 per month, and utilities cost $800 per month. In addition, the cost for insurance is $1,000 per month and depreciation on equipment is $2,500 per month. Taxes are $2,400 per month. What is the overhead for 1 week?

Salaries	$12,500
Rent	400 ($1,600 ÷ 4 weeks/month)
Utilities	200 ($800 ÷ 4 weeks/month)
Insurance	250 ($1,000 ÷ 4 weeks/month)
Depreciation	625 ($2,500 ÷ 4 weeks/month)
Taxes	400 ($2,400 ÷ 4 weeks/month)
Total overhead	$14,375/week

Practice Problems A

Calculate the overhead in the following problems. Remember not to include the cost of inventory. Show your calculations. All final answers should be shown in dollars and cents.

1. A pharmacy has a monthly cost for medication inventory of $46,725, salaries of $58,000, utilities of $2,534, rent of $770, insurance of $1,575, taxes of $7,844, depreciation of equipment of $965, and business supplies and postage of $650.

   What is the overhead cost for the pharmacy for a month?

   What is the approximate overhead cost for a year?

2. A hospital pharmacy is asked to calculate the overhead necessary to maintain safety for the patients when medications are dispensed. The following amounts would be necessary per year: salaries for pharmacists—$264,000; four pharmacy technician salaries—$22,500 each; medication inventory—$56,525 each month; utilities—$750 per month; salaries for relief pharmacists—$12,500/year; computers and software updates—$56,000 yearly; yearly liability insurance for pharmacists and pharmacy technicians—$3,500; and use of hospital space—$3,600/year.

   What is the total overhead for this hospital pharmacy for a year?

   What is the overhead for a month?

3. A pharmacist needs to know how much income each month is necessary to meet the overhead for the business he owns. The expenses are salaries of $72,000 per year for the pharmacist, $27,500 per year each for two pharmacy technicians, $560,430 per year for inventory costs, $5,600 per year for utilities and rent, $27,500 per year for equipment replacement, and taxes and other business expenses of $1,560 per month.

   What is the overhead for this pharmacy per month?

   What is the overhead for the pharmacy for a year?

4. A retail pharmacy wants to ensure that sufficient income is being obtained for a new branch that has just opened. The monthly expenses are $6,500 for the pharmacist's salary, total of $1,250 for two pharmacy technicians who both work part-time while in school, $25,340 for inventory, $560 for taxes, business expenses of $980, utilities and rent of $11,500, and payment for equipment of $4,500 per month.

   What is the total amount of overhead for a month?

   What is the overhead for a year?

5. A pharmacy needs to compute the amount of overhead the store has in a year. The salaries are $54,000 per month, rent is $1,250 per month, utilities are $22,500 per year, inventory is $86,950 per month, equipment costs $60,000 per year in replacements, supplies are $1,250 per month, and miscellaneous expenses are $1,550 per month. The depreciation rate is $950 per month.

   What is the overhead for a year?

   What is the overhead for a month?

MARKUP

The **markup amount** is the difference in the **purchase cost** of the drug and the **selling price** of the same drug. The formula is as follows:

   Markup = Selling price − Purchase cost

Markup rates on brand name drugs are generally lower than the markup rate on generics. For instance, if a brand name antibiotic, such as Keflex, costs $100 and has a 6% markup ($100 × 0.06 = $6), the cost to the customer is $106. A generic for the same drug, cephalexin, may cost $40 with a 25% markup ($40 × 0.25 = $10), so the cost to the customer is $50. Pharmacies have higher profit margins available with generics than they do with brand name drugs.

EXAMPLE 17.2

A prescription sells for $35.60, and the cost is $29.90. What is the markup?

   Markup = $35.60 − $29.90

   Markup = $5.70

Practice Problems B

Calculate the markup on the following problems:

1. A medication has a selling price of $56 and a cost of $45.

   What is the markup?

2. A medication has a selling price of $34.50 and a cost of $15.60.

   What is the markup?

3. A medication has a selling price of $43.50 and a cost of $39.90.

   What is the markup?

4. A medication has a selling price of $10.20 and a cost of $9.20.

   What is the markup?

5. A medication has a selling price of $125 and a cost of $93.50.

   What is the markup?

Markup Percentage

The **markup percentage** or **gross margin** is calculated by dividing the markup by the cost and then multiplying by 100. Markup percentages provide information about which prescription medications have the greatest percentage of profit. The formula is as follows:

$$\text{Markup percentage} = (\text{Markup} \div \text{Purchase cost}) \times 100$$

EXAMPLE 17.3

A medication costs the pharmacy $29.90 and is sold for $35.60. What is the markup percentage?

Markup = $35.60 − $29.90 = $5.70

Markup percentage = ($5.70 ÷ $29.90) × 100 = 19%

TECH NOTE

If the selling price is more than twice the purchase cost, the markup percentage will always be over 100%.

Practice Problems C

Calculate the percentage of markup in the following problems. Show your calculations. Round all final answers to tenths.

1. A medication has a selling price of $56 and a purchase cost of $45.

   What is the markup percentage?

2. A medication has a selling price of $34.50 and a cost of $15.60.

   What is the markup percentage?

3. A medication has a selling price of $43.50 and a cost of $39.90.

   What is the markup percentage?

4. A medication has a selling price of $10.20 and a cost of $9.20.

   What is the markup percentage?

5. A medication has a selling price of $125 and a cost of $93.50.

   What is the markup percentage?

6. A medication has a selling price of $45 and a cost of $42.

   What is the markup percentage?

7. A medication has a selling price of $27.90 and a cost of $23.60.

   What is the markup percentage?

8. A medication has a selling price of $33.75 and a cost of $30.

   What is the markup percentage?

9. A medication has a selling price of $12.90 and a cost of $9.20.

   What is the markup percentage?

10. A medication has a selling price of $255 and a cost of $193.50.

    What is the markup percentage?

Copyright © 2019 by Elsevier, Inc. All rights reserved.

DISCOUNTS

A **discount or markdown** may be applied to prescriptions, over-the-counter (OTC) drugs, or other merchandise. The markdown price is calculated by subtracting a **discount percentage**, a percentage of the original selling price of the item, which lowers the price the customer pays. Discounts and markdowns are used as an incentive to encourage customers to purchase items by realizing a savings on the original selling or retail price. Markdowns and discounts may be in the form of manufacturers' coupons or special discounts for reasons such as senior citizens' initiatives. The amount of the discount is *always* based on the selling price, not on the cost of the item. The item must be marked up for sale first, and then a discount can be applied. A discount *decreases* the sale price; markup is based on the pharmacy's purchase price. The formulas for discounts are as follows:

Discount amount = Selling price × Discount percentage

Discounted price = Selling price − Discount amount

When discounts are given based on manufacturers' or other coupons, the amount of the coupon should be subtracted from the selling price and the coupon placed in the cash drawer to be used at the end of the day to balance the cash drawer.

EXAMPLE 17.4

A medication that sells for $45.00 has a manufacturer's coupon for 15% off as an incentive to try the medication. What is the cost to the patient after the use of the discount coupon?

Hint: Change percentage to a decimal number for each calculation.

Discount amount = $45.00 × 0.15 = $6.75

Discount price = $45.00 − $6.75 = $38.25

An alternative to finding the discount amount and subtracting from the original price is to consider how much of the total cost the customer will need to pay and multiply by that decimal. In Example 17.4, with a 15% discount, the customer will pay the remaining 85% of the cost (100% − 15% = 85%). The customer will pay $45.00 times 0.85, which equals $38.25.

Discounts may also be offered to a pharmacy from the wholesaler for timely payment of the invoice. For example, the invoice may say 8% discount if paid by the 15th of the month. The supplier may also discount certain medications or provide a discount for bulk purchases. These discounts provide a way for pharmacies to increase their profits.

TECH NOTE
The customer discount is always calculated from the sale price, not the pharmacy's purchase cost, or the pharmacy would lose money.

Practice Problems D

Calculate the discounted prices in the following problems. Show your work. Remember that the discounted price will always be lower.

1. A patient has a manufacturer's discount coupon in the amount of 25% for a new prescription. The selling price is $42.50.

   What is the discount amount?

   What is the price of the prescription after the discount?

2. An ad in the local paper offers ⅓ off a medication that is taken regularly by one of your customers. *Hint: Multiply by the fraction ⅓ as opposed to changing it to a decimal.* The patient brings in the coupon for the medicine that costs $33.

   What is the discount amount?

   What is the price of the medication after the discount?

3. A drug supplier offers a deal that will provide a 25% discount for 10 tubes of a new dermatologic preparation. The cost for the 10 tubes is $525.

   What is the discount amount?

   What is the discounted price for these tubes of medication?

4. An older patient on a fixed income comes to the pharmacy with a new prescription. The pharmacist tells the patient that he will provide a 12% discount for the medication, which costs $65.

   What is the discount amount?

   What is the price of the prescription after the discount?

5. An insurance company has a contract with the pharmacy to provide a 5% discount for any prescription for its members. A prescription has a retail price of $75.40.

   What is the discount amount?

   What discounted price should be charged to the insured?

6. A retail pharmacy has advertised a 35% off sale on all pain relievers during the first 2 weeks of April. Tylenol's regular price is $7.59 and Aleve's price is $8.29.

   What is the discounted price for each of these OTC products? Perform these calculations by multiplying by 0.65 (the 65% balance that the customer will have to pay) to go directly to the discounted price. Verify your answers by determining the discount amount and subtracting from the selling price.

   Tylenol:

   Aleve:

7. An ad in the local paper offers 30% off an antacid with a regular price of $4.54.

   What is the discounted price for the product?

8. A manufacturer's coupon offers a 20% discount on cough syrup. The retail price is $5.79.

   What is the discounted price for the cough syrup?

9. A manufacturer offers a discount of 40% on the first prescription of a hypolipidemic agent that sells for $75 retail.

   What is the price of the prescription after the discount?

10. A pharmacy bought an OTC medication at 30% less than the usual wholesale price of $12.00 for 100 tablets.

    What is the discounted price?

    The usual retail price is $22 for 100 tablets and the pharmacist wants to offer a 25% discount to the patients as a means to bring in more customers.

    What is the discounted price of 100 tablets for the patient?

    How much would the pharmacy make on one 100-tablet bottle in this situation?

GROSS INCOME

The **gross income** (sometimes referred to as **gross profit**) is the difference in the sales price and the cost of the inventory with no other expenses of the business considered. This usually is calculated for the total income of the business.

   Gross income = Sales – Cost of inventory

EXAMPLE 17.5

If a pharmacy's sales were $200,000 and its purchases were $175,000, its gross profit would be $25,000.

Practice Problems E

Calculate the following problems. A month should be considered 4 weeks.

1. A pharmacy has sales of $1,253,000 with a cost of inventory of $1,125,566.

   What is the gross profit?

2. A pharmacy sells $25,420 a week with a monthly cost of inventory of $19,986.

   What is the gross profit?

3. A pharmacy has an income of $31,567 for the month of June.

   If this monthly income remains constant for a year, and the inventory costs for that year are $299,599, what is the year's gross profit?

4. A pharmacy that is open 7 days a week has sales amounting to $6,500/day with inventory costs of $5,990/day.

   What is the weekly gross profit?

5. The bank requests the gross profit of a store for a quarter. The sales are $65,432/month and inventory costs are $64,120/month.

   What is the gross profit for the quarter?

NET INCOME

Net income (sometimes referred to as the bottom line or **net profit**) is the gross profit minus the overhead. It is the difference between the sales and all of the costs related to the business (inventory and overhead). A positive net income is necessary for the business to remain fiscally sound.

Net income = Sales – (Inventory + Overhead)

Because sales minus inventory is gross profit, this can be simplified to:

Net income = Gross income – Overhead

Using Example 17.5, if the overhead for the same store was $18,000 for the month, the net income would be $25,000 – $18,000 = $7,000.

EXAMPLE 17.6

A pharmacy has monthly sales of $425,000, inventory purchases of $310,000, salaries and wages of $60,000, utilities of $2,500, insurance of $1,100, and maintenance of $775.

What is the gross income (sales – inventory cost)?

$425,000 – $310,000 = $115,000

What is the overhead for the month (all expenses excluding inventory)?

$60,000 + $2,500 + $1,100 + $775 = $64,375

What is the net income (gross income – overhead)?

$115,000 – $64,375 = $50,625

Practice Problems F

Calculate the gross income, overhead, and net income in the following examples.

1. A retail pharmacy has monthly sales of $204,300. Inventory purchases were $177,700, salaries and wages were $21,350, utilities were $1,750, rent was $1,800, insurance was $750, and repairs were $900.

   What is the gross income for the month?

   What is the total overhead for the month?

   What is the net income?

2. A retail chain location has monthly sales of $354,740. Inventory purchases were $317,600, salaries and wages were $27,000, utilities were $2,400, rent was $3,800, insurance was $1,200, and repairs were $80.

   What is the gross income for the month?

   What is the total overhead for the month?

   What is the net income?

3. A hospital pharmacy's charges to patients are $454,000 for a month. Inventory purchases were $377,400, salaries and wages were $26,000, utilities allocated to the pharmacy were $850, licenses were $450, and supplies were $1,900.

   What is the gross income for the month?

   What is the total overhead for the month?

   What is net income?

4. A retail pharmacy has monthly sales of $174,080. Inventory purchases were $146,220, salaries and wages were $16,200, utilities were $1,950, rent was $1,400, insurance was $800, and repairs were $270.

   What is the gross income for the month?

   What would be the total overhead for the month?

   What would be the net income?

5. A retail pharmacy has monthly sales of $379,300. Inventory purchases were $317,300, salaries and wages were $31,400, utilities were $2,675, rent was $3,500, insurance was $1,400, and supplies were $775.

   What is the gross income for the month?

   What is the total overhead for the month?

   What is the net income?

INSURANCE REIMBURSEMENT

Insurance or third-party reimbursement plays a major role in a pharmacy's income. The pharmacy signs contracts with insurance carriers for predetermined reimbursement amounts that may be specific to a medication or calculated based on the average wholesale price. To receive reimbursement, a pharmacy submits a claim electronically. On receipt of the claim, the insurance company processes it according to the terms of the contract, supplies the pharmacy with the proper amount to charge the customer, and submits reimbursement, a process called **adjudication**. Most third-party reimbursements are based on **average wholesale price (AWP)**, markup or markdown rates, and a **dispensing fee**.

Average Wholesale Price

AWP is based on the national average cost of medication purchased from a wholesale market. A pharmacy may not actually pay AWP for medications because discounts are provided to pharmacies that order large quantities of drugs or for payment of invoices within a specified time. Fast-selling medications are often ordered in large quantities to obtain these discounts, thus increasing the profit on prescriptions. Today most patients have third-party payers (insurance companies) that reimburse the pharmacy for their prescriptions.

Applying a Markup or Markdown

In many instances, insurance companies provide reimbursement based on AWP plus a percentage of AWP, which is noted as AWP + %AWP. In other instances, reimbursement is based on AWP less a percentage of AWP, which is noted as AWP − %AWP. Applying a markdown to a prescription uses the same process as offering a discount. Applying a markup is the opposite. To apply a discount, multiply the discount percent (in decimal form) by the AWP and *subtract* this discount amount from the AWP. To apply a markup, multiply the markup percent (in decimal form) by the AWP and *add* this markup amount to the AWP.

Dispensing Fees

Dispensing fees may vary by insurance companies and medications prescribed depending on the contract. The fees are a means of providing reimbursements for overhead expenses.

The following formula is used to determine insurance reimbursement:

Reimbursement of prescription = AWP ± Percentage of AWP allowed + Dispensing fee

Reimbursement of prescription = AWP ± (%AWP) + Dispensing fee

EXAMPLE 17.7

AWP for a drug is $64 for a 30-day supply.

Insurance percentage is +15%

$64.00 × 0.15 = $9.60

Professional or dispensing fee is $3

Reimbursement = $64 + $9.60 + $3 = $76.60

The profit would be $12.60 ($76.60 − $64.00) if the pharmacy purchased the medication at AWP. If the pharmacy was able to purchase this medication for less than the AWP due to discounts, the profit would be greater.

EXAMPLE 17.8

A pharmacy purchases 1,000 tablets of medication at the wholesale price of $112. The wholesale distributor allows a 10% discount on invoices paid within 10 days. The payment is made according to the discount.

The AWP for this medication is $140.00/1,000 tablets.

Insurance reimbursement is AWP *less* (minus) 5% plus a $5 dispensing fee.

A prescription is written for 60 tablets.

1. What is the discounted wholesale price for 1,000 tablets?

$112 − ($112 × 0.10)

$112 − $11.20 = $100.80

2. What is the price for 60 tablets at the discounted wholesale cost?

$$\frac{\$108.80}{1{,}000 \text{ tabs}} = \frac{x}{60 \text{ tabs}} \quad x = \$6.53$$

$6.53 for 60 tablets at the discounted wholesale cost

3. What is the AWP for 60 tablets?

$$\frac{\$140.00}{1{,}000 \text{ tabs}} = \frac{x}{60 \text{ tabs}} \quad x = \$8.40$$

$8.40 for 60 tablets at AWP

4. Calculate the amount billed to insurance.

$8.40 − (5% × $8.40) + $5

$8.40 − (0.05 × $8.40) + $5

$8.40 − ($0.42) + $3 = $12.98

5. Calculate profit or loss on the prescription with insurance reimbursement.

$12.98 − $6.53 = $6.45

> **TECH NOTE**
> Remember that when changing a percentage into a decimal, anything less than 10% will have a zero in the tenths place. For example, 5% is 0.05, whereas 50% is 0.5.

Practice Problems G

Calculate the following problems indicating the formula used.

1. A prescription has an AWP of $25.60. The insurance percentage is +18% AWP. The professional dispensing fee is $3.50.

   Total reimbursement:

   Profit:

2. A compounded prescription has a total AWP of $35.65. The insurance percentage is +9% AWP. The professional dispensing fee is $7.50.

   Total reimbursement:

   Profit:

3. A prescription has an AWP of $7.90. The insurance percentage is +12% AWP. The professional dispensing fee is $5.

   Total reimbursement:

   Profit:

4. An antibiotic prescription for 10 days has an AWP of $46.50. The insurance percentage of payment is +7.5% AWP. The professional dispensing fee is $12.50.

   Total reimbursement:

   Profit:

5. A prescription for a month's supply of medication has an AWP of $120. The insurance percentage is −2% on monthly prescriptions. Professional dispensing fees are increased to $15 for this medication.

   Total reimbursement:

   Profit:

   Using the same AWP, change the insurance percentage to +3% AWP with a professional dispensing fee of $7.75.

   Total reimbursement:

   Profit:

   Which of these two means of reimbursement would be most advantageous to the pharmacy?

6. A maintenance drug prescription has an AWP of $15.20. The insurance percentage is +9% AWP. The professional dispensing fee is $5.23.

   Total reimbursement:

7. A compounded prescription has a total AWP of $49.90. The insurance percentage is +7% AWP. The professional dispensing fee is $13.

   Total reimbursement:

8. A 7-day prescription of a medication taken three times daily has an AWP of $14.45. The insurance percentage is –5% AWP. The professional dispensing fee is $6.

   Total reimbursement:

9. A topical ointment prescription for 14 days has an AWP of $32.40. The insurance percentage of payment is +12.25% AWP. The professional dispensing fee is $9.

   Total reimbursement:

10. A prescription for a 90-day supply of medication has an AWP of $190. The insurance percentage is +6% AWP. The professional dispensing fee is $18.

    Total reimbursement:

    Using the same AWP, change the insurance percentage to –1.5% AWP with a professional dispensing fee of $21.

    Total reimbursement:

    Which of these two means of reimbursement would be most advantageous to the pharmacy?

CAPITATION

Capitation refers to a contract between the pharmacy and the third-party payer to provide medications to the insured patient. **Capitation fees**, usually paid on a monthly basis, are a set amount of money paid to the pharmacy by a third party for a person whether the person receives a single prescription, multiple prescriptions, or no prescriptions. All prescriptions presented must be filled even if the cost exceeds the fee provided to the pharmacy. This type of reimbursement may provide the pharmacy with a loss during a 1-month period but can provide a profit over several months depending on the individual's prescription costs.

Profit (or Loss) on prescriptions = Capitation fee − Prescription costs

TECH NOTE
On financial statements, amounts that signify losses are often placed within parentheses.

EXAMPLE 17.9

The pharmacy accepts a capitation fee of $225 for a senior citizen who has multiple monthly standing prescriptions, most of which are available as generic drugs.

The wholesale cost for the monthly drug supplies are $9.50, $27, $65, and $42 = $143.50.

Profit (or Loss) = $225 − $143.50 = $81.50 (Profit for the month)

However, the next month the person has a severe sinus infection requiring additional prescriptions of $45 and $55 for antibiotics, $15 for a decongestant, and $26.50 for pain medication. The patient still receives her regular medications as scheduled. What is the profit or loss for month 2?

Extra costs = $45.00 + $55.00 + $14.00 + $26.50 = $141.50

Profit (or Loss) = $143.50 for maintenance medications
 + 141.50
 ─────
 $285.00

Profit (or Loss) = $225 − $285.00 = −$60.00 (Loss for the month)

Writing a number in parentheses ($60.00) indicates a loss.

What is the profit or loss over the 2-month time period?

Total capitation fees for 2 months = $450 ($225 × 2)
Total cost of medications   − 428.50 ($143.50 + $285)
Profit (or Loss) $21.50 Profit

Practice Problems H

Calculate the profit or loss using the capitation fee supplied. Show your work.

1. A pharmacy agrees to a monthly capitation fee of $175 for a patient who has standing prescriptions of $43 and $27. This month, the person had two other prescriptions for $35 and $18.

   What is this month's profit or loss?

2. The pharmacy agrees to a capitation fee of $425 for a family of four. Prescriptions for the family in 1 month are $12.50, $25, $30, and $62.50.

   What is this month's profit or loss?

3. A capitation fee for a year for a patient is $1,800. Prescriptions for this person for routine medications cost $25, $30, and $15 per month.

   What would be the profit or loss for these medications for the year?

   If this patient had additional prescriptions for acute conditions for $56 twice, $75 twice, and $85 once, what would be the annual profit or loss?

4. The capitation fee accepted by the pharmacy for a child is $125 per month. The child has a total of $1,650 in prescriptions for the year.

   Did the pharmacy have a profit or loss? _____

   What is the profit or loss?

   Would it be advantageous for the business to recalculate the capitation fee for this child if the expected costs for prescriptions were to remain the same?
   _____

5. A pharmacy is asked to accept a capitation fee of $350/month for an elderly patient who had six routine prescriptions of $25, $40, $35, $15, $80, and $75 monthly. Additional medications for acute conditions this month were $120, $25, and $160.

   What is the monthly profit or loss?

INVENTORY MANAGEMENT

An inventory is a list of all stock *available for sale* by a business on a specific date. Inventories may be taken at separate times for different sections of a store or pharmacy. Controlled drugs are normally inventoried more often than other medications depending on the protocol of the particular business and state and federal regulations.

In many cases, perpetual inventories are automatically maintained using computer programs. Restocking occurs on a continual basis with this type of system because the computer submits the order to the wholesaler electronically as stock is used or purchased by customers. As medication is sold it is subtracted from inventory, and when medication is received it is added to the inventory. A **par** or reorder level is determined by sales history. For seasonal medications, such as antihistamines and flu vaccines, the par level may need to be increased at certain times of the year. To maintain the inventory flow and minimize the need for extra shelf space, replacements for medications should arrive shortly before they are needed for use.

Number to reorder = Par or reorder level − Medication in stock

TECH NOTE

A **PAR** (periodic automatic replenishing) level is set in some pharmacies that have the capability of reordering medications automatically as they are used.

EXAMPLE 17.10

The par level or reorder point for amoxicillin during the winter is 1,500 capsules. Prescriptions for 1 day show dispensing 750 capsules. The bottle of 1,000 capsules has been opened and appears to be about half full. If the medication is available in 100-capsule, 500-capsule, and 1,000-capsule bottles, what should be ordered?

Number to reorder = 1,500 − 500 = 1,000 capsules

The approximate AWP costs are $25/100 capsules, $95/500 capsules, and $156/1,000 capsules. The cost per capsule for the 100-capsule size is 25¢, the 500-capsule size is 19¢, and the 1,000-capsule size is 15.6¢. The order should be one bottle of 1,000 capsules because the cost is less with this size and fewer larger containers require less storage space.

The original par level would suggest ordering one bottle of 1,000 capsules; however, with what seems to be the increased seasonal use of the medication, the technician may want to consult with the pharmacist about increasing the par level temporarily and ordering an additional 1,000 at the better price.

Practice Problems I

Calculate the amount of product to order for the medications in the following problems. The pharmacist desires the most efficient stock replacement using the lowest AWP cost of the medication. Round prices to tenths of a cent if necessary. Show your work.

1. The par level for the loop diuretic furosemide 20 mg is 400 tablets. The inventory available is 50 tablets. Available sizes of medication are as follows: 30 tablets for $3.90; 90 tablets for $9.90; 100 tablets for $12.00; and 500 tablets for $40.

    How many tablets are needed to replenish the stock?

    What is the cost per tablet for each size container? 30, 90, 100, 500

    What is the most appropriate size to order considering cost? _____

    How many containers of this size should be ordered? _____

2. The par level for the inotropic agent digoxin 0.25 mg is 200 tablets. The inventory is 25 tablets. The available medications from the wholesaler are 25 tablets for $6.50; 50 tablets for $7.50; and 100 tablets for $14.00.

    How many tablets are needed to replenish the stock?

    What is the cost per tablet for each size container? 25, 50, 100

    What is the most cost efficient stock medication size? _____

    How many containers of this size should be ordered? _____

3. The par level for the thyroid hormone levothyroxine 0.1 mg is 225 tablets. The inventory available is 75 tablets. Available sizes of medications with the wholesale cost for each are as follows: 50 tablets for $4.75; 100 tablets for $8.50; and 250 tablets for $12.50.

   How many tablets are needed to replenish the stock?

   What is the cost per unit for each size container? 50, 100, 250

   What is the most cost-efficient stock medication size? _____

   How many containers of this should be ordered? _____

4. The par level for the nonsteroidal antiinflammatory medication ibuprofen 800 mg is 1,500 tablets. The inventory available is 250 tablets. The available medications from the wholesaler are 100 tablets for $7.50; 200 tablets for $13.75; and 500 tablets for $27.45.

   How many tablets are needed to replenish the stock?

   What is the cost per unit for each size container? 100, 200, 500

   Which is the most cost-efficient stock medication size? _____

   How many containers of this size should be ordered? _____

5. The par level for the antidepressant Paxil 20 mg is 400 tablets. The inventory available is 180 tablets. Available sizes of medications are as follows: 40 tablets for $9.20; 90 tablets for $17.10; 150 tablets for $24.00; and 250 tablets for $37.50.

   How many tablets are needed to replenish the stock?

   What is the cost per unit for each size container? 40, 90, 150, 250

   What is the most cost-efficient stock medication size? _____

   How many containers should be ordered? _____

INVENTORY TURNOVER RATE

Inventory **turnover rate** is the frequency at which inventory is sold and replaced over a specified time period. The turnover rate is important for setting par levels of medications. This number helps the pharmacy determine whether inventory should be increased or decreased, thus controlling the amount of cash that is tied up in inventory. The turnover rate is the total value of inventory ordered over a specific time period, such as 1 month, 6 months, or 1 year, divided by the average value of inventory on hand. The formula for turnover rate is as follows:

Inventory turnover rate = Total purchases over a given time ÷ Average inventory value

EXAMPLE 17.11

A pharmacy spends $2,450,000 per year for inventory. The average inventory value is $350,000.

Turnover rate = $2,450,000/year ÷ $350,000

Turnover rate = 7 times per year

Practice Problems J

Calculate the inventory turnover rate in the following situations. Round all answers to tenths. Show your work.

1. A pharmacy has an average inventory of $225,000. The purchases for 6 months are $1,237,500.

   What is the turnover rate for this pharmacy for 6 months?

2. A pharmacy has an average inventory of $125,000. The purchases for 6 months are $2,250,000.

   What is the turnover rate for this pharmacy for 6 months?

3. A hospital has an average inventory of $70,000. The purchases for the past 2 months are $270,000.

   What is the turnover rate for 2 months?

4. A pharmacy has an average inventory of $22,500. The purchases for the year are $775,200.

   What is the turnover rate for this pharmacy for the year?

5. A pharmacy maintains an average inventory of $120,000. The pharmacist is concerned that he keeps too much stock. He spends $870,000 per year for medications. He likes a turnover rate of 2.5 every 2 months or less.

   What is his approximate turnover rate every 2 months?

   Is he maintaining the turnover rate that he desires? _____
   What is his turnover rate per year?

   How can the pharmacist increase his turnover rate?
   _____

DAILY CASH REPORT

Retail pharmacies may require technicians to prepare a daily **cash flow** report to verify that the payments received during the day balance with the amount of money in the cash drawer. This procedure varies for different pharmacies depending on how the store accounts for coupons, credit card payments, and discounts.

Posttest

Answer the following questions, rounding to dollars and cents. When calculating for a month use 4 weeks as the typical month and 28 days as the typical number of days per month.

1. The pharmacy spends $10,587.43 a week for medications. Salaries for the two registered pharmacists total $12,360 for the 4-week period. Rent is $1,825 per month, utilities are $1,450 per month, telephone is $576.08 per month, liability insurance on the building is $254 per month, professional malpractice insurance is $243 per month per pharmacist, and taxes paid are $3,856 per month. The total for pharmacy technicians is $2,650 per week. Depreciation on equipment is $4,320 per month.

    What is the overhead each month?

    If the pharmacy has an average income of $3,460 per day, what is the *gross* profit or loss for 1 month?

    If the pharmacy has an average income of $3,460 per day, what is the *net* profit or loss for 1 month?

2. A pharmacy buys new shelving costing $34,000 to be depreciated over 5 years. $2,500 for installation of the shelves should be added to the cost.

    What is the annual depreciation for the shelving?

Posttest, cont.

3. A pharmacy received an order of 1,000 tablets for $560.

   What is the cost of 50 tablets with a markup of 45%?

   What is the selling price per tablet with this markup?

   What is the selling price based on price per tablet for a prescription of 75 tablets?

4. During the past year, the pharmacy spent $1,600,000 for inventory supplies. The average inventory value during the past year was $250,000.

   What is the inventory turnover?

5. The pharmacy has announced a 25% off sale on all generic medications for the last Friday of the month. A customer arrives and wants to buy the following generic OTC medications with a retail cost as shown:

   acetaminophen (Tylenol) $7.99

   multiple vitamins $10.75

   docusate sodium (Colace) $9.99

   neomycin cream $6.50

   What is the discounted price for acetaminophen?

   What is the discounted price for multiple vitamins?

   What is the discounted price for docusate sodium?

   What is the discounted price for neomycin cream?

   What are the customer's savings on the entire purchase?

Continued

Posttest, cont.

6. A medication has an AWP of $75.60 for 50 tablets. The contract with the third-party payer is AWP + 15% AWP + $7.85 dispensing fee for a prescription for 50 tablets.

    What is the total that should be billed to the insurance company?

    If 100 tablets of the medication were purchased for $152.50 with a 15% discount for payment made within 10 days, what is the cost to the pharmacy for the above prescription?

    What is the profit from insurance reimbursement in this case?

7. A pharmacy has a capitation contract with an insurance company to pay the pharmacy $250 a month for an elderly patient who takes multiple medications. The patient takes prescriptions costing the pharmacy $7.68, $15.98, $46.32, and $48.21.

    If these are the only prescriptions obtained in a month, what is the monthly profit from the prescriptions for this patient?

    If the patient adds prescriptions costing $24.89, $50.65, and $12.50 to be taken on a regular basis, what is the profit or loss per month?

8. The par level for reorder of Enablex (darifenacin) for overactive bladder is 500 tablets. The pharmacy technician takes an inventory on Monday for reorder on Tuesday. The count is 125 tablets. The medication is available in bottles of 250 tablets.

    How many bottles should be ordered?

Posttest, cont.

9. Joseph is on an insurance plan that pays AWP + 12.5% AWP with a dispensing fee of $12.75. He brings prescriptions to the pharmacy for medications with an AWP of $34.50, $12.35, and $5.35.

   What is the amount to be charged to the third-party payer for the prescription with AWP of $34.50?

   What is the profit on this prescription if it cost the pharmacy $29.50?

   What is the amount to be charged for the prescription with an AWP of $12.35?

   What is the profit if this prescription cost the pharmacy $15.45?

   What is the amount to be charged for the prescription with an AWP of $5.35?

   What would be the profit on this prescription if the medication costs the pharmacy $5.69?

   Which prescription provides the highest gross profit?

Continued

Posttest, cont.

10. A pharmacy has depreciation of $4,325/month, inventory costs of $2,678.36 for an average week, utilities of $1,025.25 per month, telephone bill of $568 per month, and salaries of $4,500 a week for the pharmacist and $1,500 a week for two pharmacy technicians. The income for the month is $65,342.

   What is the total overhead expense for the month?

   What is the net profit or loss for the month?

   What is the discount amount for 1 week if the pharmacy uses a 20% markup on inventory and *then* offers it to the customers with a 5% discount?

REVIEW OF RULES—EQUATION REVIEW

Annual Depreciation
- Annual depreciation = Cost ÷ Estimated time of use in years

Overhead
- All expenses required for doing business *except the cost of inventory.*

Markup Amount
- Markup amount = Selling price − Purchase cost

  or

  Markup amount = Purchase cost × Markup percentage (written as a decimal)

Markup Price
- Markup price = Purchase cost + Markup amount

Markup Percentage
- Markup percent = (Markup ÷ Cost) × 100

Profit/income or Loss (Typically Income Includes Total of All Business Transactions)

- Gross profit (or loss) = Sale price of merchandise − Purchase cost of inventory
- Net profit (or loss) = Gross profit − Overhead

Discounts

- Discount amount = Selling price × Discount percentage (written as a decimal)
- Discounted price = Selling price − Discount amount

Insurance Reimbursements

- Reimbursement of prescription = AWP ± Percentage of AWP + Dispensing fee
- Insurance profit (or loss) = Reimbursement amount − Purchase cost
- Capitation profit or loss = Capitation fee − Medication costs

Par Levels

- Needed inventory = Par level − Amount on shelf

Inventory Turnover Rate

- Inventory turnover rate = Total purchases over a given time ÷ Average inventory value

APPENDIX

Extra Practice Problems

Chapter 1

Write the meaning of the following abbreviations.

1. ID _____
2. q6h _____
3. SUBCUT _____
4. ac _____
5. liq _____
6. qod _____
7. hs _____
8. qh _____
9. ASAP _____
10. am _____
11. ung _____
12. L _____
13. g _____
14. lot _____
15. IT _____
16. PV _____
17. SL _____
18. Q8h _____
19. Tbsp _____
20. pc _____
21. mL _____
22. c̄ _____
23. AD _____
24. ↑ _____
25. po _____
26. OU _____
27. rep _____
28. NPO _____
29. syr _____
30. oz _____
31. # or lb _____
32. c _____
33. pt _____
34. mcg _____
35. mg _____
36. pr _____
37. STAT _____
38. qs _____
39. kg _____
40. gal _____
41. OTC _____
42. ad lib _____
43. aa̅ _____
44. IV _____
45. bid _____
46. prn _____
47. tab _____
48. fl or f _____
49. tsp _____
50. gtt _____
51. supp _____
52. DAW _____
53. Rx _____
54. < _____
55. top _____
56. U _____
57. NKDA _____
58. TO _____
59. q week _____
60. IM _____

61. qd _____
62. tid _____
63. cr _____
64. qid _____
65. qt _____
66. m _____
67. gr _____
68. s̄ _____
69. VO _____
70. OS _____
71. " _____

72. Which three of the above abbreviations are on TJC Official "Do Not Use List"?
_____

Chapter 2

Round decimal answers to nearest hundredth if necessary/reduce all fractions to simplest terms.

1. 12 • 14 =
2. 13 ÷ 1.1 =
3. 43.2 • 3.6 =
4. 4.21 • 4.8 =
5. 53.6 ÷ 1.6 =
6. 7.2 ÷ 0.9 =
7. 43.61 − 12.68 =
8. 3.91 + 8.78 =
9. 831 − 6.32 =
10. 43.71 + 2.6 =
11. $\frac{1}{4} - \frac{1}{6} =$
12. $\frac{3}{8} + \frac{1}{4} =$
13. $\frac{5}{8} + \frac{5}{10} + \frac{2}{5} =$
14. $\frac{5}{16} - \frac{3}{32} =$
15. $\frac{3}{11} \cdot \frac{4}{6} =$
16. $\frac{5}{8} \cdot \frac{1}{2} =$
17. $1\frac{2}{3} \cdot \frac{5}{6} =$
18. $\frac{3}{4} \div \frac{1}{2} =$
19. $\frac{4}{5} \div \frac{5}{8} =$
20. $2\frac{1}{3} \div 7 =$

21. If 480 mL of medication is available in stock and a prescription calls for ¼ of this amount, how many milliliters of the medication are needed to fill the prescription?

22. A patient wants 1/2 of a prescription that costs $45. What is the cost to the patient?

23. A customer buys front merchandise that costs $2.98, $5.36, $1.69, and $3.45. How much change should be given to the customer from a 20-dollar bill?

24. A patient is ordered to take three 75 mg tablets each morning. How many milligrams is this?

25. A patient is prescribed 16 oz of medication with instructions to use 1/16 of the bottle at bedtime every night. How much should be used each night?

Convert the following percents to decimals.

26. 33% =

27. 1.5% =

28. 100% =

29. 14% =

30. 230% =

Convert the following percents to fractions and reduce to lowest terms.

31. 50% =

32. 4% =

33. 0.25% =

34. 76% =

35. 320% =

Convert the following decimals to percents.

36. 6.8 =

37. 0.3 =

38. 0.01 =

39. 0.75 =

40. 1.0 =

Convert the following fractions to percents.

41. $\dfrac{1}{2} =$

42. $\dfrac{3}{4} =$

43. $\dfrac{1}{8} =$

44. $\dfrac{3}{10} =$

45. $\dfrac{1}{3} =$

Convert the following fractions to decimals.

46. $\dfrac{1}{3} =$

47. $\dfrac{2}{3} =$

48. $\dfrac{3}{25} =$

49. $\dfrac{3}{2} =$

50. $\dfrac{5}{6} =$

Convert the following decimals to fractions and reduce to lowest terms.

51. 0.5 =

52. 0.8 =

53. 0.02 =

54. 0.96 =

55. 0.001 =

Express the following as ratios in lowest terms.

56. 2 mg : 14 mg

57. 0.6%

58. 20 : 200

59. $\dfrac{3}{6}$

60. 50 cents to 1 dollar

Solve the following proportions for x. Round to the nearest hundredth if necessary.

61. 6 is to 12 as 5 is to x

62. 5 is to 15 as x is to 45

63. 13 : 39 :: 1 : x

64. $\dfrac{20 \text{ mg}}{1 \text{ tab}} = \dfrac{60 \text{ mg}}{x}$

65. $\dfrac{250 \text{ mg}}{5 \text{ mL}} = \dfrac{750 \text{ mg}}{x}$

Calculate the following rounding to the hundredths place if necessary.

66. What is 10% of 25?

67. What is 25% of 14?

68. What is 50% of 180 mL?

69. 14 is what percent of 28?

70. 3 is what percent of 15?

71. 45 is what percent of 180?

72. 30 is 25% of what number?

73. 50 is 80% of what number?

74. 0.5% of 500 mL of a preparation must be cherry flavoring. How many mL of cherry flavoring are needed?

75. A patient wants 20% of their prescription of 180 capsules. How many capsules should you prepare?

Chapter 3

Change the following to either Roman numerals or Arabic numbers as appropriate.

1. xli
2. 93
3. xlv
4. 72
5. cxxix
6. 59
7. CD
8. 25
9. XCIX
10. 2018

Change the following to 12 or 24-hour time as appropriate.

11. 11:40 AM
12. 7:17 PM
13. 1200
14. 0030
15. 1:35 AM
16. 2:03 AM
17. 2112
18. 8:00 AM
19. 0622
20. 4:32 PM

Convert the following temperatures to Celsius or Fahrenheit as appropriate.

21. 102.6° F

22. 90° C

23. 89.6° F

24. 14.2° C

25. 32° F

26. 98.6° F

27. 5° C

28. 100° F

29. 8° C

30. 10° F

Answer the following.

31. A physician wants medication to be given at 6:00 AM, 2:00 PM, and 10:00 PM. What are these times on the 24-hour clock?

32. The hospital uses the 24-hour clock, but the nurse remembers hanging an IV at noon to run over 8 hours. When should the next one be due?

33. If a medication is given at 9:30 AM and the next dose is to be given in 6 hours, what is the time for administration using the 24-hour clock?

34. The temperature in a patient's room is 22.5° C. What is the temperature in Fahrenheit?

35. If a prescription specifies xxx tablets, how many should be dispensed?

36. A prescription requires iv ounces of a medication. How many ounces of medication should be supplied?

37. A patient's temperature was measured at 40° C. What is this in ° F? Would this be cause for alarm?

38. A prescription is written for gr v of one medication to be combined with gr vi of another. How many grains will there be in total?

39. A medicine is scheduled for administration at 8:00 AM, 12:00 PM, 4:00 PM, and 8:00 PM. How should the nurse record these times in the patient's chart?

40. An IV needs to be hung at 0630, 1430, and 2230. What are these times using the 12-hour clock?

41. The pharmacy has the thermostat set at 72° F. What is the temperature in Celsius?

42. If a medication is given at 8:30 AM and the next dose is to be given in 4 hours, what is the time for administration on the 24-hour clock?

Chapter 4

Rewrite the following using the appropriate numerals and abbreviations (or numerals and symbols with the apothecary system).

1. twenty five milligrams
2. forty milliequivalents
3. ten grains
4. three teaspoonful
5. four fluid ounces (apothecary system)
6. two hundred pounds
7. six cups
8. 250 micrograms
9. 2 drops
10. 8 fluid drams
11. two and one half pints
12. three and one half liters
13. six and one half drams
14. three and one fourth drams
15. ten and one half milliliters
16. nine minims
17. two and two thirds quarts
18. one hundredth grain
19. sixteen fluid ounces (apothecary system)
20. forty units

Complete the following equivalencies

21. 1 Tbsp = _____ tsp
22. 1 qt = _____ pt
23. 1 g = _____ mg
24. 1 L = _____ mL
25. fl℥ i = _____ fl ʒ
26. 1 kg = _____ g
27. 1 gal = _____ qt
28. 1 mg = _____ mcg
29. 1 oz = _____ Tbsp
30. 1 c = _____ oz

Chapter 5

Answer the following, making sure to use the appropriate numerals and symbols for each system. Be sure to use leading zeros and avoid trailing zeros. Show your work.

1. 8 oz = _____ #
2. 3 Tbsp = _____ oz
3. 5′ = _____ ″
4. 6 tsp = _____ Tbsp
5. 10 gtt = _____ mL
6. 500 mg = _____ g
7. 6 qt = _____ gal
8. 3.2 L = _____ mL
9. 0.5 mL = _____ L
10. 2 Tbsp = _____ tsp
11. 144 oz = _____ pt
12. 0.025 g = _____ mg
13. 12 tsp = _____ Tbsp
14. 16 oz = _____ c

15. 4½ Tbsp = _____ tsp
16. ʒ xxiv = ʒ _____
17. ʒii = ɱ _____
18. 0.001 kg = _____ mg
19. 2 oz = _____ c
20. 250 mL = _____ L

21. Premarin (conjugated estrogens) for hormone replacement therapy is available in 0.625 mg tablets. How many micrograms is this?

22. A prescription is written for flʒ iv. How many flʒ would this be?

23. A physician orders a medication be mixed in 6 oz of water before drinking. How many cups of water should be used to prepare the medication?

24. A compounded prescription calls for 0.005 g of powdered medication. How many mg should be measured?

25. A prescription for a foot soak calls for 1,500 mL of water to be added to 1 g of powder. How many liters of water should be added?

26. An order is written 0.02 g of medication to be taken qid. How many mg are needed for one dose?

27. A medication is available in 250 mg tablets. How many g is this?

28. Lanoxin (digoxin) for congestive heart failure is available as 0.125 mg per tablet. How many micrograms is this?

29. A physician orders Glucophage (metformin) 500 mg twice a day with meals for a Type II diabetic. How many grams will the patient take in one day?

30. A compounded prescription calls for 1 liter of fluid. One fourth of this amount is water. How many mL of water are needed?

31. A patient is 6¼ feet tall. How many inches is he?

32. A patient is taking 500 mg of amoxicillin every 8 hours for bronchitis. How many grams is the patient receiving per day?

33. A patient is prescribed 1 g of antibiotic per day in 4 divided doses. How many milligrams is the patient to receive per dose?

34. A doctor recommends drinking eight eight-ounce glasses of water per day. How many gallons is this?

35. A formulation for a batch of antiseptic calls for 14 quarts of water. How many gallons is this?

Chapter 6

Answer the following, making sure to use the appropriate numerals and symbols for each system. Be sure to use leading zeros and avoid trailing zeros. Show your work.

1. 3 tsp = _____ mL
2. 50 gtt = _____ mL
3. 110# = _____ kg
4. 2 pt = _____ mL
5. 240 mL = _____ qt
6. 100 gtt = _____ mL
7. codeine gr iss = _____ mg
8. gr 1/60 = _____ mg
9. 168# = _____ kg
10. 1 c = _____ mL
11. 120 mL = _____ pt
12. 220 # = _____ kg
13. 4 Tbsp = _____ mL
14. 5′8″ = _____ cm
15. 325 mg of aspirin = gr _____
16. 10 oz = _____ mL
17. 2 tsp = _____ mL
18. 2 Tbsp = _____ mL
19. 12 kg = _____ #
20. 37.5 mL = _____ Tbsp

21. An adult places a NTG SL tablet gr 1/150 under his tongue for chest pain. How many milligrams is this?

22. If a patient is prescribed 30 mL of medication, how many tablespoons would this be?

23. A patient is to take 30 mL of an antacid. How many teaspoons should the patient take?

24. A child weighs 68 #. How many kilograms does the child weigh?

25. A female is 5′5″ tall. What is her height in centimeters?

26. Three fourths of a pint of medication is on the shelf. How many milliliters are left in the container?

27. A prescription requires 90 mL of Zantac (ranitidine) for GERD (gastroesophageal reflux disease). How many ounces are needed to fill this prescription?

28. A medication order in a hospital reads Tylenol (acetaminophen) gr xv ASAP for headache. How many milligrams is this?

29. A prescription calls for 6 oz of cough medicine. How many mL is this?

30. A premature baby weighs 5½ #. How many *grams* is this?

Chapter 7

Write the instructions, as they should appear on the patient's label. Remember to use the metric system with liquids and use numerals instead of writing out the words.

1. Rx: doxycycline 100 mg
   Sig: i tab po bid × 7d
   Stock available: doxycycline 100 mg tablets (antibiotic)

2. Rx: Lanoxin (digoxin) 0.25 mg
   #30
   Sig: i tab daily in am if P ↑60 bpm
   Stock: Lanoxin 250 mcg tablets (for congestive heart failure)

3. Rx: Keppra (levetiracetam) 500 mg
   #60
   Sig: i tab po bid
   Stock: Keppra 500 mg tablets (anticonvulsant)

4. Rx: amoxicillin suspension 250 mg/5 mL
   150 mL
   Sig: 1 tsp tid until gone
   Stock: amoxicillin 250 mg/5 mL for oral suspension 150 mL bottle (antibiotic)

5. Rx: Prozac (fluoxetine) 20 mg
   #90
   Sig: i cap po qam
   Stock: fluoxetine 20 mg capsules (antidepressant)

6. Rx: Synthroid (levothroxine) 25 mcg
   #90
   Sig: i tab qam ā eating c̄ full glass of water
   Stock: Synthroid 25 mcg tablets (thyroid replacement)

   _____

7. Rx: Zocor (simvastatin) 5 mg
   #30
   Sig: i tab po qpm c̄ low fat snack
   Stock: Zocor 5 mg tablets (antihypercholesterolemic)

   _____

8. Rx: Zyban (bupropion) 150 mg
   #60
   Sig: i tab qam and i tab 8 hours later × 7 weeks
   Stock: Zyban 150 mg tablets (smoking cessation aid)

   _____

9. Rx: diltiazem 30 mg
   #120
   Sig: i tab qid ac and at bedtime
   Stock: diltiazem 30 mg tablets (for angina – chest pain)

   _____

10. Rx: Xanax (alprazolam) 0.25 mg
    #60
    Sig: i to ii tabs bid prn anxiety
    Stock: alprazolam 0.25 mg tablets

    _____

11. Rx: Xalatan (latanoprost ophthalmic)
    Sig: i gtt OU qpm
    Stock available: Xalatan Ophthalmic 2.5 mL bottle (for glaucoma)

    _____

12. Rx: Temovate (clobetasol) cream 0.05%
    Sig: apply to aā bid
    Stock available: clobetasol 0.05% cream (steroid for itching) 30 g tube

    _____

13. Rx: Levaquin (levofloxacin) 250 mg
    Sig: i tab qd × 5d
    Stock available: levofloxacin 250 mg tablets (antibiotic)

    _____

14. Rx: Ventolin HFA
    Sig: 2 puffs po 15-30 min ā exercise
    Stock available: Ventolin HFA (albuterol) 1.8 g Oral Inhaler (for asthma)

    _____

15. Rx: Humulin R
    10 mL
    Sig: 15 units SUBCUT tid ac
    Stock available: Humulin R 10 mL vial

    _____

Interpret the following medication orders. Remember interpreting is only writing the order without abbreviations.

16. acetaminophen gr x q6h prn fever

    _____

17. Norco 5/325 q6h × 24h post-op

    _____

18. cephalexin suspension 500 mg po q12h

    _____

19. Vistaril 50 mg IM STAT

    _____

20. Discontinue amoxicillin; start Bactrim DS po bid

    _____

21. Lunesta 1 mg po at bedtime prn sleep

    _____

22. labetalol 5-10 mg IV q4h prn BP > 150/90

    _____

    _____

23. cefazolin 500 mg IM q8h

24. furosemide 80 mg po qam

25. Singulair 10 mg qpm

26. Reglan 10 mg po qid 30 min ac and at bedtime

27. digoxin 0.25 mg po qam

28. Epogen 20 units/kg SUBCUT on Mon, Wed, Sat

29. Narcan 0.2 mg IV stat; may rep until desired response up to 0.8 mg total

30. cefazolin 1 g IV 1 hr pre-op and q8h post-op × 24 h

Answer the following questions about the labels.

31.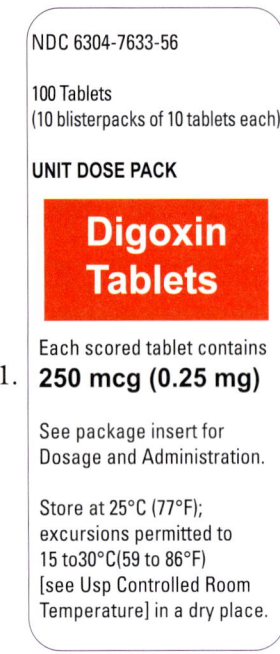

What is the type of packaging for this medication? _____

How many tablets are found in the total package? _____

What is the strength of the medication in mcg? _____ in mg? _____

What are the storage requirements of the medication? _____
_____

What is the dosage form of the medication? _____

32.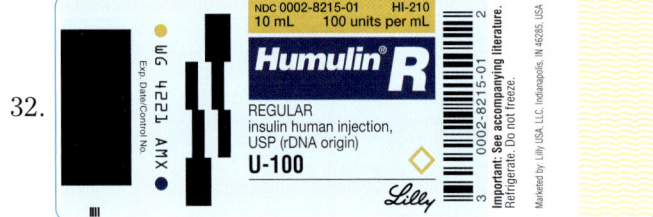

What is the dosage form of this medication? _____

Who manufactures this medication? _____

What type capsules are found in this container? _____

How many capsules are in the container? _____

Chapter 8

Determine the dose to administer. Assume generic substitution is permitted.

1. Dose ordered: Avapro 300 mg
   Stock available: irbesartan 150 mg tablets

2. Dose ordered: Cardura 2 mg
   Stock available: doxazosin 1 mg tablets

3. Dose ordered: ampicillin 250 mg
   Stock available: ampicillin 125 mg capsules

4. Dose ordered: Decadron 0.75 mg
   Stock available: dexamethasone 1.5 mg tablets

5. Dose ordered: Accupril 5 mg
   Stock available: quinapril 5 mg tablets

6. Dose ordered: aspirin 325 mg
   Stock available: aspirin gr v tablets

7. Dose ordered: Robaxin (methocarbamol) 1,500 mg
   Stock available: methocarbamol 500 mg tablets

8. Dose ordered: Protonix (pantoprazole) 40 mg
   Stock available: Protonix 20 mg tablets

9. Dose ordered: Paxil (paroxetine) 10 mg
   Stock available: Paxil 20 mg tablets

10. Dose ordered: Accupril (quinapril) 7.5 mg
    Stock available: Accupril 5 mg tablets

Determine the dose to administer and write directions, as they should appear on the patient's label.

11. Prescription: Lyrica (pregabalin) 150 mg bid
    Stock available: Lyrica 75 mg capsules (anticonvulsant)

12. Prescription: Relafen (nabumetone) 1 g qd with or without food for arthritis pain
    Stock available: Relafen 500 mg tablets

13. Prescription: Adipex-P (phentermine) 18.75 mg bid one hour before breakfast and dinner
    Stock available: Adipex-P 37.5 mg tablets (weight loss agent)

14. Prescription: Zyloprim 200 mg q8h for severe gout
    Stock available: allopurinal 100 mg tablets

    _____

15. Prescription: Elavil 40 mg at bedtime
    Stock available: amitriptylline 10 mg tablets (antidepressant)

    _____

16. Prescription: Zithromax (azithromycin) 500 mg po now, then 250 mg po qd × 4d
    Stock available: azithromycin 250 mg tablets (antibiotic)

    _____

    _____

17. Prescription: Elavil 10 mg po tid and 20 mg at bedtime
    Stock available: amitriptylline 10 mg tablets (antidepressant)

    _____

18. Prescription: Seroquel (quetiapine) 50 mg po at bedtime on first day, 100 mg po at bedtime on second day, 200 mg po at bedtime on third day, and then 300 mg po at bedtime
    Stock available: quetiapine 50 mg tablets (antipsychotic)

    _____

    _____

    _____

19. Prescription: Klonopin (clonazepam) 0.25 mg po bid
    Stock available: clonazepam 0.5 mg tablets (antianxiety/anticonvulsant)

    _____

20. Prescription: Namenda (memantine) 10 mg po bid
    Stock available: Namenda 10 mg tablets (Alzheimer's agent)

    _____

Chapter 9

1. Order: Vibramycin oral suspension 100 mg
   Stock strength available: doxycycline 25 mg/5 mL suspension
   What is the volume of the daily dose?

2. Order: phenobarbital elixir 15 mg
   Stock available: phenobarbital 20 mg/5 mL elixir
   What is the *measurable* volume of medication for this dose?

3. Order: Benadryl elixir 50 mg
   Stock available: diphenhydramine elixir 12.5 mg/5 mL
   What is the volume for one dose?

4. Order: acetaminophen suspension 400 mg
   Stock available: Children's acetaminophen liquid suspension 160 mg/5 mL
   What is the volume for the dose?

5. Order: cephalexin 375 mg tid
   Strength dispensed: cephalexin 250 mg/5 mL oral suspension
   What volume of medication should be taken per dose

6. Order: Pepcid (famotidine) oral suspension 30 mg bid
   Strength dispensed: famotidine 40 mg/5 mL oral suspension
   What is the *measurable* volume of medication for this dose?

7. Order: methylphenidate solution 5 mg bid before breakfast and lunch for ADHD
   Strength dispensed: methylphenidate oral solution 10 mg/5 mL
   What volume of medication should be taken per dose?

8. Order: Colace (docusate sodium) 60 mg
   Strength available: docusate sodium syrup 20 mg/5 mL
   What is the volume for the dose?

9. Order: Dynapen (dicloxacillin) 125 mg
   Strength available: dicloxacillin suspension 62.5 mg/5 mL
   What is the volume for the dose?

10. Order: Diflucan (fluconazole) 25 mg
    Strength available: fluconazole suspension 10 mg/mL
    What is the volume for the dose?

Determine the dose to administer and write directions, as they should appear on the patient's label.

11. Prescription: Prozac (fluoxetine) 30 mg po qam
    Strength available: fluoxetine oral solution 20 mg/5 mL

    _____

12. Prescription: Lanoxin (digoxin) 0.125 mg po qam
    Stock strength: Lanoxin Elixir 50 mcg/mL

    _____

13. Prescription: Zantac (ranitidine) 45 mg po bid 30 min ac
    Stock strength: Zantac syrup 15 mg/mL

    _____
    _____

14. Prescription: nitrofurantoin 100 mg po qid with food × 7d
    Stock available: nitrofurantoin oral suspension 25 mg/5 mL

    _____
    _____

15. Prescription: Septra DS i po q12h × 10d (patient requires liquid medications)
    Stock available: Septra DS tablets: 800 mg sulfamethoxazole and 160 mg trimethoprim
    Oral Susp: 200 mg sulfamethoxazole and 40 mg trimethoprim /5 mL

    _____

16. Prescription: nystatin 400,000 units po ½ dose in each side of mouth qid, swish as long as possible and swallow
    Stock available: nystatin oral suspension 500,000 units/5 mL

    ___

    ___

    ___

17. Prescription: amoxicillin 300 mg po q8h
    Stock available: amoxicillin 125 mg/5 mL oral suspension

    ___

18. Prescription: penicillin V potassium 62.5 mg po qid
    Stock available: penicillin V potassium 125 mg/5 mL oral suspension

    ___

19. Prescription: Risperdal (risperidone) 3 mg po qd
    Stock strength: risperidone 1 mg/mL

    ___

20. Prescription: griseofulvin 500 mg po q12h with a high fat snack × 6 mo
    Stock strength: griseofulvin oral suspension 125 mg/5 mL

    ___

    ___

Chapter 10

1. Medication order: gentamicin 5 mg IM
   Stock strength: gentamicin 20 mg/2 mL injection
   What volume of medication should be administered?

   What size syringe should be used for administration? ___

2. Medication order: diazepam 10 mg IM
   Stock strength: 5 mg/mL injection
   What volume of medication should be administered?

   What size syringe should be used for administration? ___

3. A physician orders Acthar Gel 40 Units IM
   Stock strength: Acthar Gel 80 units/mL
   What volume of medication should be administered?

   What syringe should be used for administration? _____

4. Medication order: KCl 5 mEq
   Stock available: potassium chloride injection 10 mEq/5 mL vial
   What volume of medication should be administered?

   What syringe should be used for administration? _____

5. Medication order: penicillin 250,000 units
   Strength: The vial is reconstituted to 500,000 units/mL.
   What volume of medication should be administered?

   What syringe should be used for administration? _____

6. Medication order: meperidine 50 mg and promethazine 25 mg IM stat
   Strengths available: meperidine 100 mg/mL and promethazine 25 mg/mL
   What volume of meperidine should be administered?

   What volume of promethazine should be administered?

   What the total dose volume of this order? _____

7. Medication order: codeine sulfate 48 mg IM stat
   Stock available: codeine sulfate 60 mg/mL.
   What volume of medication should be administered per dose?

   What syringe should be used for administration? _____

8. Medication order: Vitamin B-12 0.25 mg subcut
   Stock strength: cyanocobalamin (B-12) 10,000 mcg/10 mL.
   What volume of medication should be administered?

   What syringe should be used for the administration? _____

9. Medication order: prochlorperazine 6 mg IM
   Stock strength: prochlorperazine injection 5 mg/mL
   What volume of medication should be administered?

   What size syringe should be used for administration? _____

10. Medication order: prochlorperazine 10 mg IM, rep q 3 to 4 hours prn
    Stock strength: prochlorperazine injection 5 mg/mL
    What volume of medication should be administered?

    What size syringe should be used for administration? _____

11. Medication order: gentamicin 15 mg IM
    Stock strength: gentamicin 20 mg/2 mL injection
    What volume of medication should be administered?

    What size syringe should be used for administration? _____

12. Medication order: aminophylline 65 mg IV
    Stock strength: aminophylline 25 mg/mL injection
    What volume of medication is needed?

    What size syringe should be used for administration? _____

13. Medication order: Ativan (lorazepam) 1 mg IM
    Stock strengths available: lorazepam injection 2 mg/mL and 4 mg/mL
    Which strength should be chosen for the smallest volume per dose? _____
    How much is needed using this strength?

    Lorazepam requires a 1:1 dilution with normal saline or sterile water for injection to facilitate IM administration.
    How much normal saline needs to be added to the above dose? _____
    What size syringe should be used for administration? _____

14. Medication order: Lasix (furosemide) 10 mg IM
    Stock strength: furosemide injection 40 mg/4 mL
    What volume of medication should be administered?

    What size syringe should be used for administration? _____

15. Lanoxin (digoxin) 0.125 mg IV
    Strength available: Lanoxin Injection 500 mcg/2 mL
    What volume of medication should be administered?

    What size syringe should be used for administration? _____

16. Medication order: Dilaudid 1-2 mg IM q 2-3h prn for severe pain
    Stock available: 1 mL ampules of Dilaudid (hydromorphone) Injection in the following strengths: 1 mg/mL, 2 mg/mL, and 4 mg/mL
    Interpret the order:
    _____
    _____

    Considering the fact that Dilaudid is a CII medication that requires documentation if any is wasted, which ampule should be chosen for the 1 mg dose? _____

    What volume is needed from this ampule for the 1 mg dose? _____

17. Medication order: Dilaudid 750 mcg IM stat
    Stock available: 1 mL ampules of Dilaudid (hydromorphone) Injection in the following strengths: 1 mg/mL, 2 mg/mL, and 4 mg/mL
    What volume of medication would be administered using the 1 mg/mL strength?

    What volume of medication would be administered using the 2 mg/mL strength?

    What volume of medication would be administered using the 4 mg/mL strength?

    Which of the above strengths will provide a dose that is most exact (does not require rounding to a measureable dose? _____

    How many mcg would each of the other strengths provide once rounded to a measurable dose?

18. Medication order: Solu-Medrol 75 mg IM stat
    Stock available: Solu-Medrol (methylprednisolone sodium succinate) 125 mg/2 mL Inj
    What volume of medication should be administered?

    What size syringe should be used for administration? _____

19. Valium (diazepam) 3 mg IM
    Stock available: diazepam injection 5 mg/mL
    What volume of medication should be administered?

    What size syringe should be used for administration? _____

20. Medication order: Zosyn 3.375 g IV infusion over 30 min q6h
    Stock strength: Zocyn Injection (3 g piperacillin/0.375 g tazobactam) *This medication appears different than most combination products since the strength of the two ingredients are listed together as 3.375 g*
    Interpret the order:

    _____

    _____

    Direction for reconstitution: Add 15 mL of sterile water for injection to completely dissolve the powder, then qs (add a sufficient quantity) with 0.9% sodium chloride for injection to 50 mL.
    What volume will then contain the required dose to be infused? _____

21. Medication order: streptomycin 300 mg IM daily. Use the following label:

    Streptomycin Sulfate, USP
    Equivalent to 5.0 g of Streptomycin Base
    5.0 g
    For intramuscular use only

    Recommended Storage in dry form. Store below 86°F (30°C)
    Sterile reconstituted solutions should be protected from light and may be stored at room temperature for four weeks without significant loss of potency.

    Knowledge Pharmaceuticals
    St. Louis, MO 63043

    Usual Daily Dosage
    Adults: Varies, consult package insert
    Adult average single injection 0.5 – 1.0 g

mL diluent added	mg/mL of solution
9.0 mL	400 mg/mL

    The dry powder is dissolved by adding Water for injection, USP or Sodium Chloride Injection, USP in an amount to yield the desired concentration.
    Patient: _____
    Room No: _____
    Date Diluted: _____

    What volume of diluent should be added to the vial? _____
    What diluent should be used for this reconstitution? _____

    _____

    What is the dosage strength of the medication following reconstitution? _____
    What are the storage requirements following reconstitution?

    _____

    _____

    What volume of medication should be administered per dose?
    What syringe should be used for the administration? _____

22. Medication order: Zithromax 500 mg IV qd × 2 days; follow with 500 mg po × 5 days

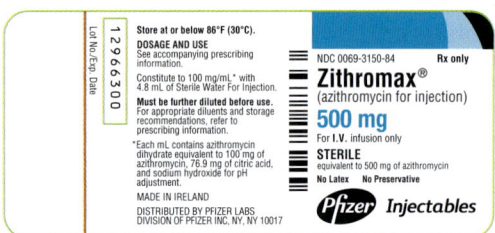

What volume of diluent should be added to the vial? _____

What diluent should be used for reconstitution? _____

What is the dosage strength of the medication following reconstitution? _____

What is the additional requirement before using?
_____

What volume of medication should be used for each daily dose?

Chapter 11

Calculate the following. Remember to round to the nearest hundredth if the answer is less than 1 mL and tenths if the answer is greater than 1 mL.

1. A physician orders Humulin 70/30 50 units subcut qam and Humulin R 32 units subcut qpm

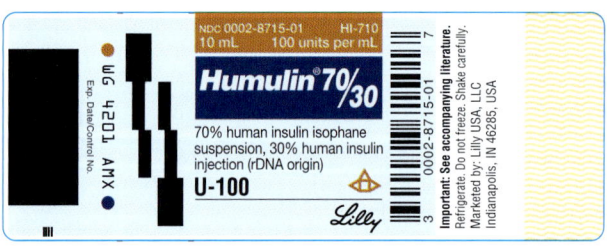

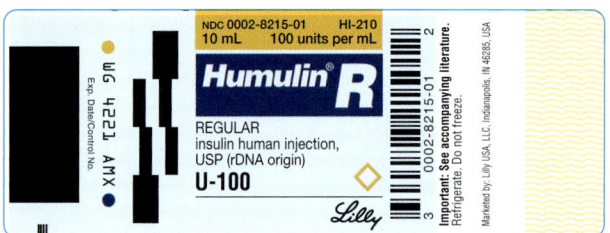

How many units of the Humulin 70/30 dose are regular insulin? _____

What are the total units of regular insulin that the patient receives in a day? _____

What size syringe should be used for administration of the morning dose? _____

What size syringe should be used for administration of the evening dose? _____

2. Medication order: Humulin R 85 units as an IV additive
   Stock available: 10-mL vial of Humulin R U-100
   How many mL of Humulin R U-100 are needed? _____

3. Dose ordered: Humulin R 20 units subcut qam

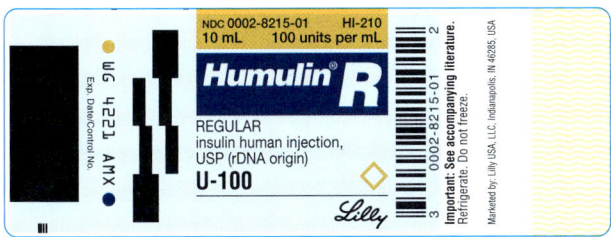

   What size insulin syringe should be used for administration of the dose? _____

4. Prescription: Humulin R 10 units and Humulin N 25 units subcut qam

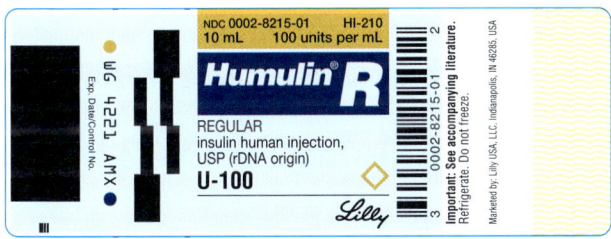

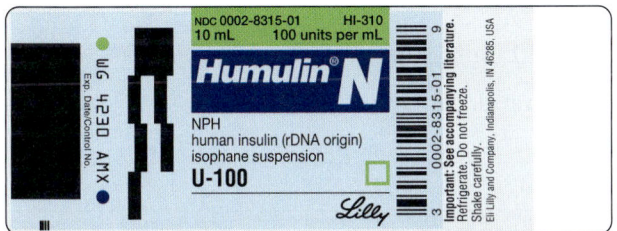

   What volume (mL) of Regular insulin is needed per dose? _____
   What volume (mL) of NPH insulin is needed per dose? _____
   What total volume is needed if they are drawn in the same syringe? _____
   What is the proper procedure for drawing them up in the same syringe? _____
   _____

Mark the amount of regular insulin needed on the first syringe, the amount of NPH insulin needed on the second, and the *total* amount of insulin needed on the final syringe.

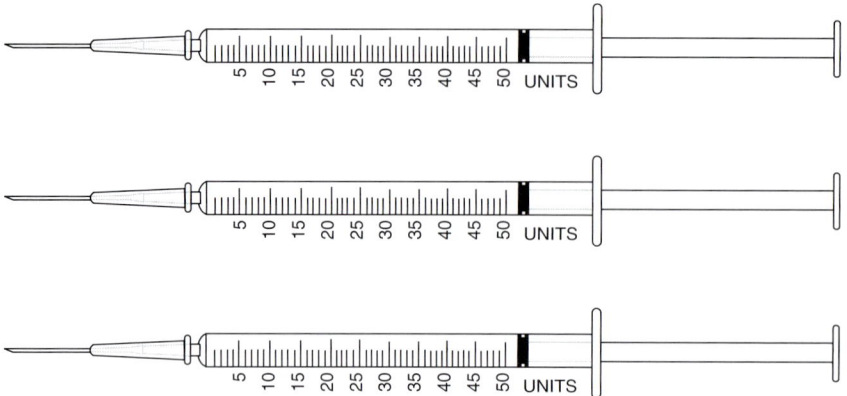

5. Prescription: Lantus 20 units subcut qam
   Stock strength: Lantus (insulin glargine injection) 100 units/mL (10 mL vial)
   Only a 1-mL TB syringe is available. The physician approves its use in this instance.

   How many mL should be administered? _____

6. Prescription: 18 units of regular insulin and 35 units of NPH subcut qam
   Strengths available: as shown in question #4

   What size insulin syringe must be used to draw them up as a single injection? _____

7. Medication order: add 40 units of insulin to the IV

   What is the only type of insulin that can be used in this instance? _____

8. Order: Lantus 10 units and Humulin R 40 units subcut qam

   List the syringe(s) needed for the morning dose. _____

   Explain your answer. _____
   _____

9. Lantus (insulin glargine) is manufactured as U-100 insulin with 100 units/mL
   Toujeo (insulin glargine) is manufactured as U-300 insulin with 300 units/mL.
   If a patient is stabilized on 30 units of Lantus qd, theoretically, what would be the equivalent dose in mL of Toujeo? _____

10. A physician orders Humulin 70/30 40 units subcut qam
    How many units of regular insulin does the patient receive per day?

    How many units of NPH insulin does the patient receive per day?

Use the following labels for the questions about heparin dosing.

A.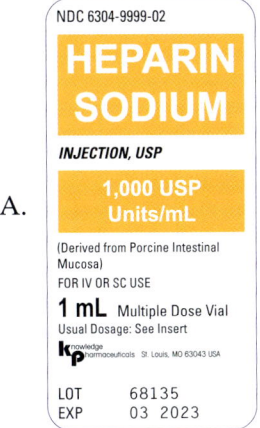

B.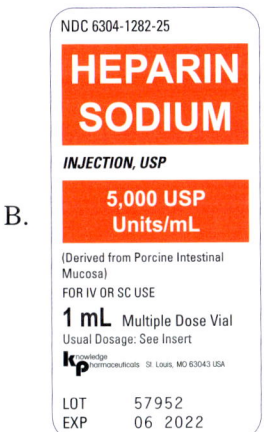

C.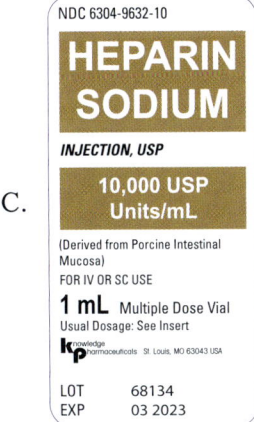

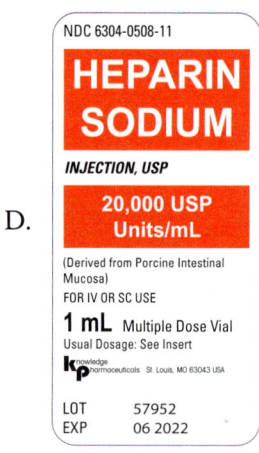

D.

11. Medication order: heparin 350 units subcut
    Stock strength: heparin sodium 1,000 USP units/mL
    What is the volume of the dose to be given?

12. Medication order: heparin 2,500 units subcut
    Which of the stock strengths above would provide the smallest dose volume with the most accuracy (without having to round the answer). _____

    How many mL are needed to provide the appropriate dose using the chosen strength?

    Indicate this volume on the following syringe:

    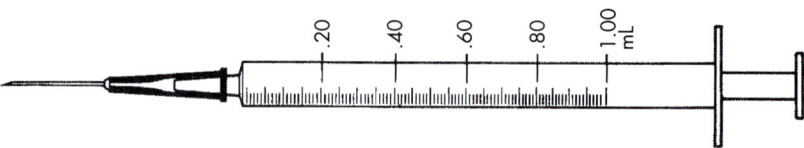

13. Medication order: Fragmin 4,000 International units subcut
    Supplied: FRAGMIN (dalteparin) 10,000 units/mL (9.5 mL vial)
    What volume of medication should be given to this patient?

    Show the dose on the following syringe:

    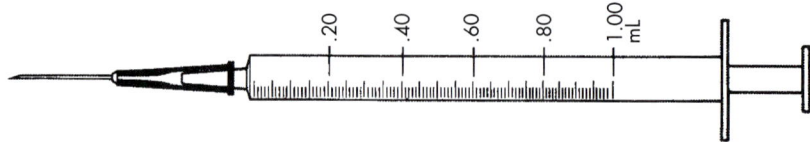

14. Medication order: heparin sodium 16,000 units subcut stat
    Which of the stock strengths above would provide the smallest dose volume? _____
    What volume should be administered to the patient?

15. Medication order: heparin 12,000 units subcut
    Which of the stock strengths above would provide the smallest dose volume? _____
    Show the correct dose on the syringe below using the chosen strength.

    What volume should be administered to the patient?

    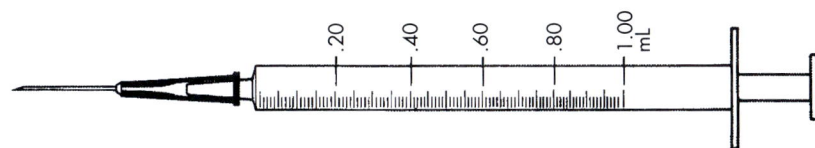

16. Medication order: heparin 400 units subcut
    Calculate the volume needed for this dose using each of the above strengths.
    A

    B

    C

    D

    Which of the strengths would provide the most accurate dose? _____

17. Medication order: heparin 4,000 units subcut
    Stock strength: use vial C above
    What volume should be administered to the patient?

18. Medication order: Fragmin 1,600 International units subcut stat
    Supplied: FRAGMIN 10,000 units/mL (9.5 mL vial)
    What volume of medication should be administered?

    If this is the first dose taken from the vial, what volume is left in the vial? _____
    Show the correct dose on the following syringe.

    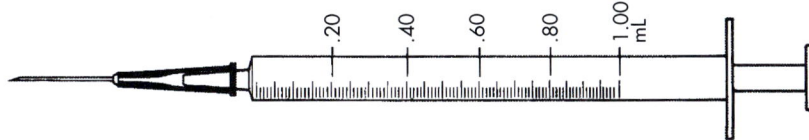

19. Medication order: heparin 14,000 units subcut
    Stock strength: use vial D above
    What volume should be administered to the patient?

20. Medication order: heparin 800 units subcut
    Stock strength: use vial A above
    What volume should be administered to the patient?

Chapter 12

Identify which method to use (Clark's Rule, Fried's Rule, Young's Rule, Body Weight, or BSA) and calculate the answers. Round to the hundredth if the dose is less than 1 mL and tenth if over 1 mL. Pay close attention to how both the order and the questions are presented as in per day or per dose. Also pay attention to how the medication is ordered in terms of once a day, bid, single dose, divided doses, etc.

1. An 8-month old child is to take a medication with a normal adult dose of 75 mg/*dose*.
   What method should be used? _____
   What is the approximate dose that should be given to the infant?

2. A child weighs 30 lb and the normal adult dose is 50 mg tid.
   What method should be used? _____
   What is the approximate dose for the child?

3. A 46-lb child is 30″ tall. The adult dose of a medication is 15 mg.
   What method should be used? _____
   What is the approximate dose for the child?

4. A 12-year-old child is to take a medication bid. The normal adult dose is 200 mg/*dose*.
   What method should be used? _____
   What is the approximate strength of medication that the child should receive per dose?

   What is the total strength of medication the child should receive in a day?

   If the stock liquid medication strength is 125 mg/5 mL, what volume of medication is required per dose?

5. A 68-pound child is to receive a medication tid. The normal adult dose is 90 mg/day.
    What method should be used? _____
    What is the strength of one dose for the child?

    What is the total strength of the medication the child should receive in a day?

    If the medication is available as 10 mg/5 mL, what volume of mediation should the child receive per dose?

6. A 64-pound child is ordered a medication with an adult dose of 60 mg tid.
    What method should be used? _____
    What is the approximate dose for the child?

7. A 22 lb child is to receive 0.05 mg/kg/day in *two divided* doses.
    What method should be used? _____
    What is the total strength of medication that the child should receive per *day*?

    What is the strength of medication that the child should per *dose*?
    The medication is available as 1 mg/mL.

    What volume of medication should the child receive per *dose*?

8. A physician orders an initial dose of vancomycin of 15 mg/kg for a 187-pound male.
    What method should be used? _____
    How many mg are needed?

9. A female with breast cancer is prescribed paclitaxel 175 mg/m^2 IV over 3 hours every 3 weeks for 4 doses. Her BSA is 1.6 m^2. Paclitaxel is supplied in 6 mg/mL strength.
    What method should be used? _____
    How many mg should she receive?

    How many mL are required for this dose?

    This amount is to be further diluted to 500 mL with 5% dextrose.
    What is the final strength in mg per mL?

10. Medication order: aminophylline 20 mg/kg/*day* for a 72-lb child in *divided doses* q6h
    What method should be used? _____
    Stock strength: aminophylline oral solution 105 mg/5 mL
    How many mL are needed per dose?

11. Prescription: nitrofurantoin 7 mg/kg/*day* given in four *divided doses* for a 39 lb-child
    Stock strength: nitrofurantoin oral suspension 25 mg/5 mL
    What method should be used? _____
    What is the total strength of the medication the child should receive in a day?

    What is the strength of one dose for the child?

    How many mL are needed per dose?

12. Prescription: griseofulvin 10 mg/kg/*day* for a 45-lb child for nail fungus
    Stock strength: griseofulvin oral suspension 125 mg/5 mL
    What method should be used? _____
    What is the strength of one dose for the child?

    How many mL are needed per dose?

13. A 165-lb male is ordered a medication at 10 mg/kg/*dose* q8h
    The stock strength is 300 mg/2 mL
    What method should be used? _____
    How many mL are needed per dose?

14. Medication order: doxorubicin 60 mg/m² IV push q21d (patient's BSA is 1.6 m²)
    Stock sizes available: doxorubicin 50 mg/25 mL vial and 200 mg/100 mL vial for inj
    What method should be used? _____
    How many mL are needed per dose?

    Which size vial(s) should be used to waste the least amount of medication? _____

15. Prescription: Cefzil q12h for a 37.5-lb child/ Adult dose 500 mg q12h
    Stock strength: Cefzil (cefprozil) 125 mg/5 mL oral suspension
    What method should be used? _____
    How many mL are needed per dose?

16. Prescription: Cefzil q12h for a 4-year-old child/ Adult dose 500 mg q12h
    Stock strength: Cefzil (cefprozil) 125 mg/5 mL oral suspension
    What method should be used? _____
    How many mL are needed per dose?

17. Prescription: Cefzil q24h for a 37.5-lb child at a rate of 7.5 mg/kg q12h
    Stock strength: Cefzil (cefprozil) 125 mg/5 mL oral suspension
    What method should be used? _____
    How many mL are needed per dose?

18. Prescription: amoxicillin for a 6-month-old infant /usual adult dose 500 mg qid
    Stock strengths available: amoxicillin 125 mg/5 mL oral suspension
    What method should be used? _____
    How many mL are needed per dose using this strength?

19. Prescription: Lanoxin elixir for a 40-lb child based on 6 mcg/kg/*day* in two *divided doses*
    Stock strength: Lanoxin (digoxin) Pediatric Elixir 50 mcg (0.05 mg)/mL
    What method should be used? _____
    How many mL are needed per dose?

20. A physician orders medication A 100 mg tid for a 60-lb child with a BSA of 0.85 m^2.
    Medication A can be dosed at 118 mg/m^2 *tid* or 10–12 mg/kg/*day* in 3 *divided doses*
    What *dose* would be given if calculated using BSA?

    Is the ordered dose adequate for the child? _____
    Calculate the range for one *dose* using body weight.
    What is the range? _____
    Is the ordered dose within this range? _____

Chapter 13

Answer the following. Consider one month to be 30 days unless otherwise noted.

1. A physician orders Lasix 20 mg qam
   The available medication Lasix (furosemide) 20 mg tablets
   How many tablets are needed for a 1-month supply?

2. A physician orders Valium 7.5 mg at bedtime.
   The available medication is Valium (diazepam) 5 mg tablets
   How many tablets are needed for a 1-month supply?

3. A physician orders Actos 30 mg qd
   The available medication is Actos (pioglitazone) 15 mg tablets
   How many tablets are needed for a 90-day supply?

4. A physician orders Prozac 60 mg qd
   The stock available is Prozac (fluoxetine) 20 mg capsules
   How many capsules would be needed for a 90-day supply?

5. Prescription: methylphenidate solution 10 mg/5 mL
   Sig: 5 mg bid ac breakfast and lunch for ADHD
   How much is needed for a 30-day supply?

6. Prescription: cephalexin 175 mg po q6h X 7d
   Stock available: cephalexin oral suspension 125 mg/5 mL 200 mL
   How many mL are needed for the entire dosage?

   How many bottles should be reconstituted for dispensing (at the time of pick up)?

7. A vaccine contains 2 units/0.5 mL.
   How many 2-unit doses are available in one 5-mL multi-dose vial?

8. A prescription is received for regular insulin 14 units tid pc. What is the days' supply in one 10-mL vial of Humulin R U-100? *(round days' supply down to nearest whole number)*

9. Prescription: Timoptic 0.25% gtt ii right eye bid with 6 refills
   Stock available: timolol 0.25% ophthalmic solution 5 mL and 10 mL
   What is the days' supply in the 5 mL container?

   What is the days' supply in the 10 mL container?

   For sterility purposes the medication should only be used for 4 weeks after opening. Which size should be dispensed? _____

10. Medication order: amoxicillin 250 mg po qid X 7 days
    Stock available: 250 mg capsules
    How many capsules are needed to fill this prescription?

11. An 11-lb infant is to receive erythromycin 40 mg/kg/day in 4 divided doses x 10 days. The medication strength available is erythromycin oral suspension 200 mg/5 mL. How many mg should be given per dose?

    What is the measurable volume to be given per dose?

    How many mL are needed to fill this prescription?

12. A physician orders phenobarbital elixir gr ½ tid
    The available medication strength is phenobarbital elixir 20 mg/5 mL.
    How many doses are in a 480 mL stock bottle? *(use gr i = 60 mg)*

    What is the days' supply to enter for insurance purposes?

13. A physician prescribes cephalexin 125 mg q6h for 10 days.
    How many days would one 100-mL bottle of 125 mg/5 mL cephalexin last?

    How many bottles should be reconstituted for dispensing (at the time of pick up)?

14. Prescription: Tylenol #3 i-ii tabs q4-6h prn pain #60
    Stock available: Tylenol #3: acetaminophen 300 mg and codeine 30 mg/tablet
    What is the days' supply if the maximum amount is taken daily?

    The daily limit of acetaminophen should not exceed 4,000 mg.
    What amount of acetaminophen would this patient receive in one day at the maximum dosage for the prescription?

15. Prescription: Amoxicillin 500 mg 4 times a day for 7 days
    Stock available: Amoxil (amoxicillin) 250 mg/5 mL
    How many mL are needed to fill this prescription?

16. A consumer purchases Benadryl (diphenhydramine) elixir over the counter. The strength of the medication is 12.5 mg diphenhydramine/5 mL.
    How long will the 4-ounce bottle last if she takes 25 mg every night.

What is the days' supply for the following prescriptions? Use the maximum possible doses for all calculations.

17. 280 mL to be taken 5 mL bid
    Days supply: _____

18. 180 tablets to be taken ii tid
    Days supply: _____

19. 480 mL to be taken 1 oz qhs
    Days supply: _____

20. 36 tablets to be taken i-ii q4h prn
    Days supply: _____

21. Rx: Motrin (ibuprofen) 600 mg #120
    Sig: i q6h with food
    Days supply: _____

22. Rx: Xanax (alprazolam) 0.25 mg #60
    Sig: i to ii tabs bid prn anxiety
    Days supply: _____

23. Rx: diltiazem 30 mg #360
    Sig: i tab qid ac and bedtime
    Days supply: _____

24. Rx: Xalatan (latanoprost ophthalmic) 2.5 mL
    Sig: i gtt OU qpm
    Days supply: _____

25. Prescription: Ventolin HFA 60 MDI (metered dose inhalations)
    Sig: ii inh po q4-6h
    Days supply: _____

Chapter 14

1. How many g of dextrose are in 250 mL of D5W?

2. How many g of sodium chloride are in 1,000 mL of ½ NS?

3. How many g of amino acids are in 300 mL of 5.5% Travesol (amino acids)?

4. If 12 g of medication are dissolved in 100 mL of solution, what is the percent strength?

5. How many mL of a 25% solution will provide 5 g of active ingredient?

6. If a 1 g vial of powdered medication is diluted to 10 mL, what is the strength in mg/mL?

7. What is the percent strength of a 50 mg/mL solution?

8. How many g of zinc oxide are needed to prepare 30 g of a 1.5% zinc oxide ointment?

9. What is the concentration in mg/mL of a 1:2,000 solution?

10. What is the weight in mg of NaCl in 100 mL of 0.06% NaCl?

11. What is the percent strength of a 6 mg/mL v/v solution?

12. What is the ratio strength of a 4 mg/mL v/v solution?

13. How many mL of a 0.5% solution can be prepared with only 100 mg of active ingredient?

14. How many grams of active ingredient are in 60 g of a 2.5% ointment?

15. How many g of amino acid are in 300 mL of 8.8% Travesol (amino acids)?

16. How many mL of 50% dextrose are needed to provide 200 g of dextrose?

17. How many g of active ingredient are needed to prepare 250 mL of a 10% solution?

18. How many 400 mg capsules are needed to prepare 120 mL of a 40% solution?

19. How many grams of magnesium sulfate are present in a 50 mL vial of 50% magnesium sulfate injection?

20. How many mg of active ingredient are needed to prepare 60 g of a 1:2,500 w/w ointment?

21. How many grams of Neosporin powder are needed to prepare 2 liters of a 1:1,000 w/v bladder irrigation?

22. Convert 1:20,000 to percentage strength.

23. What is the percentage strength of a 1:100 w/v solution?

24. Convert 1:100,000 w/v to percentage strength.

25. What is the percentage strength of a solution containing 25 g of active ingredient in 500 mL of total solution?

Chapter 15

Solve the following. Round to tenths unless otherwise noted.

1. Order: 30 g of 0.5% ointment. The available active ingredient is 10% ointment.

   How many grams of 10% ointment will be needed to prepare 30 g? _____

   How many grams of petroleum will be needed to prepare 30 g? _____

2. Prepare 400 mL of 6% solution from a stock solution of 7.5% and water.

   How many milliliters of the stock solution are needed? _____

   How many milliliters of the solvent (water) are needed? _____

3. Prepare 15 g of 0.5% ointment from a stock ointment of 2.5% and petrolatum

   How many g of 2.5% ointment will be needed? _____

   How many g of petrolatum will be needed? _____

4. Prepare 1 liter of 15% dextrose from a 50% dextrose solution.

   How many mL of 50% dextrose (stock solution) are needed? _____

   How many mL of solvent (water) are needed? _____

5. What is the percentage strength of the resultant solution if 250 mL of a 10% solution is combined with 750 mL of water? (*Hint: start with determining the "desired" volume*)

6. How much water should be added to 300 mL of a 25% solution to make a 10% solution?

7. If 500 mL of a 1:1,000 solution is diluted to 1,000 mL, what is the ratio strength of the new solution?

8. How much of a 4% solution is needed to make 120 mL of a 1:200 solution?

9. Order: 10 mL of 25 mg/mL solution
   Stock on hand: 60 mL of 100 mg/mL solution *(Hint: not all of the stock will be needed)*

   How many milliliters of the stock solution are needed? _____

   How many milliliters of the solvent (water) are needed? _____

10. If 60 mL of a 15% solution is diluted to 100 mL, what is the percentage strength of the resultant solution?

11. Order: ophthalmic suspension to contain 100 mg in 5 mL
    Stock on hand: 5% ophthalmic suspension in normal saline

    How much 5% suspension is needed? _____

    How much sterile normal saline solution is needed? _____

12. Prepare 250 mL of a 4% solution from a 3% solution and an 8% solution.

    How many mL of 8% solution are needed? _____

    How many mL of 3% solution are needed? _____

13. Prepare 30 g of 1 % ointment from 0.5% ointment and 5% ointment.

    How many g of 5% ointment are needed? _____
    How many g of 0.5% ointment are needed? _____

14. Prepare 400 mL of 6% Travesol solution from 5.5% Travesol and 8.8% Travesol.

    How many mL of 8.8% Travesol are needed? _____
    How many mL of 5.5% Travesol are needed? _____

15. An order for 750 mL of 1:25 solution is to be prepared from 1:100 and 1:20 stock solutions.

    How many milliliters of 1:20 solution are needed? _____
    How many milliliters of 1:100 solution are needed? _____

16. White Ointment, USP contains 5 parts white wax and 95 parts white petrolatum. How many grams of each are needed to prepare 180 g?

    white wax: _____   white petrolatum: _____

17. How much of each ingredient is needed to prepare 30 g of the following? (*do not round*)

    | Ingredient A | 500 mg |
    | Ingredient B | 10 g |
    | Cream Base | 109.5 g |

    What is the percent strength of ingredient A? (*round to nearest tenth*)

18. How much urea is needed to prepare 18 g of the following formulation?

    Urea   20 g
    Propylene glycol   20 mL
    Cream base   qs to 60 g

19. How much of each ingredient is needed to prepare 240 mL of the following syrup?

    Sucrose   85 g
    Cherry flavoring   2 mL
    Purified water   qs ad 100 mL

    What is the percent strength of the sucrose?

20. How many *grams* of each ingredient are needed to make 90 glycerin suppositories from the following formulation?

    Glycerin Suppositories #20

    Glycerin   36 g
    Sodium stearate   3.6 g
    Water   1.8 mL (same as 1.8 g since the specific gravity of water is 1)

    Glycerin:

    Sodium stearate:

    Water:

    What is the percentage of glycerin in this preparation? (*round to nearest whole number*)

Chapter 16

Round all drip rates to the nearest whole number. Round other answers to tenths if necessary. Figure time in minutes and then convert to hours and minutes.

1. A physician orders 1,000 mL of D5NS to infuse over 8 hours. How many mL will be delivered per hour?

    How much dextrose is in one liter of D5NS?

    How many g of dextrose will the patient receive in 2 hours?

    What weight of NaCl will the patient receive in 2 hours?

    If the drop factor is 20 gtt/mL, what is the drip rate?

2. A physician orders 2 L of D5NS to infuse at 8 mL/min with a drop factor of 20 gtt/mL. How many drops per minute should the patient receive?

    How long will it take for the fluids to infuse in hours and minutes?

3. Medication order: 500 mL D5-1/2-NS to infuse over 6 hr with a drop factor of 10 gtt/mL.
   What is the weight of dextrose in the solution?

    What is the weight of NaCl in the solution?

    What is the flow rate in mL/hr?

    What is the drip rate in gtt/min?

4. Medication order: cimetidine 300 mg in D5W, total volume 75 mL to run over 2 hours. Using a drop factor of 60 gtt/mL, what is the drip rate for these fluids?

    How many milligrams of cimetidine will the patient receive in 20 minutes?

5. Medication order: ampicillin 1,250 mg in D5W IVPB, total volume 100 mL, q8h to infuse over 1 hour with a drop factor of 10 gtt/mL.
   What is the drip rate for these fluids?

   How many milligrams of ampicillin will the patient receive in 45 minutes?

6. A physician orders regular insulin 400 units/250 mL NS to infuse over 5 hours.
   What volume of fluids should be infused every hour?

   How many units of insulin will the patient receive each hour?

   If the infusion set is 20 gtt/mL, what is the flow rate of the infusion?

7. Medication order: dopamine 200 mcg/150 mL D5W to run at 1 mcg/min
   The drop factor is 20 gtt/mL.
   What is the drip rate for the medication?

   How long will it take for the fluids to infuse in hours and minutes?

   How many micrograms of dopamine will the patient receive in 30 minutes?

8. Order: 1,000 mL D5NS with 40 mEq KCL to infuse over 10 hr.
   How many hours will the IV last?

   How many mEq of KCl will the patient receive in 2 hours?

9. Order: vancomycin 400 mg/100 mL IVPB over 4 hours with an infusion set of 20 gtt/mL.
   What is the flow rate in mL/hr?

   What is the drip rate in gtt/min?

10. Order: ampicillin 1 g/100 mL to run over 30 min q6h with a drop factor of 15 gtt/mL
    What is the drip rate?

11. How many hours will it take to infuse 500 mL D5W run at 40 gtt/min with a drop factor of 15 gtt/mL? (*round to nearest hour*)

12. How many hours will a 1 L IV last if run at:
    50 mL/hr

    100 mL/hr

    125 mL/hr

13. If a 1,500 mL IV is hung at 0830 at a rate of 100 mL/hr, when will the next bag be due?

14. Order: One liter of DNS to be administered at 20 gtt/min with a drop factor of 30 gtt/mL
    How many hours would this IV run?

    What volume should be left when it is time to change the IV?

15. A physician orders Cefobid (cefoperazone) 1g in D5NS with a total volume of 250 mL to run over 30 minutes q12h.
    What is the flow rate in mL/hr?

16. A physician orders heparin sodium 6,000 units in 500 mL of D5LR to run at 1,000 units/hr with a drop factor of 10 gtt/mL.
How many drops per minute should the patient receive?

How many hours will the IV run?

17. A compounded TPN has 400 mL of 8.8% Travesol (amino acid), 300 mL of 50% dextrose, 100 mL of lipids, and 200 mL of sterile water.

What is the final concentration of Travesol?

What is the final strength of the dextrose?

Use the following stock strengths for the next 3 questions.

TPN Additive		Stock Strengths Available
Potassium chloride		2 mEq/mL
Sodium chloride	14.6%	2.5 mEq/mL
Calcium gluconate	10%	4.65 mEq/10 mL
Magnesium sulfate	50%	40.6 mEq/10 mL
Sodium acetate		2 mEq/mL
Sodium phosphates	45 mM/15 mL	60 mEq/15 mL
Potassium acetate	19.6%	2 mEq/mL
Potassium phosphate	15 mM/5 mL	4.4 mEq/mL
Humulin R insulin		100 units/mL
Vitamin C		250 mg/2 mL
Folic Acid		5 mg/mL

18. Calculate the following TPN order from the stock available.
    Calculate the amounts needed for each of the following ordered additives.
    Potassium chloride (KCl) 80 mEq

    Sodium chloride (NaCl) 45 mEq

    Magnesium sulfate 24 mEq

    Trace elements   3 mL

    MVI   10 mL

    Humulin R insulin 60 units

    What is the total volume of the additives?

    Base Solutions Ordered
    10% Travesol   1,000 mL
    50% Dextrose   1,000 mL
    Sterile water for injection   500 mL

    What is the total volume of the TPN?

    How many grams of amino acids are in this TPN?

    How many g of dextrose are in this TPN?

    What is the final concentration of Travesol (amino acid)?

    What is the final concentration of dextrose?

    If it is hung at 0800 and runs at 125 mL/hr, when will the next bag be due?

19. The following TPN to be run over 24 hours is for a 20-pound infant. Calculate the following from the stock strengths available.

    Calculate the amounts needed for each ordered additive.
    Potassium chloride 2.5 mEq/kg

    Sodium chloride 2.5 mEq/kg

    Magnesium sulfate 0.5 mEq/kg

    What is the total volume of the additives?

    Base Solutions Ordered

5.5% Travesol	200 mL
20% Dextrose	150 mL

    What is the total volume of the TPN?

    How many grams of amino acids are in this TPN?

    How many g of dextrose are in this TPN?

    What is the final concentration of Travesol (amino acids)?

    What is the final concentration of dextrose?

20. Calculate the following TPN order from the stock strengths available.

    Calculate the amounts needed for each of the following ordered additives.
    Potassium chloride 15 mEq

    Sodium chloride 10 mEq

    Magnesium sulfate 250 mg

    Sodium phosphates 20 mEq

    Vitamin C 500 mg

    Folic Acid 10 mg

    Trace elements   5 mL

    MVI-12   10 mL

    What is the total volume of the additives?

    Base Solutions Ordered
    Travesol (amino acids) 30 g

    Dextrose 200 g
    Sterile water for injection qs ad 1,000 mL

    Base Solutions Available
    Travesol 8.8%
    Dextrose 50%

    Round the following two answers to whole numbers.

    How many milliliters of 8.8% Travesol are needed to provide 30 grams of amino acids?

    How many milliliters of 50% dextrose are needed to provide 200 g of dextrose?

    How many mL of sterile water are needed?

    Run at 100 mL/hr

    If it is hung at 0600, when will the next IV be due?

Chapter 17

Perform the following business math calculations. Round answers to tenths or appropriate dollars and cents.

1. The pharmacy offers a 1% senior citizen discount on all prescriptions.
   What is the cost to a senior citizen for a $54.00 prescription?

2. The pharmacy marks up private pay prescriptions 35%.
   What will be charged for a prescription that costs the pharmacy $ 14.98?

3. A pharmacy accidently ordered 100 bottles of mouthwash at $4.49 each instead of 10. In order to reduce inventory, they offered a 20% discount after marking the bottles up 40%.
   What is the sale price for one bottle of mouthwash after the discount?

   How much profit will the pharmacy make on all 100 bottles?

4. The wholesaler offers a 7% discount if the invoice is paid within 10 days of delivery.
   How much could be saved on a $22,643 invoice?

5. The pharmacy buys a new computer for $9,000. The expected time of use is 4 years.
   What is the amount of depreciation for the computer for one year?

6. A pharmacy is under contract with an insurance company for AWP plus 10% with a $7.00 dispensing fee.
A prescription for 30 tablets has an AWP of $1.05 per tablet. The pharmacy buys this medication at AWP less 10% for payment within 10 days of invoice.
How much does the pharmacy pay for 30 tablets with the discount?

What is the amount that should be billed to the insurance company?

What is the profit on this medication for the pharmacy based on AWP?

7. A prescription for 60 tablets has a cost of $0.55 per tablet. This medication sells for $55.00.
What is the markup on this prescription?

What is the markup percentage on this prescription?

8. The pharmacy is under contract with an insurance company for a customer based on a capitation fee of $255 per month.
The customer had three prescriptions filled today for $10.50, $65.00, and $45.00.
If the customer already had prescriptions filled this month for $25.00, $46.00, and $32.50, what is the amount of profit or loss for the pharmacy?

9. A customer buys 2 bars of soap, aspirin, and a box of tissue. He has a coupon for the soap for $0.50 off two bars that sell for $2.50 each. The aspirin sells for $8.99 for 250 tablets.
The tissue is on sale for 15% off the usual price of $1.89 a box.
What is the customer's price for all three items?

The customer reminds you that today is senior citizen discount day and he qualifies for the 10% discount.
What is the total that should now be charged to the customer?

You have already entered the original amount without the discount in the cash drawer before the person reminds you of the senior citizen discount.
How much should you refund to the person from the cash drawer?

10. The pharmacist asks you to compute the overhead for the pharmacy for the month.
    The salary for the pharmacist is 3,700.00 twice a month.
    The two pharmacy technicians are each paid $3,400 per month.
    Inventory costs per week average approximately $12,000.00 for medications while front end merchandise averages about twice that much per month.
    Rent for the building is $950.00 per month; professional malpractice insurance is $255.00 per month, utilities average about $1,450.00 per month; supplies are about $672.00 per month; and miscellaneous expenses average about $565.00 per month.
    What is the overhead for a month?

11. The pharmacy purchases a medication for $86.00 for 100 tablets. The pharmacy must have a 45% markup on these tablets because the medication is not ordered on a regular basis.
    What is the cost for a prescription for 60 tablets for a customer who has no insurance?

    The pharmacist approves as 20% discount for this customer to help with the cost.
    What is the amount of the discount?

    What is cost to the customer after the discount has been applied?

    If the pharmacy took advantage of the wholesaler's 8% discount by paying the invoice in 10 days, but did not pass this on to the customer, what is the profit on this prescription?

12. An insurance company allows AWP minus 10% plus a $15.00 dispensing fee.
    The customer brings in a prescription for 60 tablets with an AWP of $5/tablet
    What should be charged to the insurance company?

13. A pharmacy technician is responsible for inventory in the pharmacy department.
    The following medication is needed:
    Cogentin (benztropine): Inventory is 75 tablets. Par is 750 tablets.
    How many tablets are needed to reach par?

    The available stock bottles of medication from the wholesaler are 1,000 tablets for $1,250.00, 500 tablets for $650.00, and 100 tablets for $140.00.
    What purchase would come closest to meeting the par level (within a 10% margin)?

    How much would this order cost the pharmacy if they took advantage of a 7% discount for paying the invoice within 10 days?

14. A patient brings the following prescriptions to the pharmacy:
    (A) The first prescription is for 75 tablets at $0.70 per tablet.
    (B) The second prescription is for 90 tablets that cost $1.10 per tablet.
    (C) The third prescription is for 25 capsules at $2.50 per capsule.
    The markup on each of the prescriptions is 25%. Because this person does not have insurance the pharmacist offers a 15% discount on the most expensive and 10% on the other two prescriptions.
    What is the cost to the pharmacy for prescription A?

    What is the cost to the pharmacy for prescription B?

    What is the cost to the pharmacy for prescription C?

    What is the cost to the patient for prescription A prior to discount?

    What is the cost to the patient for prescription B prior to discount?

    What is the cost to the patient for prescription C prior to discount?

    What is the final cost of prescription A with the allowable discount?

    What is the final cost of prescription B with the allowable discount?

    What is the final cost of prescription C with the allowable discount?

15. What is the percentage markup on a prescription based on a wholesale cost of $16.75 and a selling price of $31.50?

16. A compounded prescription has a wholesale price of $21.28. The insurance company will pay AWP + 15% with a $9.00 dispensing fee.
How much will the pharmacy be reimbursed from the insurance company?

What is the pharmacy's profit on the compounded prescription?

17. A pharmacy had a monthly income of $132,987. The inventory for the month was 42,033, salaries and wages were 26,577, and rent, utilities, and insurance costs were $4,200.
What was the net income (or loss) for this month?

18. An insurance company reimburses the pharmacy for AWP – 5% with a dispensing fee of $14.00.
A patient brings in a prescription for 60 capsules with an AWP of $0.75 each.
What is the total amount to be billed to the insurance company?

What is the profit for the pharmacy?

19. A pharmacy has an average inventory value of $500,000 at any given time. The total amount spent on inventory in a year is $2,000,000.
What is the inventory turnover rate for the year?

20. A pharmacy purchases aspirin at an AWP of $3.00 for 100 tablets.
Mark the price up by 45% and then offer a 25% discount.
What is the price of the medication after the 45% markup?

What is the selling price after the 25% discount?

What profit would the pharmacy make on 10 bottles of 100?

ANSWERS TO APPENDIX

Extra Practice Problems

Chapter 1
3. subcutaneous
6. every other day
9. as soon as possible
12. liter
15. intrathecal
18. every eight hours
21. milliliter
24. increase
27. repeat
30. ounce
33. pint
36. rectal
39. kilogram
42. as desired
45. twice a day
48. fluid
51. suppository
54. less than
57. no known drug allergies
60. intramuscular
63. cream
66. meter
69. verbal order
72. qod, U, and qd

Chapter 2
3. 155.52
6. 8
9. 824.68
12. $\frac{5}{8}$
15. $\frac{2}{11}$
18. $1\frac{1}{2}$
21. 120 mL
24. 225 mg
27. 0.015
30. 2.3
33. $\frac{1}{400}$
36. 680%
39. 75%
42. 75%
45. 33.3%
48. 0.12
51. $\frac{1}{2}$
54. $\frac{24}{25}$
57. 3:500
60. 1:2
63. x = 3
66. 2.5
69. 50%
72. 120
75. 36 caps

Chapter 3
3. 45
6. LIX
9. 99
12. 1917
15. 0135
18. 0800
21. 39.22° C
24. 57.56° F
27. 41° F
30. −12.22° C
33. 1530
36. 4 oz
39. 0800, 1200, 1600, 2000
42. 1230

Chapter 4
3. gr x
6. 200 # (or 200 lb)
9. 2 gtt
12. 3.5 L
15. 10.5 mL
18. gr $\frac{1}{100}$
21. 3
24. 1,000
27. 4
30. 8

Chapter 5
3. 60″
6. 0.5 g
9. 0.0005 L
12. 25 mg
15. 13½ tsp
18. 1,000 mg
21. 625 mcg
24. 5 mg
27. 0.25 g
30. 250 mL
33. 250 mg

Chapter 6
3. 50 kg
6. 5 mL
9. 76.4 kg
12. 100 kg
15. gr v
18. 30 mL
21. 0.4 mg
24. 30.9 kg
27. 3 oz
30. 2,500 g

Chapter 7
3. Take 1 tablet by mouth 2 times a day
6. Take 1 tablet every morning before eating with a full grass of water

9. Take one tablet four times a day before meals and at bedtime
12. Apply to affected area 2 times a day
15. Inject 15 units subcutaneously 3 times a day before meals
18. cephalexin suspension 500 mg by mouth every 12 hours
21. Lunesta 1 mg by mouth at bedtime as needed for sleep
24. furosemide 80 mg by mouth every morning
27. digoxin 0.25 mg by mouth every morning
30. cefazolin 1 g intravenously 1 hour before surgery and every 8 hours after surgery for 24 hours

Chapter 8

3. 2 capsules
6. 1 tablet
9. ½ tablet
12. Take 2 tablets every day with or without food for arthritis pain
15. Take 4 tablets at bedtime
18. Take 1 tablet by mouth at bedtime on day 1, take 2 tablets by mouth at bedtime on day 2, take 4 tablets by mouth at bedtime on day 3, and then take 6 tablets by mouth at bedtime

Chapter 9

3. 20 mL
6. 3.8 mL
9. 10 mL
12. Take 2.5 mL by mouth every morning
15. Take 20 mL by mouth every 12 hours for 10 days
18. Take 2.5 mL by mouth 4 times a day

Chapter 10

3. 0.5 mL; 1-mL TB syringe
6. 0.5 mL; 1 mL; 1.5 mL
9. 1.2 mL; 3-mL syringe
12. 2.6 mL; 3-mL syringe
15. 0.5 mL; 1-mL TB syringe
18. 1.2 mL; 3-mL syringe
21. 9 mL; Water for Injection, USP or Sodium Chloride for Injection, USP; 400 mg/mL; Protect from light and can be stored at room temperature for 4 weeks without significant loss of potency; 0.75 mL; 1-mL TB syringe

Chapter 11

3. 30-unit insulin syringe
6. 100-unit insulin syringe
9. 0.1 mL
12. 10,000 units/mL; 0.25 mL

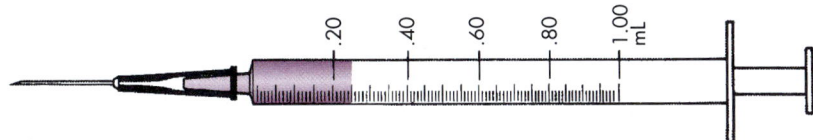

15. 20,000 units/mL; 0.6 mL;

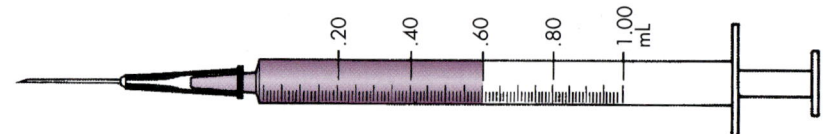

18. 0.16 mL; 9.34 mL;

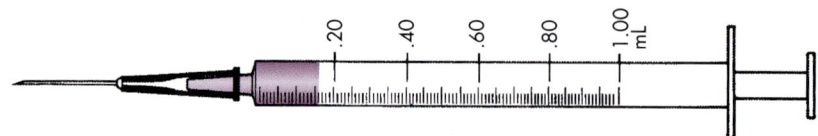

Chapter 12
3. Clark's Rule; 4.6 mg
6. Clark's Rule; 25.6 mg
9. BSA; 280 mg; 46.7 mL; 0.56 mg/mL
12. Body weight; 204.5 mg; 8.2 mL
15. Clark's Rule; 5 mL
18. Fried's Rule; 0.8 mL

Chapter 13
3. 180 tablets
6. 196 mL; 1 bottle
9. 25 days; 50 days; 5 mL
12. 64 doses; 21 days
15. 280 mL
18. 30 days
21. 30 days
24. 25 days

Chapter 14
3. 16.5 g
6. 100 mg/mL
9. 0.5 mg/mL
12. 1:250
15. 26.4 g
18. 120 capsules
21. 2 g
24. 0.001%

Chapter 15
3. 3 g of 2.5% ointment; 12 g of petrolatum
6. 450 mL
9. 2.5 mL stock solution; 7.5 mL water
12. 50 mL of 8% solution; 200 mL of 3% solution
15. 562.5 mL of 1:20 solution; 187.5 mL of 1:100 solution
18. 6 g

Chapter 16
3. 25 g dextrose; 2.25 g NaCl; 83.3 mL/hr; 14 gtt/min
6. 50 mL/hr; 80 units of insulin per hour; 17 gtt/min
9. 25 mL/hr; 8 gtt/min
12. 20 hr; 10 hr; 8 hr
15. 500 mL/hr
18. 40 mL KCl; 18 mL NaCl; 5.9 mL $MgSO_4$; 3 mL Trace elements; 10 mL MVI; 0.6 mL Humulin R; 77.5 mL; 2,577.5 mL; 100 g amino acids; 500 g dextrose; 3.9% Travesol; 19.4% dextrose; 0437 the following day

Chapter 17
3. $5.03; $54
6. $28.35; $41.65; $13.30
9. $15.10; $13.59; $1.51
12. $285.00
15. 88%
18. $56.75; $11.75

ANSWER KEY

Chapter 1
Practice Problems A
3. nothing by mouth
6. four times a day
9. bedtime
12. microgram
15. grain
18. every hour
21. intramuscular
24. prescription; take
27. sufficient quantity
30. ointment
33. elixir
36. dram
39. by mouth
42. every evening
45. daily
48. every

Basic Math Skills Proficiency Self-Test
3. 1.59
6. $13.11
9. 8 5/8
12. XXX
15. 2 2/9
18. 2/5
21. 5 1/12
24. 1/150
27. 3.5
30. 3 7/8
33. 21 capsules
36. 60
39. 5,500 mg
42. 24.2
45. 20
48. $26.10

Chapter 2
Pretest
3. 11,008
6. 308.9
9. 2 1/8
12. 21/40
15. 10
18. 1 4/15
21. 12
24. 6.13
27. 1.75
30. 1/3
33. 24
36. $\frac{44}{100} = \frac{11}{25}$
39. 0.33
42. 37.5 mL
45. 42.5%

Practice Problems A
3. 150 g
6. 8,500 mL
9. 75 mL
12. 225 mg
15. 40 mL

Practice Problems B
3. 8,700
6. 85,250
9. 74
12. 40
15. 2,500 mg

Practice Problems C
3. 7; 15

Practice Problems D
3. 8 3/4
6. 3
9. 1 1/2 tablets
12. 23/8
15. 33/7
18. 9/2 tablet
21. 1 1/4
24.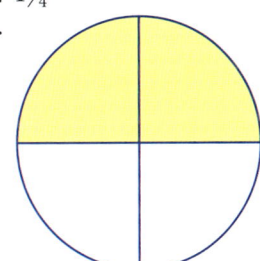

Practice Problems E
3. 2/3
6. 1/4
9. 1/2

Practice Problems F
3. 5/7
6. 3/15 = 1/5
9. 1 7/9
12. 65/77
15. 1/2 tsp
18. 1
21. 1 5/24 tsp
24. 9/16 oz

Practice Problems G
3. 3/8
6. 4/15
9. 8 13/15
12. 10 61/72
15. 8/15
18. 1 5/16
21. 2 1/12
24. 125 tablets

Practice Problems H
3. six and seven hundred fifty-one thousandths
6. thirty-five ten thousandths
9. seventy-eight hundredths

Practice Problems I
3. 36.45
6. 8.24
9. 3.6
12. 3.1
15. 2.5 mL
18. 14

Practice Problems J
3. 1363.08
6. $153.59
9. 2.81
12. $10.10
15. 2 mg
18. $76.10; $3.90

Practice Problems K
3. 42.5
6. 8.25
9. 7.5 mg
12. 2,000 mg
15. 61.25 mg

Practice Problems L
3. 5
6. 0.25
9. 310.75
12. 211.2 mg
15. $85.10

Practice Problems M
3. 33/100
6. 5/100; 1/20
9. 1,244/10,000; 311/2,500

543

Practice Problems N
3. 0.8
6. 0.83
9. 0.63

Practice Problems O
3. $^{125}/_{100}$; $1\frac{1}{4}$
6. $^{80}/_{100}$; $\frac{4}{5}$
9. $^{12.5}/_{100}$; $\frac{1}{8}$
12. $^{0.025}/_{100}$; $\frac{1}{4,000}$
15. $\frac{5}{4} \times \frac{1}{100}$; $\frac{5}{400}$; $\frac{1}{80}$

Practice Problems P
3. $^{200}/_5$; 40
6. $^{700}/_3$; 233.33
9. $^{300}/_4$; 75
12. $^{400}/_5$; 80

Practice Problems Q
3. 0.78
6. 3.25
9. 0.32
12. 12.45
15. 0.0006
18. 0.0013

Practice Problems R
3. 2.5
6. 550
9. 1040
12. 15
15. 46.7

Practice Problems S
3. 5:25; 1:5
6. 95:100; 19:20
9. 325:10,000; 13:400
12. 36:100; 9:25
15. 6:48; 1:8
18. 2:50; 1:25

Practice Problems T
3. yes
6. yes
9. no

Practice Problems U
3. 25
6. $5
9. 21 capsules
12. 56 tablets
15. 2 mL

Practice Problems V
3. 45
6. 81

9. 5.12 oz
12. $3.75
15. 24.5 tablets
18. 8%

Posttest
3. 66.35
6. 4.18
9. $\frac{49}{24}$; $2\frac{1}{24}$
12. $\frac{3}{40}$
15. $\frac{24}{12}$; 2
18. 4.93
21. 0.56
24. 1.83
27. $5\frac{33}{100}$
30. 3:5
33. 250 mg:5 mL; 50 mg:1 mL
36. $\frac{60 \text{ tabs}}{1 \text{ month}} = \frac{x}{3 \text{ months}}$; $x = 180$ tabs
39. 9 tablets
42. 125 capsules

Chapter 3
Pretest
3. liv
6. xcv
9. 8
12. 97
15. $37\frac{1}{2}$
18. $44\frac{1}{2}$
21. 0001
24. 0146
27. 11:02 AM
30. 11:57 PM
33. 4:45 PM
36. 40.3°C
39. 38°C
42. 39.2°C
45. −12.2°C
48. 33.6°C

Practice Problems A
3. xxi
6. ix
9. lxxv
12. xxxv
15. xxxiii ss

Practice Problems B
3. 19
6. 66
9. 95
12. $37\frac{1}{2}$
15. 99

Practice Problems C
3. 0615
6. 0345
9. 0655
12. 2020
15. 2359
18. 12:01 PM
21. 4:15 PM
24. 7:05 AM
27. 8:20 PM
30. 9:45 AM

Practice Problems D
3. 1.7°C
6. 93.2°F
9. 37°C
12. 37.9°C
15. 118.8°F
18. 37.9°C; yes

Posttest
3. $93\frac{1}{2}$
6. xxxvi ss
9. lxxv
12. 125
15. clxv
18. 4:25 PM
21. 12:45 AM
24. 1210
27. 1526
30. 6:35 AM
33. 82.2°C
36. 212°F
39. 35.6°F
42. 95.4°F; yes
45. 0600; 1200; 1800; 2400
48. 1630

Chapter 4
Pretest
3. gram
6. inch
9. milliequivalent
12. teaspoon
15. pound
18. $1\frac{1}{2}$ tsp
21. 1,000 units

24. 1,000
27. viii (8)
30. 4

Practice Problems A
3. 2
6. 16
9. teaspoon
12. pint

Practice Problems B
3. mL
6. gram
9. milliliter

Practice Problems C
3. pound

Posttest
3. 3 tsp
6. fl℥ x
9. 12.5 mg
12. 2½ qt
15. 4 c
18. 110 # or 110 lb
21. 40 mEq
24. 8
27. Tbsp
30. mg

Chapter 5
Pretest
3. 5
6. i
9. 1½
12. 1,560
15. 2,500
18. 5,000,000,000
21. 18
24. 32

Practice Problems A
3. 1½
6. 5
9. 1¼
12. 1½
15. 180
18. 80
21. 1½ Tbsp
24. 4 c

Practice Problems B
3. 4,000
6. 500

9. 0.05
12. 6,540,000
15. 50,600
18. 3.5
21. 0.005
24. 300,000
27. 0.25 mg
30. 1.5 g

Practice Problems C
3. 1/15
6. xl (40)

Posttest
3. 120
6. 1¼
9. 0.0125
12. ½
15. 2
18. ½
21. 0.0405
24. 3
27. 0.075
30. 4
33. 4
36. 32
39. 0.6
42. 2½
45. 2,500
48. fl℥ 64
51. 0.025 g
54. 6 tsp

Chapter 6
Pretest
3. 4.4
6. 10
9. iv
12. ii
15. v
18. 0.4
21. ½
24. 15.2
27. 60
30. 2

Practice Problems A
3. 5
6. 15
9. 2.2
12. 20

Practice Problems B
3. xvi ♏
6. 24 ♏
9. 64
12. v
15. 3 Tbsp; every 3 to 4 hours as needed

Practice Problems C
3. 15
6. 720
9. 2½
12. ¾
15. 30
18. 152.4

Practice Problems D
3. ¼
6. 0.5
9. 30
12. 45,000
15. 15 mg; no

Posttest
3. 45
6. 1/100
9. 3.8
12. viii
15. 1/600
18. ix
21. ii s̄s̄
24. 7
27. 5.2
30. gr 1/150

Chapter 7
Pretest
3. Take 1 tablet by mouth every morning as needed for swelling
6. Take 2 tablets by mouth now, then take 1 tablet by mouth daily on days 2 through 5
9. Take 1 tablet by mouth 3 times a day
12. Take 1 tablet by mouth daily with evening meal or at bedtime with a snack for hyperlipidemia

15. Take ½ to 1 tablet by mouth every 4 to 6 hours as needed for anxiety or muscle spasms
18. metoprolol 50 mg by mouth two times a day

Practice Problems A
3. Zoloft 50 mg, 30 tablets, one tablet by mouth daily with morning meal; take 1 tablet by mouth daily with morning meal
6. Allegra 180 mg, 30 tablets, one tablet by mouth daily; Take 1 tablet by mouth daily
9. Fosamax 70 mg, 4 tablets, one tablet by mouth on same day every week; Take 1 tablet by mouth once a week on the same day every week
12. Glucotrol XL 10 mg, 30 tablets, one tablet by mouth with morning meal; Take 1 tablet by mouth daily with morning meal

Practice Problems B
3. cephalexin 500 mg by mouth every 8 hours for 3 days
6. albuterol sulfate two puffs every 4 hours for shortness of breath
9. Levothroid 100 micrograms by mouth every day with morning meal
12. hydrocodone/acetaminophen 7.5/325 by mouth every 6 hours as needed for pain
15. furosemide 40 mg by mouth every morning as needed for swelling

Posttest
3. Dilantin 100-mg capsules, 120 capsules, four capsules by mouth now, then one capsule by mouth four times a day; Take 4 capsules by mouth now; then take 1 capsule by mouth 4 times a day
6. Take 1 tablet by mouth every 4 to 6 hours as needed
9. meperidine 75 mg and Phenergan 25 mg intramuscularly every 4 to 6 hours as needed for extreme pain
12. Tagamet 300 mg intramuscularly now
15. digoxin 250 mcg by mouth every morning with pulse over 60
18. 40 mEq; 20 mL; Hospira; solution for injection; MUST BE DILUTED BEFORE USE

Chapter 8
Pretest
3. 1 tablet
6. ½ tablet
9. 2 capsules
12. 1 tablet
15. 1 tablet

Practice Problems A
3. 2 capsules
6. ½ tablet
9. 3 tablets

Practice Problems B
3. 3 capsules
6. 2 tablets
9. 4 tablets

Posttest
3. 2 tablets
6. 1 tablet
9. 1 tablet
12. 200 mg; 2 tablets; 100 mg; 1 tablet

Chapter 9
Pretest
3. 10 mL
6. 7.5 mL; 1½ tsp
9. 2.5 mL; ½ tsp

Practice Problems A
3. 2.5 mL; ½ tsp
6. 2.5 mL; ½ tsp; 5-mL dose spoon, 3-mL or 5-mL oral syringe
9. 10 mL; 5 mL; 3.3 mL
12. 0.6 mL,

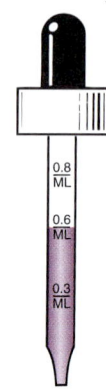

Practice Problems B
3. 150 mL; water; 90 mL; 60 mL; add water in two portions, shake well; 125 mg/5 mL; store in refrigerator, shake well, discard after 14 days; 14 days; 15 mL

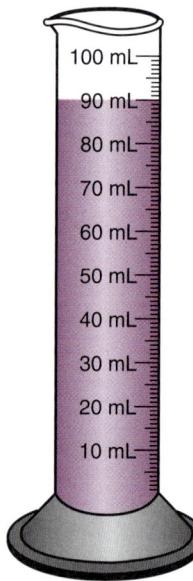

Posttest

3. 10 mL; 2 tsp; indicate volume on medicine cup

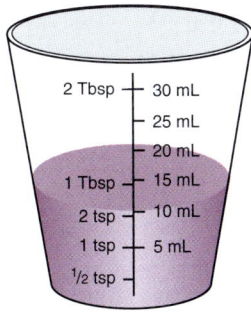

6. Zantac syrup 75 mg two times a day, 30 minutes before meals; 5 mL; 1 tsp; indicate volume on utensils

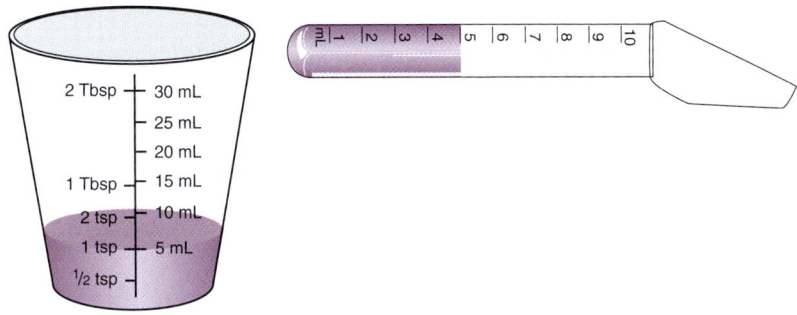

9. 3 mL; 1.5 mL

Chapter 10

Pretest

3. meperidine 40 mg intramuscularly immediately for pain; 0.8 mL
6. codeine phosphate ½ grain subcutaneously every 4 hours as needed; 1 mL

Practice Problems A

3. 1.8 mL
6.

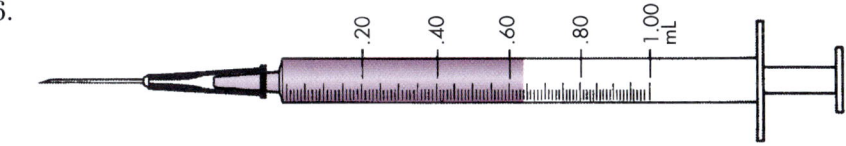

9.

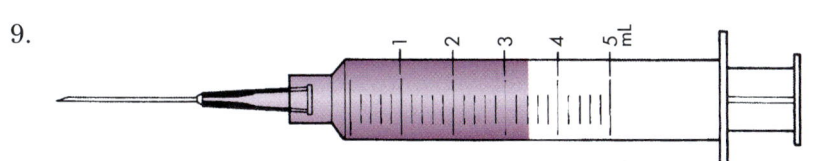

Practice Problems B

3. tobramycin (Nebcin) 60 mg intramuscularly every 8 hours; 1.5 mL

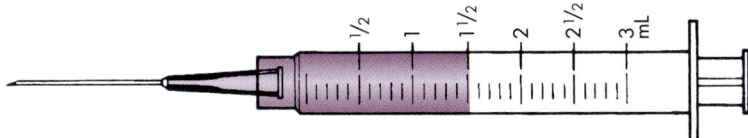

6. Cogentin 1.5 mg intramuscularly daily; 1.5 mL

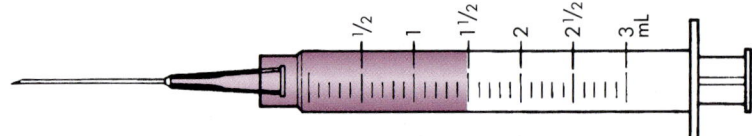

9. hydroxyzine 75 mg and meperidine 50 mg intramuscularly immediately; 1.5 mL hydroxyzine; 0.5 mL meperidine

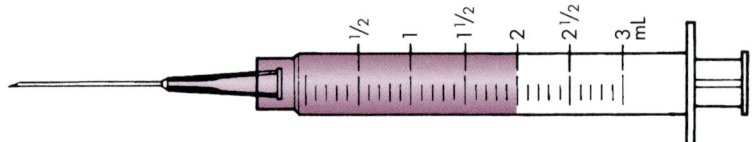

12. Solu-Cortef 125 mg intramuscularly immediately; 1 mL

Posttest
3. Solu-Medrol 37.5 mg intramuscularly now; 0.6 mL

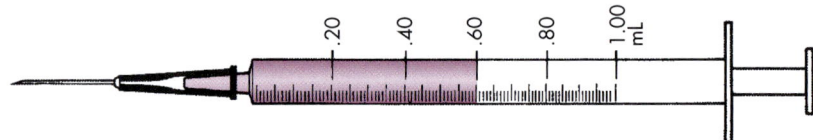

6. digoxin 0.1 mg intramuscularly now and then once daily; 0.25 mg/mL; 0.4 mL
9. meperidine 50 mg intramuscularly every 4 hours as needed for pain; 0.67 mL; 0.5 mL; meperidine 100 mg/mL

Chapter 11

Pretest
3. 0.5 mL; 9.5 mL (50-unit insulin syringe)

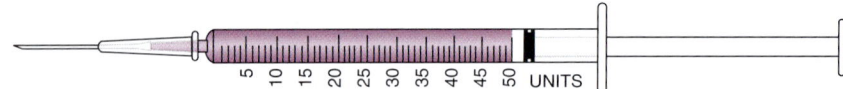

6. B; 0.85 mL; 1-mL TB syringe (1-mL TB syringe)

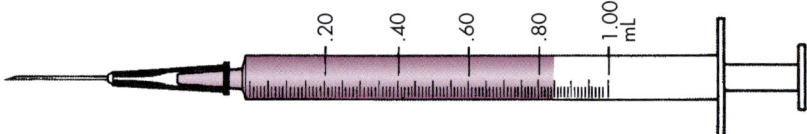

9. Inject 14 units subcutaneously three times a day before meals; 30-unit insulin syringe

Practice Problems A
3. C; C
6. B; A
9. D and B; C; 31 units; 21 units
12. D; B; NPH 28 units; Regular 12 units

Answer Key 549

Practice Problems B

3. 0.4 mL

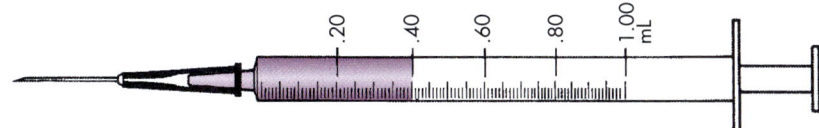

6. 0.75 mL

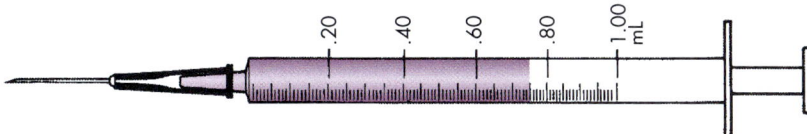

9. A; 0.75 mL

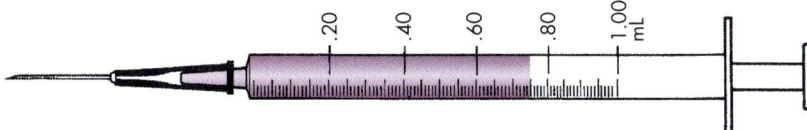

12. 0.6 mL

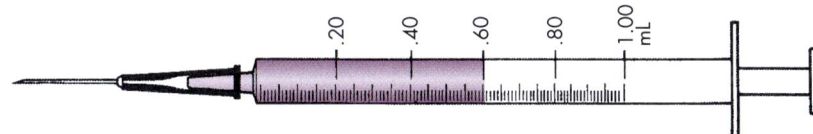

15. 0.3 mL

Posttest

3. 0.5 mL; 1-mL TB syringe

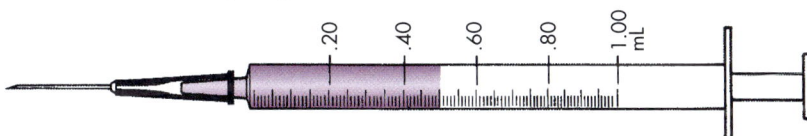

6. C: Draw Regular before NPH

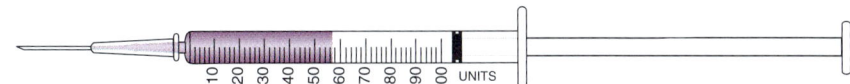

9. 0.3 mL (1-mL TB syringe)

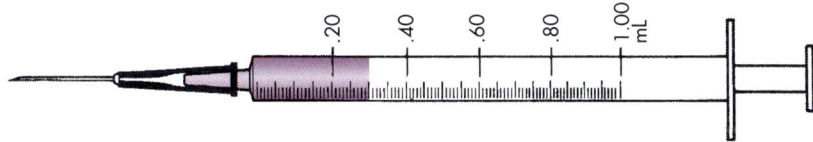

Chapter 12

Pretest

3. 25 mg tid
6. 127.3 mcg; 2.5 mL
9. 22 mg q6–8h prn; 8.8 mL; yes

12. 15.1 mL; 15 mL; 1 Tbsp

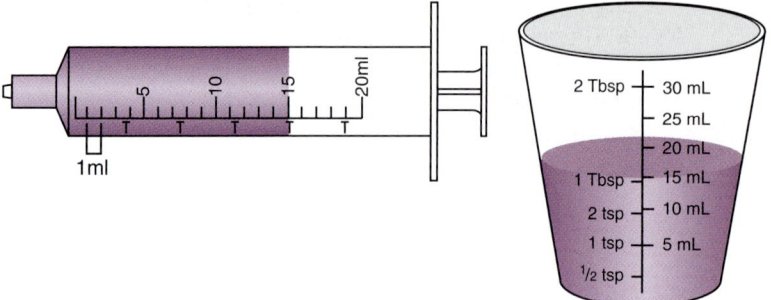

15. 153.4 mg; 3.8 mL; 306.8 mg/day

Practice Problems A

3. 34.09 kg

Practice Problems B

3. 2.5 mL; ½ tsp

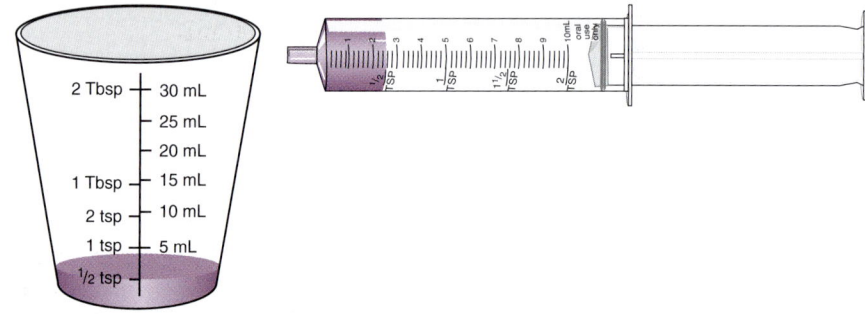

6. 4 mL
9. 9.8 mg; one tablet
12. 45.5 mg; 2.5 mL; ½ tsp
15. 25 mg; 0.5 mL

Practice Problems C

3. 10 mg; 4 mL

Practice Problems D

3. 0.29 m^2

Practice Problems E

3. 1.34 m^2; 3.94 mg; 3.9 mL
6. 23.53 mg; 2.4 mL
9. 810 mg; two tablets

Practice Problems F

3. 2 mg; 0.2 mL

Posttest

3. 0.95 m^2; 279.41 mg; 250 mg/5 mL; 5.6 mL
6. 136.36 mg; 6.5 mL
9. Fried's; 13 mg; 0.41 mL
12. 1.75 mg; 17.5 mL; 0.44 mL
15. 113.75 mg; 56.9 mL; 75-mL vial
18. Clark's rule; 183.33 mg; 7.3 mL

Chapter 13

Pretest

3. Topamax 25 mg, 4 tablets twice a day for 1 month; 240 tablets; Take 4 tablets 2 times a day for 1 month
6. 15 tablets; 12.5 mg; Take ½ tablet by mouth every day
9. 10 mL; 7.5 mL; 5 vials; 5 vials are needed for 45 mL because each vial contains 10 mL
12. 60 tablets; Take 1½ tablets by mouth every morning and ½ tablet by mouth at bedtime

Practice Problems A

3. 56 capsules; Take 2 capsules by mouth 4 times a day for 7 days
6. amoxicillin 500 mg, 2 times a day for 10 days; 40 capsules; Take 2 capsules 2 times a day for 10 days
9. 2 vials; 1.5 mL
12. 31 tablets; Take 2 tablets by mouth now, then take 1 tablet by mouth daily

Practice Problems B

3. 7 doses; 4 containers; Take 4 capsules by mouth daily, 1 hour before a meal for tuberculosis
6. 50; Take 2 tablets 3 times a day after meals

Practice Problems C

3. 10 days; 120 tablets; Take 4 tablets by mouth daily
6. 31 days; Altace 5 mg #62, one tablet twice a day for blood pressure
9. 7 days; Take 1 tablet 4 times a day until gone
12. 2 days; 4 containers; Take 10 mL by mouth 2 times a day for 10 days
15. 7.5 mL; 16 doses; 4 days
18. 90 days; 45 tablets; Take 1 tablet every morning and ½ tablet every evening

Posttest

3. 8 patches; Apply 1 patch twice a week
6. Cipro 500 mg #20, one tablet twice a day; 10 days
9. 8 days
12. 15 days
15. 56 capsules; Take 2 capsules by mouth 2 times a day for 14 days
18. 240 mL

Chapter 14

Pretest

3. 12.5 g
6. 0.2 g Zephiran chloride in 100 mL of total solution; 1 g
9. 50 mg
12. 25 mL

Practice Problems A

3. 3 g; 25 g
6. 2.5 g
9. 16.5 g

Practice Problems B

3. 0.5 g glycerol in 100 mL of solution: 5 mg/mL
6. 0.3 g ciprofloxacin in 100 mL of solution; 7.5 mg
9. 10 g calcium gluconate in 100 mL of solution; 1 g; 4.65 mEq
12. 375 g; 750 g; 187.5 g
15. 3 g
18. 300 g

Practice Problems C

3. 1 g of lidocaine in 50,000 mL of solution; 0.0004 g; 400 mcg; 0.02 mg/mL
6. 0.001 g; 1 mg/mL
9. 4 mL
12. 25 mL
15. 1:250

Practice Problems D

3. 0.1%
6. 0.2%; 500 mg

Practice Problems E

3. 1:100

Posttest

3. 2.25 g epinephrine in 100 mL of total solution; 11.25 mg; 22.5 mg/mL
6. 1 g
9. 0.04 g; 0.004%
12. 1:400
15. 200 mL
18. 500 mL

Chapter 15

Pretest

3. 50 mL; 950 mL
6. 100 mL; 0 (no solvent necessary; the solution is 50% as described)
9. 10 mL; 990 mL
12. 500 mL of 0.9% NaCl; 250 mL of 0.45% NaCl
15. 0.9 g Drug A: 2.1 g Drug B; 27 g ointment base

Practice Problems A

3. 375 mL; 1,125 mL
6. 90 mL; 150 mL
9. 48 mL; 192 mL
12. 1,600 mL; 2,400 mL
15. 180 mL
18. 20 mL; 60 mL

Practice Problems B

3. 4.6 g of 25%; 15.4 g of 12%
6. 107.1 mL of 15%; 642.9 mL of 1%
9. 20 g of 15%; 30 g of 2.5%
12. 150 mL of D10W; 100 mL of D5W
15. 11 mL of 5% sodium chloride; 39 mL of 0.9% sodium chloride

18. 33.3 mL of 1:10; 66.7 mL of 1:100

Practice Problems C
3. 0.15 g of menthol; 0.18 g of phenol; 29.67 g

Practice Problems D
3. 10 mg/mL
6. 22 g mupirocin; 0.022 g betamethasone dipropionate; 0.88 g miconazole

Practice Problems E
3. 108 g glycerin; 10.8 g sodium stearate; 5.4 mL water

Posttest
3. 120 mL
6. 225 mL; 75 mL
9. 62.5 mL; 187.5 mL; seven vials
12. 62.5 mL; 187.5 mL
15. 83.3 mL of D50W; 416.7 mL of D5W
18. 50 mg

Chapter 16

Pretest
3. 188 mL/hr; 3 mL/min; 31 gtt/min
6. 6.75 g; 500 mL; 21 gtt/min
9. 1,200 mL
12. 125 min; 160 gtt/min
15. 180 mL/hr
18. 6 mL; 253 mL/hr; 42 gtt/min

Practice Problems A
3. 375 mL
6. ½ hr

Practice Problems B
3. 30 g; 25 g
6. 350 mg; 175 mg

Practice Problems C
3. 16 gtt/min; 15.6 mL/hr
6. 63 gtt/min; 187.5 mg
9. 25 gtt/min; 312.5 mg
12. 80.9 mg; 10 gtt/min; 72.8 mg
15. 22 gtt/min; 20 mg

Practice Problems D
3. 800 min
6. 150 min; 2 hr and 30 min
9. 2.5 mL; 379 min
12. 5 hours; 30 gtt/min

Practice Problems E
3. 10 mL sodium chloride; 7.5 mL potassium acetate; 10 mL of calcium gluconate; 10 mL MVI-12; 0.25 mL (25 units) of regular insulin; 37.75 mL

Posttest
3. 4 mL; 0.9 mL/min; 52 gtt/min; 375 mg; 8 vials; 4,000 mg
6. 400 mg; 8 mL; 18 gtt/min
9. 1.5 mL/min; 1.3 mL/min
12. 15 mL; 1.1 mL/min; 1.7 mL/min
15. 0.12 mg/hr; 2 mcg/min; 240 mL; 10 gtt/min
18. 40 mL; two vials; 23 gtt/min; 90 mL/hr; 133.3 mg

Chapter 17

Note: Losses are shown in parentheses ( ).

Pretest
3. $18.37; $13.50; $31.87
6. $3,166.67
9. $26.50; ($1.00)

Practice Problems A
3. $14,901.67; $178,820

Practice Problems B
3. $3.60

Practice Problems C
3. 9%
6. 7.1%
9. 40.2%

Practice Problems D
3. $131.25; $393.75
6. $4.93; $5.39
9. $45.00

Practice Problems E
3. $79,205

Practice Problems F
3. $76,600; $29,200; $47,400

Practice Problems G
3. $13.85; $5.95
6. $21.80
9. $45.37

Practice Problems H
3. $960 annual profit; $613 annual profit

Practice Problems I
3. 150 tablets; 9.5¢; 8.5¢; 5¢; 250 tablets; 1

Practice Problems J
3. 3.9 turnovers/2 months

Posttest
3. $40.60; $0.81; $60.75
6. $94.79; $64.81; $29.98
9. $51.56; $22.06; $26.64; $11.19; $18.77; $13.08; prescription for $34.50

GLOSSARY

aa Abbreviation meaning *of each*

Active ingredients The ingredient in a medication that has the desired effect on the body

Act-O-Vial System Two-section vial divided by a seal, holding a premeasured active ingredient in the lower section and a premeasured diluent in the upper section; mixing occurs when the two sections of the vial are combined either through puncturing the seal or moving the seal through pressure; similar to Mix-O-Vial

Additives Medications added to IVs, in particular to total parenteral nutrition (TPN) solutions and peripheral parenteral nutrition (PPN) solutions; electrolytes, multiple vitamins, trace elements, Regular insulin, and other medications

Adjudication Electronic process by which insurance companies evaluate prescriptions to determine their validity and the price to charge the patient

Adolescent From 12 through 21 years*

Alligation alternate Mathematical method for determining the amount of *two* preparations of different strengths needed to prepare a required strength in between the two; aka **tic-tac-toe**

Alligation medial Calculation method by which the weighted average strength of a mixture of *two or more* preparations of known quantity and concentration may be determined

Ampule Sealed glass container that holds a single dose of medication, usually for injection

Anticoagulant Substance that stops or delays the clotting of blood

Apothecary system One of the oldest measurement systems used to calculate drug orders using measurements such as grains and minims

Arabic numerals The numbers 1, 2, 3, etc.

Assets Any property owned by the business

Auxiliary label Label added to prescriptions to provide supplementary instructions

Average wholesale price (AWP) Price that a pharmacy theoretically pays for medication; this price is theoretical because discounts, sales, and special deals may affect the actual wholesale price; this is the price basis used for insurance reimbursement

Base solution Solution for a TPN or PPN that contains carbohydrates (dextrose), protein (amino acids), and sometimes lipids (fatty acids)

Biologicals Substances made from natural sources such as human, animal, or microorganism that are used as drug treatments or to prevent or diagnose diseases; tested for potency in a biologic system

Body surface area (BSA) Measurement of total body area exposed to the environment; calculated from weight and height and expressed in square meters (m^2); used as a basis for calculating some medication doses

Buccal Between the gum and cheek; medications dissolved between the gum and cheek

Capitation fee Set amount of third-party money paid monthly to the pharmacy for a specific patient regardless of the number of prescriptions filled

Cash flow Receipts and expenses for a business

Celsius (Centigrade) System of measuring temperature; 0° is the freezing point and 100° is the boiling point of water

Child From 2 to 12 years*

Clark's rule Means of calculating a dose of medication for a child from an adult dose using weight in pounds

Complex fraction Fractions in which the numerator, denominator, or both are fractional units

Component Any of the ingredients used to compound a product

Compound A product prepared in a pharmacy to fill a prescription for a product that is *not* commercially available in the ordered dose or dosage form

Compounding formulation Similar to a recipe; list of all components needed for a particular compound

Continuous infusion Introduction of IV fluids without interruption of therapy

Conversion factor A ratio equal to 1 that is used to change one *unit* to another without changing the value of the answer

Conversion factor, time Factor needed to change from one unit of time to another such as hours to minutes; 1 hr = 60 min

Conversion factor, volume Factor needed to change from one unit of volume to another without changing the value, such as liters to milliliters; 1 L = 1,000 mL

Convert Change from one form to another

Daily cash or sales report Report made at the end of each day that summarizes the sales, discounts, and amount of cash, checks, refunds, and credit card charges that have occurred during the day's operations

Days' supply Number of days a prescription will last; important to input for insurance reimbursement

Decimal Representation of a fraction where the denominator is a power of 10 and the numerator is a number placed to the right of a decimal point

Decimal place Place values found to the right of the decimal point

Denominator Bottom number of a fraction

Depreciation Decrease in value of an asset based on total value of the asset, its estimated length of use, and its value at disposal; part of overhead

Diluent Agent that dilutes a substance; in pharmacy, the liquid added to a powder to change the powder to a liquid or the liquid used to dilute another liquid; aka **solvent**

Dilution Process of making a more concentrated preparation less concentrated by adding a diluent containing no active ingredient such as water or white petrolatum

Dimensional analysis (DA) A method used for converting between units and calculating medication doses and dosages that involves multiplying a series of fractions in an order whereby all unnecessary units are sequentially canceled until the desired unit is reached

553

Discount percent or markdown A percentage amount to be subtracted from the markup price of an item to lower the selling price

Dividend Number being divided in division

Divisor Number by which another number is divided

Dosage Size, frequency, and number of doses of medication prescribed

Dosage form Physical structure of a dose; for example: capsule, tablet, solution

Dose Amount of a medication to be administered at one time

Dose time Amount of time needed to administer medication

Dose volume Volume of medication administered at a given time

Drip rate Specific type of flow rate calculated in drops per minute; gtt/min

Drop factor Size of drop from the drip chamber; found on IV tubing (drops/mL)

Early childhood From 1 through 4 years*

Electrolytes Elements such as sodium (Na), potassium (K), magnesium (Mg), and calcium (Ca) that are necessary for normal body functions

Elixir Sweetened, flavored medication dissolved in a mixture of alcohol and water

Enteric-coated tablet Dosage form that allows medication to pass through stomach unchanged; to prevent stomach irritation or prevent degradation of the active ingredient by stomach acid

Fahrenheit System of measuring temperature; 32° is the freezing point and 212° is the boiling point of water

Flow rate Speed at which IV medications are infused into the body; aka **infusion rate**

Fraction Part of a whole number with a numerator and denominator

Fried's rule Means of calculating a dose of medication for an infant from an adult dose using age in months

Generic name Official nonproprietary name given to a drug by the U.S. Food and Drug Administration (FDA)

Graduates Containers, calibrated in the metric system, that are used to measure liquid

Gross income/gross profit Sales price of merchandise minus its purchase cost; usually refers to total income for a business

High-alert medications Medications that have a higher risk of causing significant harm to a patient if dosed or used incorrectly

Improper fraction Fraction in which the numerator is equal to or greater than the denominator; a fraction that is equal to or greater than 1

Indication Reason to prescribe a medication

Infant One month to 2 years*

Infusion Slow administration of fluids, other than blood, into a vein

Inhaler A device used to deliver medicine by breathing it in through the mouth or nose

Inscription Part of prescription indicating medication name, dosage form, strength, and quantity

International System of Units (Metric system) Internationally accepted system of measurement of mass, length, and time

International unit/Unit A *specific unit* of measurement used for biologicals; describes a standard amount of an *individual* drug that can produce a given biologic effect specific to that drug alone; a measurement of a medication's action as opposed to its weight (such as mcg, mg, g); units of one substance are *not* equivalent to the same number of units of another substance

Intradermal Into or within the dermis of the skin (ID)

Intramuscular Into or within a muscle (IM)

Intravenous Into or within a vein (IV)

Inventory List of the quantity and respective cost of merchandise in stock

Invert To turn upside down or switch positions

Large volume parenteral IV bags that are larger than 250 mL; up to 3 L

Leading zero A zero placed before the decimal point in a number that is less than 1; necessary in pharmacy to reduce possible dosing errors

Lowest term Form of a fraction in which no common number will divide into both the numerator and denominator evenly

Lyophilized Freeze-dried

Macrodrip infusion sets Infusion sets used for measuring the rate of IV fluids; macrodrip sets provide large drops (10 to 20 drops/mL) of fluid called *macrodrops*

Markup amount Difference between the selling price and the purchase cost of an item; also purchase cost times markup percentage

Markup percentage or gross margin A percentage amount added to the purchase cost of merchandise to ensure a profit; markup amount divided by the cost times 100

Markup price Purchase cost plus markup amount; becomes the selling/retail price

Measurable amount The quantity of medication that can be most accurately measured on the device available

Medication order Physician's written or verbal direction for administration of medication in an inpatient health care setting

Medication strength Concentration of active ingredient in a medication

Meniscus Curved line that develops on the upper surface of a liquid when poured into a container; always read at the bottom of the curve

Microdrip infusion sets Infusion sets used for measuring the rate of IV fluids; microdrip sets supply small drops (e.g., 60 drops/mL) called *microdrops*

Military time (International Standard Time) System of time that recognizes a 24-hour notation of hours and minutes

Milliequivalent (mEq) A type of unit used to express the concentration of electrolytes

Mixed number Number containing a whole number and a fraction

National Drug Code (NDC) Unique number on drug label that identifies manufacturer, product, and size of container

Nebulizer A device used to produce a fine spray of medication for inhalation

Net income/net profit Gross profit minus overhead; usually refers to total income for a business

Newborn From birth to 1 month

Nomogram A graphic representation of two lines marked off to height and weight and arranged so that a straightedge, used to connect the known values on these two lines, intersects the corresponding BSA measurement on another line

Nonsterile compounding The mixing of two or more components that does not require a sterile environment

Numerator Top number found in a fraction

Oral medications Medications taken by mouth (PO)

Overhead Expenses of a business, *not including cost of inventory,* such as rent, wages, utilities, insurance, license fees, depreciation, taxes paid, and other costs of doing business

Par level Minimum preset quantity of an item to be kept in stock

PAR level (periodic automatic replenishment) Predetermined point for automatic inventory reordering in a pharmacy

Parenteral Administration outside the gastrointestinal tract; mostly considered to be by injection or infusion

Parenteral nutrition IV solution used to provide nutrition to a patient; aka **hyperalimentation**

Patent Open and unobstructed as in IV lines or blood vessels

Percent Means of expressing a portion of 100 parts

Percentage strength An amount of active ingredient per 100 parts total: $x/100 = x\%$

Purchase cost Price paid by a business to obtain items for sale; also referred to as wholesale, acquisition, or inventory cost

Peripheral parenteral nutrition (PPN) IV containing a low concentration of amino acids, dextrose, electrolytes, and sometimes lipids, which is administered through a peripheral vessel

Pharmacokinetics Movement of drugs through the body; absorption, distribution, metabolism, and excretion (ADME)

Pharmacology Study of drugs, their uses, and their interactions with living systems

Pharmacotherapeutics Effects of drugs in treatment of conditions and diseases in the body

Piggyback A small-volume IV (50 to 250 mL) with added medication administered through an established IV line that is kept patent (open) by a continuous IV solution or by flushing

Powder volume Space occupied by the powdered active ingredient relative to the total volume of medication following reconstitution; aka **displacement value;** a measurement of the amount of active substance that displaces (takes the place of) some of the liquid diluent added for reconstitution

Prescription Written order by a licensed health care professional for dispensing medications

Product Number obtained by multiplying two numbers together

Profit See **Gross income/gross profit** and **Net income/net profit**

Proper fraction Fraction in which the numerator is less than the denominator; value is less than 1

Proportion Comparative relationship between the parts; one or more ratios that are compared

Purchase cost Price paid by a business to obtain items for sale; also referred to as *wholesale, acquisition,* or *inventory cost*

qs Quantity sufficient or required

qs ad Quantity sufficient to make

Quotient Answer of a division problem

Ratio Means of describing the relationship between two numbers; for example, 1:2

Ratio and proportion (R&P) A method used for *single-step* conversions between units and calculating medication doses and dosages; involves solving for two equivalent fractions using cross-multiplication and division

Ratio strength Expression of strength of weak solutions or liquid preparations; one part active ingredient in x parts total: (1:x)

Reconstitution Process of adding fluid, such as water or saline, to powdered or crystalline form of medication to make a specific liquid dosage strength

Remainder The amount left over after division

Roman numerals Letters from the Roman alphabet that are used to represent numbers, such as I for 1, V for 5, X for 10, etc.

Round To express a number to its nearest place value such as ones, tenths, hundredths, etc.

Scheduled medications Classification of medications with potential for abuse and misuse: CII, CIII, CIV, and CV

Scored tablet Tablet containing an indention for ease of breaking into equal parts

Selling price Price at which items are offered for sale to customers; also referred to as *retail price*

Signa (Sig) Part of prescription; directions for the patient—how, how much, when, how long

Solute Substance that is dissolved in a solution or semisolid

Solution Dosage form in which the medication is completely dissolved in the liquid

Solvent Substance that does the dissolving; aka **diluent**

Specific gravity The ratio of the density of a substance to the density of water when dealing with liquids in pharmacy

Standard An exact quantity agreed on for use in comparing measurements

Stock medication Medication provided by a manufacturer and kept on hand for use in preparing medication orders or prescriptions

Stock strength Strength or weight of medication available for doses

Subcutaneous Beneath the skin; medications injected into the subcutaneous tissue (Subcut)

Sublingual medications Medications placed under the tongue to dissolve (SL)

Subscription Part of a prescription that contains instructions for the pharmacist on how to compound if necessary

Superscription Part of a prescription designated with the symbol ℞, meaning, "take this drug"

Suspension Dosage form in which small particles of medication are dispersed throughout the liquid; most require shaking before dispensing and administering

Syrup Aqueous solution sweetened with sugar or a sugar substitute to disguise taste

Therapeutic range A dosage or blood concentration range that normally produces desired results; too much may be toxic and too little may not be therapeutic

Total parenteral nutrition (TPN) IV containing a high concentration of amino acids, dextrose, and sometimes lipids with electrolytes and other medications, which is administered through a large central vessel

Toxicology Study of adverse toxic reactions or toxic levels of chemicals and drugs

Trade/Brand name Proprietary name given to a medication by the manufacturer

Trailing zero A zero in the farthest right place of a number following the decimal; *not* used in pharmacy due to the increased potential for dosing errors

Turnover rate Rate at which the inventory is sold over a specified period of time

Unit A *general term* covering any quantity chosen as a standard; for a measurement to make sense, it *must* include a number and a unit; examples of units: mg, mL, teaspoon

U.S. customary system (Household system) System of measurement based on common kitchen measuring devices

Vehicle An inert component in which other components (such as the active ingredient) are mixed or dissolved (e.g., water, elixir, cream, or ointment bases); aka **diluent, solvent, base**

Vial Glass or plastic container with metal-enclosed rubber seal for injectable medications; may contain single or multiple doses

Viscosity Thickness of substance

Whole number Numeral consisting of one or more digits; number that is not followed by a fraction or decimal

Young's rule Means of calculating a dose of medication for a child from an adult dose based on age in years

---

*According to the FDA (https://www.fda.gov/RegulatoryInformation/Guidances/ucm082185.htm)

Index

Page numbers followed by "*f*" indicate figures, "*t*" indicate tables, and "*b*" indicate boxes.

A

Abbreviations
   general, 8–10
   for intravenous solutions, 330*t*
   for liquids, 7
   in pharmacology, 2–10
   for pharmacy technicians, 1–14
Accuracy, in calculation, 34
Acetaminophen, conversion factor for, 107*t*
Act-O-Vial system, 192, 193*f*
   definition of, 185
Active ingredients
   in medication, 1–2
   with percentage strength, determining the amount of, 335–341, 336*b*
Addition
   to decimals, 35–37
   definition of, 19
   to fractions, 27–29
   to whole numbers, 19–20
Additives
   definition of, 403
   in parenteral nutrition calculations, 431
Adjudication, 468
   definition of, 453
Administration, of medications
   forms of, 7
   frequency of, 6
   route of, 6
   times of, 7
Adolescence, definition of, 241, 250
Age
   Fried's rule and, 269
   medication calculation by, 241–280, 269*b*
   review of, 270
Alligation, for simple dilution, 374*f*–375*f*, 375*b*
Alligation alternate, 373–375, 374*b*–375*b*
   definition of, 354
   example of, 374, 374*f*–375*f*
Alligation medial, 376–383, 377*b*
   example of, 376–377
Amino acids, in parenteral nutrition, 431
Ampule, 188, 188*f*, 192
   definition of, 185
Annual depreciation, review of rules for, 484
Anticoagulants
   definition of, 211
   heparin sodium, 211–217, 226*b*, 234, 237
      strength of, 212, 214, 216
      syringes for, 214–216, 237
      volume of, 212, 214–216, 234, 237
   review of, 234, 234*b*
   unit calculations with, 211–240
      review of rules for, 240
Apothecary dram, 170*b*
Apothecary system, 83–84, 83*f*, 84*b*, 106
   Arabic numerals for, 83
   conversion factors for, 106*t*

Apothecary system *(Continued)*
   definition of, 73
   equivalents in, 84*t*
   household measurement and conversion between, 109–111, 110*b*
      equivalents between, 99*t*, 109*f*
   lowercase Roman numerals for, 83
   of measurement, 99–100, 99*b*
   metric system and, conversion between, 113–115, 113*b*
   pharmacology and, 8, 11
   points to remember, 84*b*
   review of rules for, 87
   for weight and volume, 75–76, 116*t*–117*t*
Arabic numerals, 61–64
   conversion of
      from Roman numerals, 63–64
      to Roman numerals, 63
Aspirin, conversion factor for, 107*t*
Assets, definition of, 453
Auxiliary label, 119
Average wholesale price (AWP), 468
   basis of, 468
   definition of, 453
AWP. *see* Average wholesale price

B

Base solution
   definition of, 403
   in parenteral nutrition calculations, 431
Basic mathematical skills, 11
   review of, 15–58
      decimals in, 32–41, 33*f*, 42*b*
      fractions in, 22–32, 22*b*–23*b*, 22*f*
      percentages in, 41–47, 52–55
      ratios in, 47–52
      whole numbers in, 19–22
   self-test of, 12–14
Biologicals, definition of, 73, 76
Body surface area (BSA). *see also* Nomogram
   definition of, 241, 250
   medication calculation by, 241–280
   review of, 270
Body weight. *see* Weight
Bottom line. *see* Net income
BSA. *see* Body surface area
Buccal, definition of, 149
Buccal tablets, 152
Business math, for pharmacy technicians, 453–485
   capitation, 473–474, 473*b*
   daily cash report, 480
   discount/markdown, 462–465, 462*b*
   gross income, 465–466
   insurance reimbursement, 468–472
   inventory management, 475–478, 475*b*
   inventory turnover rate, 478–479
   markup, 459–461
   net income, 466–468
   overhead expenses, 457–459

C

Calculations
  for dilutions, 354–402
    review of, 394, 402
    of stock medications, 361–373, 363b–364b
    using alligation, 374f–375f, 375b
  of medication
    by age, 241–280, 250b, 269b–270b
    by body surface area, 241–280, 250b, 270b
    by body weight, 241–280, 250b–251b, 253b, 270b
  of oral liquid doses, 164–184, 173b
  of oral solid doses, 149–163, 152b
Capitation fee, 473–474, 473b
  basis of, 473
  definition of, 453
Capsules, as oral medication, 151–152
Carbohydrates, in parenteral nutrition, 431
Cash drawer, balancing, 480
Cash flow, 457
  definition of, 453
Celsius, 61, 67f, 68b
  conversion of
    alternate formula for, 67–69
    from Fahrenheit, 67
    to Fahrenheit, 67
Chemicals, medications as, 1
Childhood, definition of, 241, 250
Claim, for insurance reimbursement of prescription, 468
Clark's rule
  definition of, 241
  for pediatric doses, 259–261, 259b–260b
Codeine, conversion factor for, 107t
Commas, in whole numbers, 19
Common denominator, 27–28
Complex fractions, 15, 32
Component, definition of, 354
Compound, definition of, 354
Compounding, calculations for, 354–402, 361b
  example of, 384
  review of, 394, 402
Compounding formulation
  definition of, 354, 387, 387b
  reducing and enlarging, 391–394, 392b
  example of, 391–392
Container, doses in, 294–297, 324
Continuous infusion, 413
  definition of, 403
Control number, 139
Controlled substance indicators, 139
Conversion
  apothecary system of measurement, 99–100, 99b
  of Arabic and Roman numerals, 61–64, 62b
  between Celsius and Fahrenheit, 66–69, 67f
    alternate formula for, 67–69
  decimal to fractions, 40
  decimal to percentages, 46–47
  definition of, 15
  dimensional analysis, 91–93, 91b, 108, 109b
  factors, definition of, 88
  fraction to percentage, 44–45
  fractions to decimals, 41
  between household system
    and apothecary systems, 109–111, 109f, 110b
    and metric systems, 111–113, 112f
  from larger metric numbers to smaller metric numbers, 94–95, 96b
  measurement systems and, 88–118, 104b
    review of, 100, 116
    using ratio and proportions, 90, 90b
  metric, household, apothecary measurements and, 116t–117t

Conversion *(Continued)*
  metric system, 94, 94b, 94f, 94t
    and apothecary systems, 113–115, 113b
  percentage to decimal, 45–46
  percentage to fraction, 41–43
  ratio and proportion for, 90, 90b, 108, 108b
  from smaller metric numbers to larger metric numbers, 96–98, 96b–98b
  between 12-hour and universal (military) time, 64–66, 65f
  points to remember, 65b
Conversion factors, 106–108, 107b, 107t
  for time, 403
  value of, 106b
  for volume, 403
Cubic centimeter, 80
Cup, 77t
  medication, with oral liquid medications, 167, 167f
Customary system, U. S., 73, 75–76

D

DA. *see* Dimensional analysis
Daily cash report, 480
  definition of, 453
Daily sales report, 480
Days' supply
  calculating, 298b, 324
  definition of, 297
  interpreting physicians' orders for, 281–324
    in container, 294–297, 324
      dispensing (dosage) and, appropriate quantity for, 287–293, 324
    prescription and, length of time for, 297–312, 297b–301b
    review of, 312
    review of rules for, 324
Decimal place, 33, 33f
Decimals, 32–41, 33f, 42b
  adding, 35–37
  comparing, 34
  converting
    to fractions, 40, 40b
    fractions to, 41
    to percentage, 46–47, 46b
    percentage to, 45–46
  definition of, 15
  dividing, 38–40
  as fractions, 32
  multiplying, 37–38
  rounding, 34–35, 34b
  subtracting, 35–37
Denominator, 22
  common, 27–28
  definition of, 15
Density, 76
Depreciation
  annual, review of rules for, 484
  of assets
    calculation of, 457
    formula for, 457
  calculation of, 457
  definition of, 453
Dextrose, in parenteral nutrition, 431
Diabetes mellitus, insulin for, 218
Digits, whole numbers and, 19
Diluent, 174, 361
  definition of, 164
Dilutions
  calculations for, 354–402
    review of, 394, 402
    of stock medications, 361–373, 363b–364b
    using alligation, 374f–375f, 375b
  definition of, 354

Index

Dimensional analysis (DA), 89
　for conversion of units, 91–93, 91b, 108, 109b
　　rules for using, 108b
　definition of, 88
　in dispensing (dosage) and, appropriate quantity for, 287
　for flow rates, 421, 422b
　for intravenous infusion rates, 414
　multiplication and, 91b
　oral liquid medications calculation using, 169–173
　for oral solid doses, medication calculation using, 153–156, 154b
　for pediatric doses, medication calculation using, 252b
　use of, 90
Discount/markdown, 462–465, 462b
　calculation of, 462
　definition of, 453
　review of rules for, 485
Dispensing (dosage), appropriate quantity for, 287–293, 324
Displacement value, 164, 174
Dividend, 15, 21
Division
　of decimals, 38–40
　of fractions, 30–32, 31b
　of whole numbers, 21–22
Divisor, 15, 21
"Do Not Use" List of abbreviations, of The Joint Commission, 2
Dosage, 149, 152, 152b
　calculations, basic math skills for, 11
　interpreting physicians' orders for, 281–324
　　in container, 294–297, 324
　　dispensing (dosage) and, appropriate quantity for, 287–293, 324
　　prescription and, length of time for, 297–312, 297b–301b
　　review of, 312
　　review of rules for, 324
Dosage form, 152
　definition of, 149
　of medications, 7
Dosage strength, 139
　definition of, 119
Dose, 152, 152b
　in container, 294–297, 324
　definition of, 149
　for parenteral medication, calculation of, 185–210, 193b, 195b
　　examples of, 194, 194f, 204, 204f
　　review of, 206
Dose time, definition of, 403
Dose volume, definition of, 403
Dosespoon, with oral liquid medications, 167, 167f
Drip rate, definition of, 403, 419
Drop factor, definition of, 403, 419
Drop rate, definition of, 419
Droppers, medication, with oral liquid medications, 167, 167f, 168b
Drops, 77, 77t
Drops per milliliter, 421b
Drops per minute, calculating IV flow rates in example of, 421–422
Drug. see Medication
Drug Enforcement Agency (DEA) number, on prescription, 127b

E

Early childhood, definition of, 241, 250
Ears, symbols for, 8
Electrolytes
　definition of, 73, 76
　in parenteral nutrition, 431, 432b

Elixir, definition of, 164
Enteric-coated tablet, 152
　definition of, 149
Equivalency, between household and metric systems, 92t
Equivalent fractions, 26
　changing fractions to, 27
Equivalents
　in apothecary system, 84t
　in household system, 77t
　in metric system, 80t
Excipients, 1
Expiration date, 139
Extremes, 49
Eyes, symbols for, 8

F

Fahrenheit, 61, 66–69, 67f, 68b
　conversion of
　　alternate formula for, 67–69
　　from Celsius, 67
　　to Celsius, 67
Fat, in parenteral nutrition, 431
Ferrous sulfate, conversion factor for, 107t
Five-milliliter syringes, 189, 190f
Flow rate
　calculation of, in drops per minute, 421–425
　definition of, 403, 414
Fluid, intravenous, 414
Food and Drug Administration (FDA), 1–2
Foot, 77t
Fractional values, inverted, 336b
Fractions, 22–32, 22b–23b, 22f
　adding, 27–29
　complex, 15, 32
　converting
　　to percentage, 44–45
　　percentage to, 41–43, 43b
　decimals and, 32
　　converting, 40, 40b–41b
　definition of, 15, 22
　denominator in, 22
　dividing, 30–32, 31b
　equivalent, 26
　improper, 15, 23
　multiplying, 30, 30b
　numerator in, 22
　proper, 15, 23
　reducing to lowest term, 26–27
　subtracting, 27–29
Fragmin, 235, 240
　syringes for, 235, 240
　volume of, 235
Fried's rule
　definition of, 241
　for pediatric doses, 269

G

Gallon, 77t
Generic name, 139, 139b
　definition of, 119
Graduated cylinders, 175f
Graduates, 174
　definition of, 164
Grain, 83
Gram, for weight, 79, 81f
Gross income, 465–466
Gross margin, definition of, 454
Gross profit, 457
　definition of, 454
　formula for, 465
　review of rules for, 485

H

Heparin sodium, 211–217, 226b, 234, 237
  strength of, 212, 214, 216
  syringes for, 214–216, 237
  volume of, 212, 214–216, 234, 237
High-alert medications, 211, 218
Household measurement, 106
  apothecary system and
    conversion between, 109–111, 110b
    equivalents between, 109f
  conversion factors for, 106t
  dry weight, 116t–117t
  liquid, 116t–117t
  metric conversion to, 89–93
    equivalents between, 92t
  metric system and
    conversion between, 111–113
    equivalents between, 112f
Household system, 7, 11, 76–78, 78b
  for administration of medications, 77
  definition of, 73
  drop as, 77
  expression of, 77
  of length, 77t
  points to remember, 78b
  review of rules for, 86
  of volume, 75–76, 77t
  of weight, 75–76, 77t
Humulin, 212–213, 216–217, 235–236, 238–240
  administration of, 221, 222b
  syringes for, 212, 217, 235–236, 238–239
  volume of, 212, 217, 240
Hyperalimentation, 403

I

Improper fraction, 15, 23
Inch, 77t
Income/loss, review of rules for, 485
Indication
  definition of, 119
  for medication, 127
Infant, definition of, 241, 250
Infusion
  continuous, 413
    definition of, 403
  definition of, 185
Infusion rate, 403
  calculating
    example of, 414
Infusion set, 421
  macrodrip, 403
  microdrip, 403
  types and parts of, 420f
Infusion time, intravenous, 427b
  example of, 426–427
Inhaler, definition of, 281
Injectable medications, 188, 188b
Inscription, 128f
  definition of, 119
Institute for Safe Medication Practices (ISMP), List of Error-Prone Abbreviations, Symbols, and Dose Designations of, 2
Insulin
  Humulin, 212–213, 216–217, 235–236, 238–240
    administration of, 221, 222b
    syringes for, 212, 217, 235–236, 238–239
    volume of, 212, 217, 240
  Lantus, 213
    syringes for, 213
  preparations of, approximate action of common, 219b, 221t

Insulin (Continued)
  review in, 234, 234b
  syringes, 220b, 220f
  types of, 219f
  unit calculations with, 211–240, 222b
    review of, 240
Insurance reimbursement, 468–472
  applying markup/markdown in, 469
  average wholesale price and, 468
  dispensing fees, 469–472, 470b
  review of rules for, 485
International System of Units (metric system), 73, 75–76
International unit, 73, 76b, 211, 218
Intradermal administration, 188
  definition of, 185
Intramuscular administration, 188
  definition of, 185
Intravenous administration, 188
  definition of, 185, 403, 413
Intravenous fluids
  abbreviations for, 330t
  infusion sets for, 420f
  solutes in, calculating amounts of, 330–335, 331b
Intravenous infusion time, 427b
  example of, 426–427
Intravenous (IV) medications, 413
  calculation of, 403–452
    review of, 438
Inventory
  cash flow and, 457
  cost of, 453
  definition of, 454
  net income and, 466
  perpetual, 475
Inventory control, 457
Inventory management, 475–478, 475b
Inventory turnover rate, 478–479
  calculation of, 478
  review of rules for, 485
Inverting, 30
  definition of, 15
Iron, conversion factor for, 107t

K

Kilogram, pound conversion to, 250

L

Label
  auxiliary, 119
  drug strength expressed on, 188–189, 189b
  elements of, 128, 128f
  interpretation of, 119–148
    review of, 141
    review of rules for, 148
  for solute, 355, 377
  medication, using metric system, 79, 79f
Lantus, 213
  syringes for, 213
Large-volume IV bag, 416b
Large-volume parenterals (LVPs), 190, 413
  definition of, 185
Larger metric numbers, converting to smaller metric numbers, 94–95, 96b
LCD. see Least common denominator (LCD)
Leading zero, 15, 32
Least common denominator (LCD), 15, 27
Length
  apothecary/household systems conversion for, 106t
  household measurements of, 77t
  metric equivalents of, 79, 80t
  pharmaceutical use of, 76

Lipid emulsion, in parenteral nutrition, 431
Liquid doses, oral, calculation of, 164–184, 173*b*
    review of, 180
Liquid medications, oral
    administration of, 167–173, 167*f*, 168*b*
    calculation of, 168–169, 168*b*, 170*b*
        using dimensional analysis, 169–173, 170*b*
        using ratio and proportion, 169
    reconstitution of powders into, 174–180, 174*b*, 175*f*–176*f*
Liquids, abbreviations for, 7
List of Error-Prone Abbreviations, Symbols, and Dose Designations, of Institute for Safe Medication Practices (ISMP), 2
Liter, for volume, 79, 81*f*
Lot/batch number, 139
Lowest term
    definition of, 15
    reducing fractions to, 26–27
LVPs. *see* Large-volume parenterals
Lyophilized form, 174
    definition of, 164

M

Macrodrip, definition of, 403, 419
Macrodrip infusion sets
    definition of, 403
    example of, 420*f*
Macronutrients, in parenteral nutrition, 431
Markdown/discount, 462–465, 462*b*
    applying, 469
    calculation of, 462
    definition of, 453
Markup, 459–461
    amount, 459
        definition of, 454
        review of rules for, 484
    application of, 469
    calculation of, 459
    definition of, 454
    percentage of, 460–461, 460*b*, 484
        calculation of, 460
        definition of, 454
    price
        definition of, 454
        review of rules for, 484
    profit margin and, 459
Mass, 76
Mathematical conversions, 11
Mathematical skills, 1–14
    basic, 11
    for pharmacy technician, 11
Means, 49
Measurable amount, 112*b*
Measurement, of medications, 7–8
    apothecary system, 8, 11
    household system, 7, 11
    metric system, 7, 11
    milliequivalent, 8
Measurement systems
    conversion, 88–103
        apothecary system of, 99–100, 99*b*
        household or U.S customary system, 89–93
        from larger metric numbers to smaller, 94–95, 96*b*
        review of, 100
        from smaller metric numbers to larger, 96–98, 96*b*–98*b*
        using ratio and proportions, 90, 90*b*
    conversions between, 104–118, 104*b*, 116*t*–117*t*
        review of, 116
    household measurement and conversion between, 92*t*
        equivalents between, 92*t*

Measurement systems *(Continued)*
    types of, 11
    units and equivalencies, 73–87
        apothecary, 83–84, 84*b*
        household, 76–78, 78*b*
        metric, 79–82, 82*b*
        review of, 85
Medication
    administration of
        forms of, 7
        frequency of, 6
        route of, 6
        times of, 7
    calculation of
        by age, 241–280, 250*b*, 269*b*–270*b*
        by body surface area, 241–280, 250*b*, 270*b*
        by body weight, 241–280, 250*b*–251*b*, 253*b*, 270*b*
    as chemicals, 1
    dosage form of, 139
    dosage strength of, 139
    generic name for, 139
    insurance reimbursement for, 468
    intravenous, 413
        calculation of, 403–452
    inventory management of, 475
    measurement of, 7–8
        apothecary system, 8, 11
        household system, 7, 11
        metric system, 7, 11
        milliequivalent, 8
    National Drug Code and, 139
    scheduled, 119
    seasonal, 475
    stock
        definition of, 354
        simple dilution of, 361–373, 363*b*–364*b*
    storage requirements of, 139
    total quantity of, 139
    trade/brand name for, 139
Medication cup, with oral liquid medications, 167, 167*f*
Medication dosage. *see also* Physician's order; Prescriptions
    calculation of, oral solid doses, 149–163, 152*b*
        involving different units or measurement systems, 156–159, 156*b*–157*b*
        patient safety in, 159
        review of, 160
        review of rules for, 163
        using dimensional analysis, 153–156, 154*b*
        using ratio and proportion, 152–153, 153*b*
Medication labels. *see also* Label
    interpretation of, 139–141, 139*b*–140*b*, 140*f*
    patient safety and, 139
    using metric system, 79, 79*f*
Medication orders, 127
    definition of, 119
    example of, 136*f*
    information on, 135–139
    interpretation of, 119–148
        review of, 141
        review of rules for, 148
    pharmacy technician and, 139
        responsibility of, 137*b*, 142*b*
    writing of, in Arabic and Roman numeral, 61–62
Medication strength, definition of, 325
Medicine dropper, 107*b*
    with oral liquid medications, 167, 167*f*, 168*b*
Meniscus, 167–168
    definition of, 164
    reading, 168*f*
mEq. *see* Milliequivalent
Meter, for length, 79, 81*f*

Metric system, 7, 11, 79–82, 82b, 106
    apothecary systems and, conversion between, 113–115, 113b
    conversion factors for, 106t
    conversion of, 94, 94b, 94f, 94t
    decimals in, 81
    equivalents in, 80t
    household measurement and
        conversion between, 111–113
        equivalents between, 112f
    from larger to smaller units, 94–95, 96b
    of mass, 81
    medication labels using, 79, 79f
    points to remember, 82b
    prefixes in, 79, 79b, 80f, 80t
    review of rules for, 86
    from smaller to larger units, 94–98, 96b–98b
    volume, 82, 116t–117t
    weight, 76, 116t–117t
Microdrip, definition of, 419
Microdrip infusion sets
    definition of, 403
    example of, 420f
Microgram, 80
Military time, 11, 61, 64–66
    points to remember, 65b
Milliequivalent (mEq), 8
    definition of, 73, 76
Mixed number, 15, 23
Mixtures, calculations for, 354–402
    review of, 394, 402
Multiplication
    of decimals, 37–38
    dimensional analysis and, 91b
    of fractions, 30, 30b
    of whole numbers, 20

N

National Drug Code (NDC), 139
    definition of, 119
National Formulary (NF), 1–2
NDC. see National Drug Code
Nebulizer, definition of, 281
Neonate, 241, 250
Net income, 466–468. see also Net profit
    business success and, 457
    calculation of, 466
    definition of, 454
Net profit. see also Net income
    definition of, 454
    overhead and, 466
    review of rules for, 485
NF. see National Formulary
Nitroglycerin sublingual (NTG SL) tablets, 115b
    conversion factor for, 107t
Nomogram. see also Body surface area
    for adult dose, 263f
    definition of, 241
    for pediatric doses, 261–262, 262f
    reading, 264f
    use of, 263
Nonsterile compounding, definition of, 354
Numbers. see also Arabic numerals; Roman numerals
    clinical measurements of, conversion of, 59–72
        review of, 70
Numbers, expressing, as ratios, 47–49, 48b
Numerator, 15, 22
Nutrition, parenteral, 403, 413–414
    calculations with, 432b
        example of, 432
    peripheral, 403, 431
    total, 403, 431

O

Ophthalmic medications, calculating days' supply of, 298b–299b
Oral liquid doses, calculation of, 164–184, 173b
    review of, 180
Oral liquid medications
    administration of, 167–173, 167f, 168b
    calculation of, 168–169, 168b
        using dimensional analysis, 169–173, 170b
        using ratio and proportion, 169
    reconstitution of powders into, 174–180, 174b, 175f–176f
Oral medications. see also Oral liquid medications; Oral solid doses
    absorption of, 151
    definition of, 149
    forms of, 151
Oral solid doses, calculation of, 149–163, 152b
    involving different units or measurement systems, 156–159, 156b–157b
    patient safety in, 159
    review of, 160
    review of rules for, 163
    using dimensional analysis, 153–156, 154b
    using ratio and proportion, 152–153, 153b
Oral syringes, with oral liquid medications, 167, 167f
Otic medications, calculating days' supply of, 298b–299b
Ounce, 77t
    conversion to pounds, 251, 251b
    symbols for, 92t
Overhead
    definition of, 454
    expenses, 457–459
    net profit and, 466
    review of rules for, 484

P

Pacifier, with oral liquid medications, 167, 168f
Par level, 457
    inventory management and, 475
    review of rules for, 485
Parenteral, definition of, 185
Parenteral medication
    amount of, 193
    calculation of doses for, 185–210, 193b, 195b
        examples of, 194, 194f, 204, 204f
        review of, 206
    reconstitution and, 201–206, 201b–202b, 202f–203f, 204b
    syringes for, 189–192
    weight of, 188–189
Parenteral nutrition (PN), 403, 413–414
    calculations with, 432b
        example of, 432
    peripheral, 403, 431
    total, 403, 431
Patent, definition of, 211, 226
Patient safety, medication labels and, 139
Percentage, 41–47, 331b
    calculations with, 52–55
        determining percentage of quantity in, 52–55, 53b
    converting
        to decimal, 45–46
        decimal to, 46–47
        to fraction, 41–43
        fraction to, 44–45
    definition of, 15
    of markup, 460–461, 460b, 484
        calculation of, 460
        definition of, 454

Percentage strength
    active ingredient with, determining the amount of, 335–341, 336b
    calculations with, 325–353
        review of, 348
    changing from ratio to, 345–347
    definition of, 325
    to ratio strength, 347–348
    types of, 329, 329b
Peripheral parenteral nutrition (PPN), 431
    definition of, 403
Perpetual inventory, 475
Pharmacokinetics, 127
    definition of, 119, 241, 250
Pharmacology
    abbreviations in, 2–10
    apothecary system and, 8
    course of, 11
    definition of, 1
Pharmacotherapeutics, 127
    definition of, 119
Pharmacy
    basic math skills in, 11
        self-test of, 12–14
    daily cash report in, 480
    inventory management of, 475
    inventory turnover rate in, 478
Pharmacy technicians
    abbreviations for, 1–14
    business math for, 453–485
        capitation, 473–474, 473b
        daily cash report, 480
        discount/markdown, 462–465, 462b
        gross income, 465–466
        insurance reimbursement, 468–472
        inventory management, 475–478, 475b
        inventory turnover rate, 478–479
        markup, 459–461
        net income, 466–468
        overhead expenses, 457–459
    mathematical skills for, 11
    medication orders and, 139
        responsibility of, 137b, 142b
    responsibility of, 11
    symbols for, 1–14
Phenobarbital, conversion factor for, 107t
Physician's order. *see also* Medication dosage; Prescriptions
    examples of, 136f
    interpreting of, for dosages and days' supply, 281–324
        in container, 294–297, 324
            dispensing (dosage) and, appropriate quantity for, 287–293, 324
            prescription and, length of time for, 297–312, 297b–301b
            review of, 312
            review of rules for, 324
Piggyback, 190
    definition of, 185, 403, 413
    infusion set, 413f
Pint, 77t
PN. *see* Parenteral nutrition
Pound, 77t
    converting to kilograms, 250
    household (#), 83b
Powder volume, 174
    definition of, 164
PPN. *see* Peripheral parenteral nutrition
Prefixes, in metric system, 79, 79b, 80f, 80t
Prescriptions, 127. *see also* Physician's order; Medication dosage
    average wholesale price and, 468
    calculations for, discounts/markdowns, 462

Prescriptions *(Continued)*
    components of, 127, 128f
    compounded
        preparing, 387–391, 387b
        reducing and enlarging, 391–394, 392b
    definition of, 119
    indication for, 127–139, 127b–128b, 129f
    length of time for, 297–312, 297b–301b
    medication labels and, 139–141, 139b–140b, 140f
Price
    markup
        definition of, 454
        review of rules for, 484
    selling, 459
        definition of, 454
Product, 15, 20
Proficiency self-test, for basic math skills, 12–14
Profit, 457
    gross, 457
        definition of, 454
        formula for, 465
        review of rules for, 485
    net
        definition of, 454
        overhead and, 466
        review of rules for, 485
    review of rules for, 485
Profit margin, markup and, 459
Proper fraction, 15, 23
Proportion
    calculating oral liquid medications using, 169
    for conversion of units, 90, 90b, 108, 108b
    definition, 15, 49
    expressing ratios as, 49–50
    medication calculation using, for oral solid doses, 152–153, 153b
    solving for unknowns using, 50–52, 50b
Protein, in parenteral nutrition, 431
Purchase cost, 459
    definition of, 454

Q

qs. *see* Quantity sufficient
qs ad. *see* Quantity sufficient to make
Quantity, appropriate, for dispensing (dosage), 287–293, 324
Quantity sufficient, 325, 337
Quantity sufficient to make, 325, 337
Quart, 77t
Quotient, 15, 21

R

Ratio and proportion (R&P)
    definition of, 88
    in dispensing (dosage) and, appropriate quantity for, 287
Ratio strength, 342b
    calculations with, 325–353
        review of, 348
    changing from percentage to, 347–348
    definition of, 325
    to percentage strength, 345–347
    types of, 341–342
Ratios, 47–52
    for conversion of units, 90, 90b, 108, 108b
    definition of, 15
    expressing
        numbers as, 47–49, 48b
        as proportions, 49–50
    oral liquid medications calculation using, 169

Ratios *(Continued)*
  for oral solid doses, medication calculation using, 152–153, 153*b*
  solving for unknowns using, 50–52, 50*b*
Reconstitution, 201–206, 201*b*–202*b*, 203*f*, 204*b*
  definition of, 164
  of powders, into oral liquid medications, 174–180, 174*b*, 175*f*–176*f*
Reimbursement
  insurance, 468–472
    applying markup/markdown in, 469
    average wholesale price and, 468
    dispensing fees, 469–472, 470*b*
    review of rules for, 485
  third-party, 468
Remainder, 15, 19–20
Roman numerals, 61–64, 62*b*
  conversion of
    from Arabic numerals, 63
    to Arabic numerals, 63–64
  rules for, 62
Rounding
  decimals, 34, 34*b*
  definition of, 15
  steps for, 34–35

S

Sales report, definition of, 453
Scheduled medications, definition of, 119
Scored tablet, 15, 26
Seasonal medication, 475
Self-test, of basic math skills, 12–14
Selling price, 459
  definition of, 454
Semisolids, abbreviations for, 7
Signa (Sig), 128*f*
  definition of, 119
Simple dilution, of stock medication, 361–373, 363*b*–364*b*
  example of, 362–364
Small-volume parenterals (SVPs), 413
Smaller metric numbers, converting from larger metric numbers to, 94–98, 96*b*–98*b*
Solids, abbreviations for, 7
Solute
  calculating amounts of, in intravenous fluids, 330–335, 331*b*
  definition of, 164, 325
Solution
  definition of, 164, 361
  labels of, 377
Solvent, 164, 361
Specific gravity, definition of, 73, 76
Standards, definition of, 73, 75
Stock liquids, equation for diluting, 362
Stock medication
  definition of, 354
  simple dilution of, 361–373, 363*b*–364*b*
    example of, 362–364
Stock solids, equation for diluting, 362–365
Stock strength, definition of, 149
Strengths, of medication, 114
Subcutaneous administration, 188
  definition of, 185
Sublingual medications, definition of, 149
Sublingual tablets, 152
Subscription, 128*f*
  definition of, 119
Subtraction
  of decimals, 35–37
  definition of, 19

Subtraction *(Continued)*
  of fractions, 27–29
  of whole numbers, 19–20
Superscription, 128*f*
  definition of, 119
Suspension, definition of, 164
SVPs. *see* Small-volume parenterals
Symbols
  in pharmacology, 2–10
  for pharmacy technicians, 1–14
Syringes, 189, 189*b*
  five-milliliter, 189, 190*f*
  measurement of medications in, accuracy of, 190, 190*f*–191*f*
  oral, with oral liquid medications, 167
  for parenteral medication, 189–192
  for preparation of intravenous fluids, 190*b*
  ten-milliliter, 189
  three-milliliter, 189, 189*f*
  tuberculin (TB), 189, 189*f*
  with volume of 1.7 mL, 190*f*
  with volume of 2.3 mL, 191*f*
Syrup, definition of, 164

T

Tablespoon, 77*t*
  in oral liquid medications, 167, 168*b*
Tablets, as oral medication, 151–152
Tbsp. *see* Tablespoon
Teaspoon, 77*t*
  in oral liquid medications, 167, 168*b*
Technician, pharmacy
  abbreviations for, 1–14
  mathematical skills for, 11
  responsibility of, 11
  symbols for, 1–14
Temperature, clinical measurements of, conversion of, 59–72
Ten-milliliter syringes, 189
Terminal zeros, 33
The Joint Commission (TJC), Official "Do Not Use" List of abbreviations of, 2
Therapeutic range, definition of, 185
Third-party payer, capitation and, 473
Third-party reimbursement, 468
3-in-1 formulation, parenteral nutrition, 431
Three-milliliter syringes, 189, 189*f*
Tic-tac-toe, 374*f*
Time
  conversion factor for, 403
  dose, 403
  military (24-hour) and 12-hour, conversion of, 61, 65*f*
    points to remember, 65*b*
Ton, 77*t*
Total parenteral nutrition (TPN), 431
  definition of, 403
Toxicology, 119
TPN. *see* Total parenteral nutrition
Trade/brand name, 139, 139*b*
  definition of, 119
Trailing zero, 15, 81
Tsp. *see* Teaspoon
Tuberculin (TB) syringes, 189, 189*f*
Turnover rate, 457
  definition of, 454
  of inventory, 478–479
    calculation of, 478
    review of rules for, 485
12-hour time, 64–66
24-hour time, 64–66, 65*f*
  points to remember, 65*b*

U

Units, 211, 218
    calculation
        with anticoagulants, 211–240
        with insulin, 211–240, 219b–220b, 219f–220f, 221t, 222b
        of medications, 240
    definition of, 73, 76
    dose calculation, 218
    international, 211, 218
U.S. Customary System, 73, 75–76
U.S. Department of Health and Human Services, Food and Drug Administration (FDA), 1–2
U.S. Pharmacopeia (USP), 1–2

V

Vancomycin, 427
Vials, 188, 188f, 192
    definition of, 185
Viscosity, 73
Vitamins, in parenteral nutrition, 431
Volume, 76, 168b
    apothecary/household systems, conversion for, 106t
    conversion factor for, 403
    dose, 403
    household measurements of, 77t
    household systems, conversion for, 92t
    measurement systems for, 75–76
    metric, household, apothecary system conversions and, 116t–117t
    metric equivalents of, 79, 80t
    metric systems, conversion for, 94t
Volume: volume ratio strength, 342
Volume in volume (v/v) percentage strength, 329

W

Weight. *see also* Household measurement; Metric system
    apothecary/household systems, conversion for, 106t
    household measurements of, 77t

Weight *(Continued)*
    household systems, conversion for, 92t
    measurement systems for, 75–76
    medication calculation by, 241–280, 250b–251b, 253b
        review of, 270
    metric, 76
    metric, household, apothecary system conversions and, 116t–117t
    metric conversion for, 94t
    metric equivalents of, 79, 80t
    of parenteral medications, 188–189
Weight: volume ratio strength, 341
Weight: weight ratio strength, 342
Weight in volume (w/v) percentage strength, 329, 330b
Weight in weight (w/w) percentage strength, 329
Whole number, 19–22
    addition of, 19–20
    decimal point and, 19
    definition of, 15
    division of, 21–22
    as fractions, 23b
    multiplication of, 20
    subtraction of, 19–20

Y

Yard, 77t
Young's rule
    definition of, 241
    formula for, 269

Z

Zero
    decimals and, 34
    division of, 21
    leading, 15, 32
    multiplication of, 20
    terminal, 33
    trailing, 15, 81